Cardiopulmonary Anatomy and Physiology

Essentials for Respiratory Care

Cardiopulmonary Anatomy and Physiology

Essentials for Respiratory Care

THIRD EDITION

Terry Des Jardins, M.Ed., R.R.T.

Department of Respiratory Care
Parkland College
Champaign, Illinois

Delmar Publishers

an International Thomson Publishing company I(T)P®

Albany • Bonn • Boston • Cincinnati • Detroit • London • Madrid
Melbourne • Mexico City • New York • Pacific Grove • Paris • San Francisco
Singapore • Tokyo • Toronto • Washington

NOTICE TO READER AND COPYRIGHT PAGE

Cover Design: Brucie Rosch

Delmar Staff:
Publisher: Susan Simpfenderfer
Acquisitions Editor: Dawn Gerrain
Developmental Editor: Debra M. Flis
Project Editor: Coreen Filson
Production Coordinator: John Mickelbank
Art and Design Coordinator: Vincent S. Berger
Editorial Assistant: Donna L. Leto

COPYRIGHT © 1998
By Delmar Publishers
a division of International Thomson Publishing Inc.

The ITP logo is a trademark under license.

Printed in the United States of America

For more information, contact:

Delmar Publishers
3 Columbia Circle, Box 15015
Albany, New York 12212-5015

Nelson Canada
1120 Birchmount Road
Scarborough, Ontario
Canada, M1K 5G4

International Thomson Publishing Asia
221 Henderson Road
#05-10 Henderson Building
Singapore 0315

International Thomson Publishing Europe
Berkshire House
168-173 High Holborn
London, WC1V 7AA
England

International Thomson Editores
Campos Eliseos 385, Piso 7
Col Polanco
11560 Mexico D F Mexico

International Thomson Publishing—Japan
Hirakawacho Kyowa Building, 3F
2-2-1 Hirakawacho
Chiyoda-ku, Tokyo 102
Japan

Thomas Nelson Australia
102 Dodds Street
South Melbourne, 3205
Victoria, Australia

International Thomson Publishing
GmbH
Konigswinterer Strasse 418
53227 Bonn
Germany

1 2 3 4 5 6 7 8 9 10 XXX 03 02 01 00 99 98 97

Library of Congress Cataloging-in Publication Data

Des Jardins, Terry R.
   Cardiopulmonary anatomy & physiology : essentials for respiratory care/Terry Des Jardins.—3rd ed.
     p.   cm
   Includes bibliographical references and index.
   ISBN 0-8273-8256-1 (alk. paper)
   1. Cardiopulmonary system—Physiology. 2. Cardiopulmonary system—Anatomy. 3. Respiratory therapy. I. Title.
   [DNLM: 1. Respiratory System—anatomy & histology. 2. Respiratory System—physiology. 3. Cardiovascular System—anatomy & histology. 4. Cardiovascular System—physiology.   WF 101 D441c 1997]
   QP 121.D47   1997
   612.1—dc21
   DNLM/DLC
   for Library of Congress   97-8797
                                    CIP

DEDICATION

To Ken and Esther

CONTENTS

CHAPTER THREE

The Diffusion of Pulmonary Gases

3 107

11 CHAPTER ELEVEN

Cardiopulmonary Physiology of the Fetus and the Newborn   295

12 CHAPTER TWELVE

Renal Failure and its Effects on the Cardiopulmonary System   295

13 CHAPTER THIRTEEN

Aging and Its Effects on the Cardiopulmonary System 335

FOREWORD
TO THE THIRD EDITION

I am very pleased to write the foreword to the third edition of Terry Des Jardins' *Cardiopulmonary Anatomy and Physiology: Essentials for Respiratory Care.* The third edition is an even better text than its fine predecessors. A number of clinical case histories have been added that will make the basic anatomic and physiologic discussions, which are very thorough, much more relevant for students. Most students find anatomy and physiology difficult to study because these courses are taught before the student has any clinical experience, and thus the material appears to be presented in an intellectual vacuum. The case studies in the Clinical Applications section at the end of each chapter should remedy this awkward problem.

The appearance of the book has undergone significant changes. The addition of color to the fine illustrations and tables will help students by making the art much more lifelike and hence not only more pleasing to the eye but also more readily understandable. The addition of color to the tables and nomograms represents a distinct improvement.

It has been ten years since I wrote the Foreword to the first edition and it is nice to still be around to make a small contribution to the third edition.

Dr. Thomas DeKornfeld, M.D.
Ann Arbor, Michigan

PREFACE

First, it is with great pleasure that I acknowledge that all of the anatomic art illustrations, graphs, nomograms, and tables have been rendered from black and white to color in the third edition of this textbook. The addition of color to these items will, undoubtedly, facilitate and enhance the visualization—and understanding—of the material presented.

The text is designed to provide students of cardiopulmonary anatomy and physiology with accurate and complete information essential for respiratory care. The book assumes no previous knowledge of respiratory anatomy or physiology. Great efforts have been made to present a comprehensive overview of the subject matter in an organized, interesting, and readable manner. The overall layout of this book is based upon both my experiences as an educator of respiratory anatomy and physiology since 1973, and on the many things I have learned from my students. In response to personal experiences and to helpful suggestions, I have employed the following pedagogic approach.

Knowledge of a *structure* is essential to the understanding of the *function* of that structure. It therefore makes little sense to present students with physiologic details without first establishing a solid foundation in anatomy. Since most college-level anatomy courses spend only a limited amount of time on the cardiopulmonary system, respiratory care educators have generally had to cover this subject themselves. In regard to a suitable textbook, however, educators have usually found the cardiopulmonary section of college-level anatomy and physiology texts too introductory in nature. On the other hand, textbooks concentrating solely on the respiratory system have, historically, been too complex or esoteric.

To offset this problem, **Chapter One** provides the student with a thorough discussion of anatomic structures associated with the respiratory system. This chapter also features a large number of colorful illustrations. The visual impact of this chapter is intended to: (1) stimulate interest in the subject under discussion, (2) facilitate the rapid visualization of anatomic structures, and (3) help the student relate classroom knowledge to clinical experiences.

Chapters Two through **Ten** provide the major concepts and mechanisms of respiratory physiology. The discussions are comprehensive, logically organized, and, most importantly, presented at a level suitable for the average college student. When appropriate, anatomic and physiologic principles are applied to common clinical situations to enhance understanding and retention (e.g., the gas transport studies and their clinical application to the patient's hemodynamic status). In addition, a large number of colorful line drawings and tables appear throughout these chapters to assist in the understanding of various concepts and principles. Chapters Two, Three, Seven, and Nine feature several unique line drawings that relate familiar visual concepts to standard graphs and nomograms. Although I have found that the types of graphs and nomograms presented in this textbook are often difficult for students to understand at first, it is important to stress that the physiology literature uses these items extensively to impart information.

The student must understand how to read every graph and nomogram in this textbook to fully comprehend its contents.

Chapter Eleven provides the reader with the major anatomic structures and physiologic mechanisms associated with gas exchange and circulation in the fetus and newborn infant. This chapter presents the basic cardiopulmonary foundation required to understand fetal and neonatal respiratory disorders.

Chapter Twelve presents the structure and function of the renal system. It then discusses the major cardiopulmonary problems that develop when the renal system fails. This chapter is particularly important for respiratory care practitioners working with patients in the critical care unit.

Chapter Thirteen describes changes that occur in the cardiopulmonary system with age. Because the older age groups are expected to increase each year until about the year 2050, basic knowledge of this material will become increasingly important to respiratory care practitioners.

Chapter Fourteen presents the effects of exercise on the cardiopulmonary system. During heavy exercise, the components of the cardiopulmonary system may be stressed to their limits. Cardiac patients involved in exercise training after myocardial infarction demonstrate a significant reduction in mortality and major cardiac mishaps. As our older population increases, cardiovascular rehabilitation programs will become increasingly important to respiratory care practitioners.

Chapter Fifteen describes the effects of high altitude on the cardiopulmonary system. It provides a better understanding of chronic oxygen deprivation, which can then be applied to the treatment of chronic hypoxia caused by lung disease.

Chapter Sixteen provides an overview of high-pressure environments and their effect on the cardiopulmonary system. High-pressure environments have a profound effect on the cardiopulmonary system. The therapeutic administration of oxygen at increased ambient pressures (hyperbaric medicine) is now being used to treat a number of pathologic conditions.

At the end of each chapter there is a set of review questions designed to facilitate learning and retention. A new feature in the third edition is the *Clinical Application* section at the end of **Chapters Two** through **Twelve**. In this section, clinical scenarios are presented that apply several of the concepts, principles, or formulas that are presented in the chapter to actual clinical situations. In a simulated format, this section nicely facilitates the transfer of classroom material to the clinical setting.

Finally, a **glossary** is included at the end of the text. **Appendices** cover symbols and abbreviations, as well as units of measurement, commonly used in respiratory physiology. Also included is a nomogram that can be copied and laminated for use as a handy clinical reference tool in the interpretation of specific arterial blood gas abnormalities.

A student workbook and an instructor's manual to supplement this text are available from Delmar Publishers.

Terry Des Jardins, M.Ed., R.R.T.

ACKNOWLEDGMENTS

A number of colleagues and students provided important and valuable contributions in the development of the third edition of this textbook. First, I extend a most sincere thank you to Dr. Thomas DeKornfeld for his time and helpful editorial reviews of the case studies presented in the Clinical Application sections at the end of Chapters Two through Twelve. Dr. DeKornfeld made extensive editorial contributions to the first two editions of this textbook, and his constructive comments in this edition were very much appreciated.

For their valuable reviews and suggestions regarding the depth, breadth, and accuracy of all the chapters and new case studies presented in this edition, I extend a sincere thank you to the following respiratory care educators:

Allen W. Barbaro, M.S., R.R.T.
Program Director, Respiratory Care Program
Collin County Community College
McKinney, Texas

Steven Bishop, Ph.D., R.R.T.
Respiratory Care Program Director
Ozarks Technical Community College
Springfield, Missouri

Thomas J. DeKornfeld, M.D.
Emeritus Professor
University of Michigan
Department of Anesthesiology
Ann Arbor, Michigan

Beverly Edwards, B.S., R.R.T.
Department Chair, Respiratory Care Program
Florida Community College at Jacksonville
Jacksonville, Florida

Emmy L. Wishum, B.S., R.R.T.
Program Director
Respiratory Care Program
Vounteer State Community College
Gallatin, Tennessee

A special mention and gratitude go to Debra Flis, Vincent Berger, and Dawn Gerrain of Delmar Publishers for their help and efforts in the development of the third edition of this textbook. The addition of color in this textbook strongly facilitates the visualization—and understanding—of the material presented.

Terry Des Jardins, M.Ed., R.R.T.

1

THE ANATOMY OF THE RESPIRATORY SYSTEM

O B J E C T I V E S

By the end of this chapter, the student should be able to:

1. List the following three major components of the upper airway:
   —Nose
   —Oral cavity
   —Pharynx
2. List the following three primary functions of the upper airway:
   —Conductor of air
   —Prevent aspiration
   —Area for speech and smell
3. List the following three primary functions of the nose:
   —Filter
   —Humidify
   —Warm
4. Identify the following structures that form the outer portion of the nose:
   —Nasal bones
   —Frontal process of the maxilla bone
   —Lateral nasal cartilage
   —Greater alar cartilage
   —Lesser alar cartilages
   —Septal cartilage
   —Fibrous fatty tissue
5. Identify the following structures that form the internal portion of the nose:
   —Nasal septum

 • Perpendicular plate of the ethmoid bone
 • Vomer
 • Septal cartilage
   —Nasal bones
   —Frontal process of the maxilla bone
   —Cribriform plate of the ethmoid bone
   —Palatine process of the maxilla
   —Palatine bones
   —Soft palate
   —Nares
   —Vestibule
   —Vibrissae
   —Stratified squamous epithelium
   —Pseudostratified ciliated columnar epithelium
   —Turbinates (conchae)
     • Superior
     • Middle
     • Inferior
   —Paranasal sinuses
     • Maxillary
     • Frontal
     • Ethmoid
     • Sphenoid
   —Olfactory region

(continues)

—Choanae
6. Identify the following structures of the oral cavity:
—Vestibule
—Hard palate
  • Palatine process of the maxilla
  • Palatine bones
—Soft palate
—Uvula
—Levator veli palatine muscle
—Palatopharyngeal muscles
—Stratified squamous epithelium
—Palatine arches
  • Palatoglossal arch
  • Palatopharyngeal arch
—Palatine tonsils
7. Identify the location and structure of the following:
—Nasopharynx
  • Pseudostratified ciliated columnar epithelium
  • Pharyngeal tonsils (adenoids)
  • Eustachian tubes
—Oropharynx
  • Lingual tonsil
  • Stratified squamous epithelium
—Laryngopharynx
  • Esophagus
  • Epiglottis
  • Aryepiglottic folds
  • Pyriform sinuses
  • Stratified squamous epithelium
8. Identify the following cartilages of the larynx:
—Epiglottis
—Thyroid cartilage
—Cricoid cartilage
—Arytenoid cartilages
—Corniculate cartilages
—Cuneiform cartilages
9. Identify the structure and function of the following components of the interior portion of the larynx:

—False vocal folds
—True vocal folds
—Vocal ligament
—Glottis (rima glottidis)
—Epithelial lining above and below the vocal cords
10. Identify the structure and function of the following laryngeal muscles:
—Extrinsic muscles
  • Infrahyoid group
    ◦ Sternohyoid
    ◦ Sternothyroid
    ◦ Thyrohyoid
    ◦ Omohyoid
  • Suprahyoid group
    ◦ Stylohyoid
    ◦ Mylohyoid
    ◦ Digastric
    ◦ Geniohyoid
    ◦ Stylopharyngeus
—Intrinsic muscles
  • Posterior cricoarytenoid
  • Lateral cricoarytenoid
  • Transverse arytenoid
  • Thyroarytenoid
  • Cricothyroid
11. Describe the following ventilatory functions of the larynx:
—Primary function
—Secondary function (Valsalva's maneuver)
12. Describe the histology of the tracheobronchial tree, including the following components:
—Components of the epithelial lining (upper and lower airways)
  • Pseudostratified ciliated columnar epithelium
  • Basement membrane
  • Basal cells
  • Mucous blanket
    ◦ Sol layer
    ◦ Gel layer

- Goblet cells
- Bronchial glands (submucosal glands)
- Mucociliary transport mechanism
—Components of the lamina propria
  - Blood vessels
  - Lymphatic vessels
  - Branches of the vagus nerve
  - Smooth muscle fibers
  - Peribronchial sheath
  - Mast cells
    ◦ Immunologic mechanism
—Cartilaginous layer
13. Identify the location (generation) and structure of the following *cartilaginous* airways:
—Trachea
—Carina
—Main stem bronchi
—Lobar bronchi
—Segmental bronchi
—Subsegmental bronchi
14. Identify the location (generation) and structure of the following *noncartilaginous* airways:
—Bronchioles
—Terminal bronchioles
  - Canals of Lambert
  - Clara cells
15. Describe how the cross-sectional area of the tracheobronchial tree changes from the trachea to the terminal bronchioles.
16. Describe the structure and function of the following components of the bronchial blood supply:
—Bronchial arteries
—Azygos veins
—Hemiazygos veins
—Intercostal veins
17. Describe the structure and function of the following sites of gas exchange:
—Respiratory bronchioles

—Alveolar ducts
—Alveolar sacs
—Primary lobule
  - Acinus
  - Terminal respiratory unit
  - Lung parenchyma
  - Functional units
18. Discuss the structure and function of the following components of the alveolar epithelium:
—Alveolar cell types
  - Type I cell (squamous pneumocyte)
  - Type II cell (granular pneumocyte)
—Pulmonary surfactant
—Pores of Kohn
—Alveolar macrophages (Type III alveolar cells)
19. Describe the structure and function of the interstitium, including the:
—Tight space
—Loose space
20. Describe the structure and function of the following components of the pulmonary vascular system:
—Arteries
  - Tunica intima
  - Tunica media
  - Tunica adventitia
—Arterioles (resistance vessels)
  - Endothelial layer
  - Elastic layer
  - Smooth muscle fibers
—Capillaries
  - Single squamous epithelial layer
—Venules and veins (capacitance vessels)
21. Describe the structure and function of the following components of the lymphatic system:
—Lymphatic vessels
—Lymphatic nodes
—Juxta-alveolar lymphatic vessels

(continues)

22. Describe how the following components of the autonomic nervous system relate to the neural control of the lungs:
    —Sympathetic nervous system
    • Neural transmitters
    • Epinephrine
    • Norepinephrine
    • Receptors
      ◦ Beta$_2$ receptors
      ◦ Alpha receptors
    —Parasympathetic nervous system
    • Neural transmitters
      ◦ Acetylcholine
23. Identify the effect the sympathetic and parasympathetic nervous system have on the following:
    —Heart
    —Bronchial smooth muscle
    —Bronchial glands
    —Salivary glands
    —Stomach
    —Intestines
    —Eye
24. Identify the following structures of the lungs:
    —Apex of the lungs
    —Base of the lungs
    —Mediastinal border
    —Hilum
    —Specific right lung structures
    • Upper lobe
    • Middle lobe
    • Lower lobe
    • Oblique fissure
    • Horizontal fissure
    —Specific left lung structures
    • Upper lobe
    • Lower lobe
    • Oblique fissure
25. Identify the following lung segments from the anterior, posterior, lateral, and medial views:
    —Right lung segments

• Upper lobe
  ◦ Apical
  ◦ Posterior
  ◦ Anterior
• Middle lobe
  ◦ Lateral
  ◦ Medial
• Lower lobe
  ◦ Superior
  ◦ Medial basal
  ◦ Anterior basal
  ◦ Lateral basal
  ◦ Posterior basal
    —Left lung segments
• Upper lobe
  ◦ Upper division
    1) Apical-posterior
    2) Anterior
  ◦ Lower division (lingular)
    1) Superior lingula
    2) Inferior lingula
• Lower lobe
  ◦ Superior
  ◦ Anteromedial
  ◦ Lateral basal
  ◦ Posterior basal
26. Identify the following components of the mediastinum:
    —Trachea
    —Heart
    —Major blood vessels
    —Nerves
    —Esophagus
    —Thymus gland
    —Lymph nodes
27. Identify the following components of the pleural membranes:
    —Parietal pleurae
    —Visceral pleurae
    —Pleural cavity
28. Identify the following components of the thorax:
    —Thoracic vertebrae
    —Sternum

- Manubrium
- Body
- Xiphoid process
—True ribs
—False ribs
—Floating ribs
29. Describe the structure and function of the diaphragm and include the following:
    —Hemidiaphragms
    —Central tendon
    —Phrenic nerves
    —Lower thoracic nerves
30. Describe the structure and function of the following accessory muscles of inspiration:

—Scalene muscles
—Sternocleidomastoid muscles
—Pectoralis major muscles
—Trapezius muscles
—External intercostal muscles
31. Describe the structure and function of the following accessory muscles of expiration:
    —Rectus abdominis muscles
    —External abdominis oblique muscles
    —Internal abdominis oblique muscles
    —Transversus abdominis muscles
    —Internal intercostal muscles
32. Complete the review questions at the end of this chapter.

THE UPPER AIRWAY

The upper airway consists of the **nose**, **oral cavity**, and **pharynx** (Figure 1–1). The primary functions of the upper airway are (1) to act as a conductor of air, (2) to prevent foreign materials from entering the tracheobronchial tree, and (3) to serve as an important area involved in speech and smell.

THE NOSE

The primary functions of the nose are to *filter*, *humidify*, and *warm* inspired air. The nose is also important as the site for the sense of smell and to generate resonance in phonation.

The outer portion of the nose is composed of bone and cartilage. The upper third of the nose (the bridge) is formed by the **nasal bones** and the **frontal process of the maxilla**. The lower two-thirds consist of the **lateral nasal cartilage**, the **greater alar cartilage**, the **lesser alar cartilages**, the **septal cartilage**, and some **fibrous fatty tissue** (Figure 1–2, page 7).

In the internal portion of the nose there is a partition, the **nasal septum**, that separates the nasal cavity into two approximately equal chambers. Posteriorly, the nasal septum is formed by the **perpendicular plate of the ethmoid bone** and the **vomer**. Anteriorly, the septum is formed by the **septal cartilage**. The roof of the nasal cavity is formed by the **nasal bones**, the **frontal process of the maxilla**, and

Figure 1–1. *Sagittal section of human head, showing the upper airway.*

the **cribriform plate of the ethmoid bone**. The floor is formed by the **palatine process of the maxilla** and by the **palatine bones**—the same bones that form the hard palate of the roof of the mouth. The posterior section of the nasal cavity floor is formed by the superior portion of the **soft palate** of the oral cavity, which consists of a flexible mass of densely packed collagen fibers (see Figure 1–3).

Air enters the nasal cavity through the two openings formed by the septal cartilage and the alae nasi, called the **nares**, or **nostrils**. Initially, the air passes through a slightly dilated area called the **vestibule** (see Figure 1–1), which contains hair follicles called **vibrissae**. The vibrissae function as a filter and are the tracheobronchial tree's first line of defense. **Stratified squamous epithelium** (nonciliated) lines the anterior one-third of the nasal cavity (Figure 1–4A, page 8). The posterior two-thirds of the nasal cavity are lined with **pseudostratified ciliated columnar epithelium** (Figure 1–4B). The cilia propel nasal mucus toward the nasopharynx.

There are three bony protrusions on the lateral walls of the nasal cavity, called the **superior**, **middle**, and **inferior nasal turbinates**, or **conchae**. The turbinates separate inspired gas into several different airstreams. This action, in turn, increases the contact area between the inspired air and the warm, moist surface of the

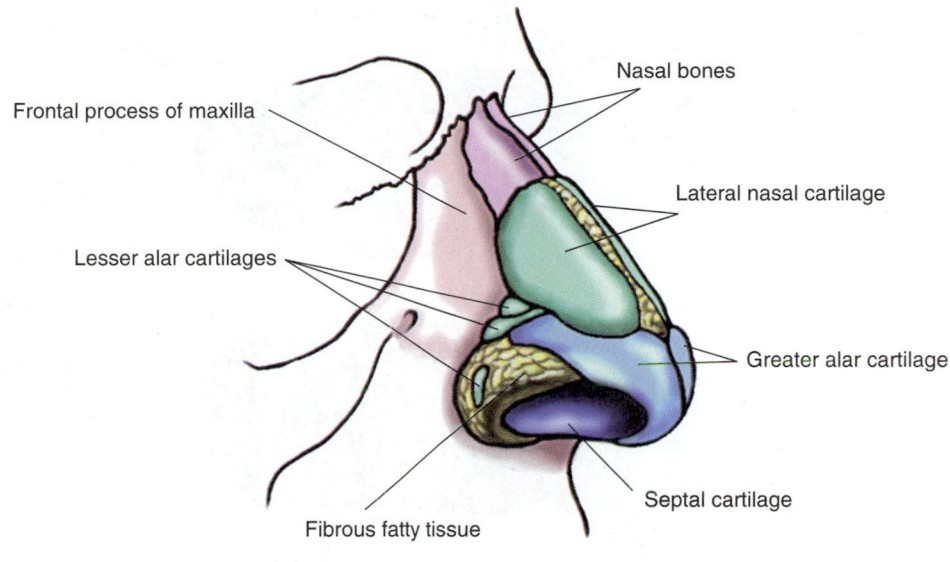

Figure 1–2. *Structure of the nose.*

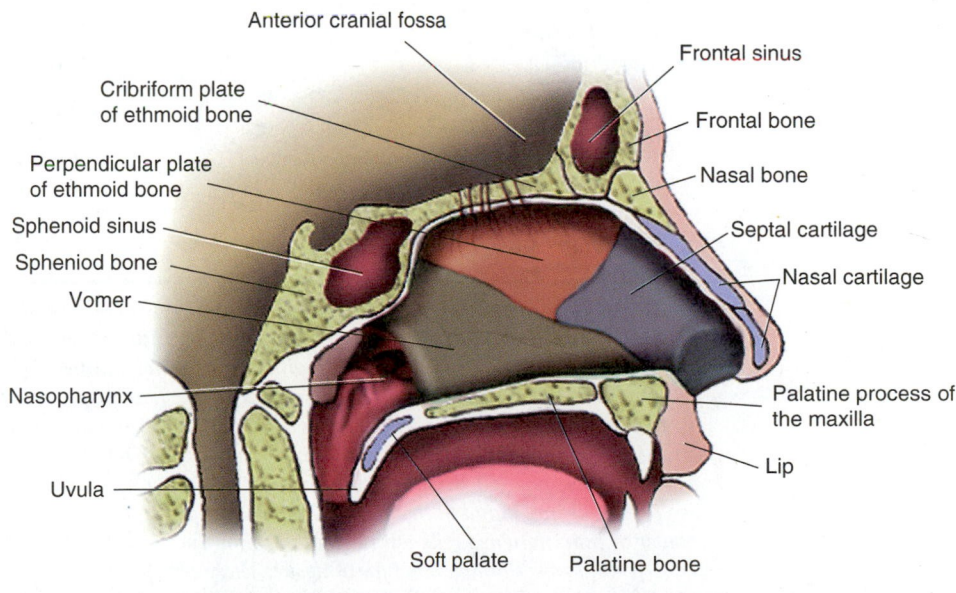

Figure 1–3. *Sagittal section through the nose, showing the parts of the nasal septum.*

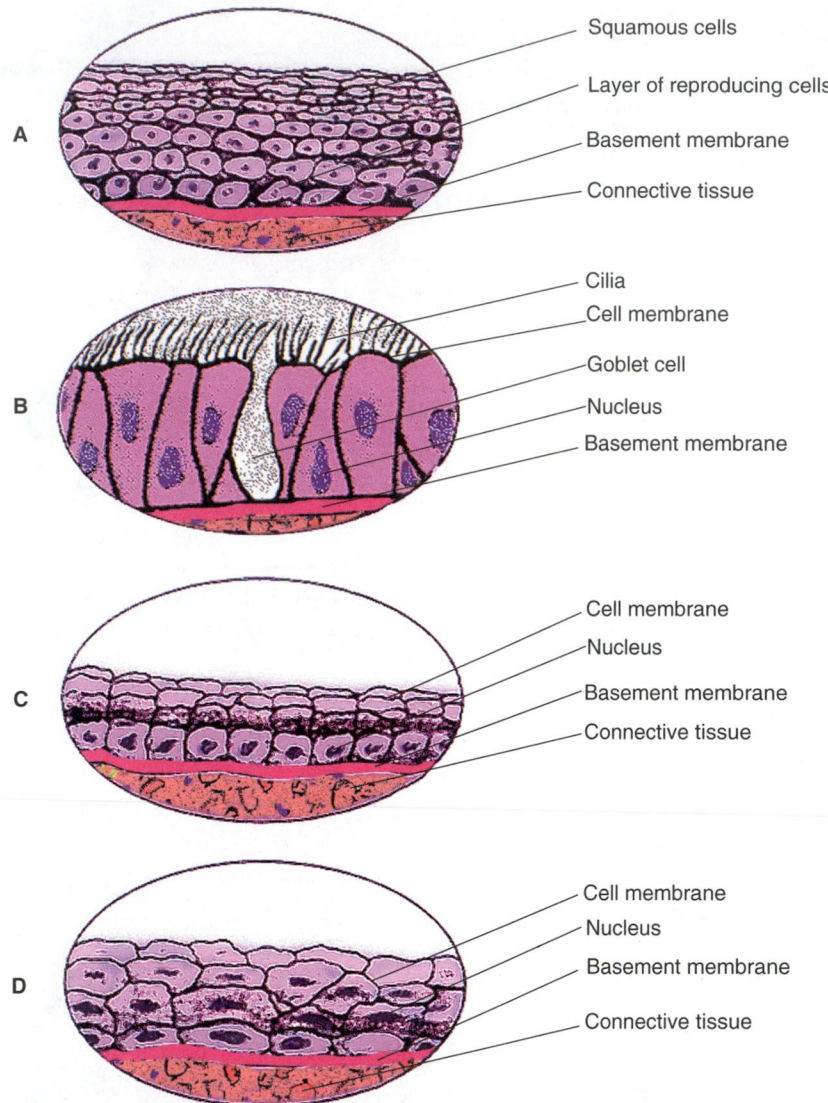

Squamous cells

Layer of reproducing cells

Basement membrane

Connective tissue

A

Cilia
Cell membrane
Goblet cell
Nucleus
Basement membrane

B

Cell membrane
Nucleus
Basement membrane
Connective tissue

C

Cell membrane
Nucleus
Basement membrane
Connective tissue

D

Figure 1–4. *A) Stratified squamous epithelium consists of several layers of cells. This tissue is found in the anterior portion of the nasal cavity, oral cavity, oropharynx, and laryngopharynx. B) Pseudostratified columnar epithelium with cilia appears stratified, because the nuclei of the cells are located at different levels. These cells have microscopic hairlike projections called cilia that extend from the outer surface. Mucus-producing goblet cells are also found throughout this tissue. Pseudostratified columnar ciliated epithelium lines the posterior two-thirds of the nasal cavity and the tracheobronchial tree. C) Simple cuboidal epithelium consists of a single layer of cube-shaped cells. These cells are found in the bronchioles. D) Simple squamous epithelium consists of a single layer of thin, flattened cells with broad and thin nuclei. Substances such as oxygen and carbon dioxide readily pass through this type of tissue. These cells form the walls of the alveoli and the pulmonary capillaries that surround the alveoli.*

nasal mucosa. The turbinates play a major role in the humidification and warming of inspired air (see Figure 1–1).

Beneath the superior and middle turbinates are the openings of the **paranasal sinuses**. The paranasal sinuses are air-filled cavities in the bones of the skull that communicate with the nasal cavity. The paranasal sinuses include the **maxillary**, **frontal**, **ethmoid**, and **sphenoid sinuses** (Figure 1–5). The paranasal sinuses provide mucus for the nasal cavity and act as resonating chambers for the production of sound. The receptors for the sense of smell are located in the **olfactory region**, which is near the superior and middle turbinates (see Figure 1–1). The two nasal passageways between the nares and the nasopharynx are also called the **choanae**.

ORAL CAVITY

The oral cavity is considered an accessory respiratory passage. It consists of the **vestibule**, which is the small outer portion between the teeth (and gums) and lips, and a larger section behind the teeth and gums that extends back to the oropharynx (Figure 1–6, page 10). The oral cavity houses the anterior two-thirds of the tongue. The posterior one-third of the tongue is attached to the hyoid bone and the mandible in the pharynx.

The roof the mouth is formed by the **hard** and **soft palate**. The hard palate is composed of the **palatine process of the maxilla** and the **palatine bones** (see

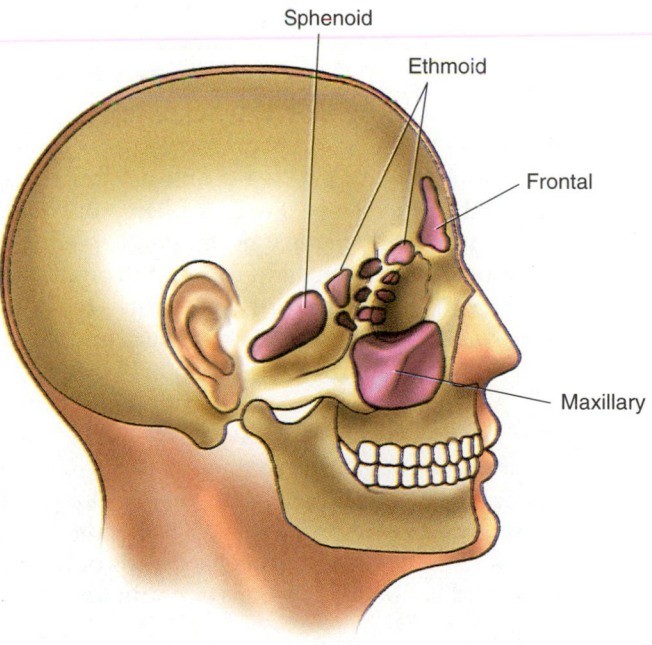

Figure 1–5. *Lateral view of head, showing sinuses.*

Figure 1–6. *Oral cavity.*

Figure 1–3). The **soft palate** consists of a flexible mass of densely packed collagen fiber that projects backward and downward, ending in the soft, fleshy structure called the **uvula** (see Figure 1–6). The soft palate closes off the opening between the nasal and oral pharynx by moving upward and backward during swallowing, sucking, and blowing and during the production of certain speech sounds. The **levator veli palatinum muscle** elevates the soft palate, and the **palatopharyngeal muscles** draw the soft palate forward and downward. The oral cavity is lined with **stratified squamous epithelium**, which is nonciliated (see Figure 1–4A).

Two folds of mucous membrane pass along the lateral borders of the posterior portion of the oral cavity. These folds form the **palatoglossal arch** and the **palatopharyngeal arch**, named after the muscles that they cover. Collectively, these arches are called the **palatine arches**. The **palatine tonsils** (faucial) are located between the palatine arches on each side of the oral cavity (see Figure 1–6). The palatine tonsils, like the pharyngeal tonsils or nasopharynx adenoids, are lymphoid tissues and are believed to serve certain protective functions.

THE PHARYNX

After the inspired air passes through the nasal cavity, it enters the **pharynx**. The pharynx is divided into three parts: the **nasopharynx**, the **oropharynx**, and the **laryngopharynx** (see Figure 1–1).

Nasopharynx

The nasopharynx is located posterior to the nasal cavity and superior to the soft palate at the back of the oral cavity. The nasopharynx is lined with **pseudostratified ciliated columnar epithelium** (see Figure 1–4B). Lymphoid tissues called **pharyngeal tonsils**, or **adenoids**, are located in the posterior nasopharynx (see Figure 1–1). An opening for the **eustachian tube** (auditory tube) is located on the two lateral surfaces of the nasopharynx. The eustachian tube connects the nasopharynx to the middle ear and serves to equalize the pressure in the middle ear.

Oropharynx

The oropharynx lies between the soft palate superiorly and the base of the tongue inferiorly (see Figure 1–1). There is also a mass of lymphoid tissue located at the root of the tongue called the **lingual tonsil**. The mucosa of the oropharynx is composed of nonciliated **stratified squamous epithelium** (see Figure 1–4A).

Laryngopharynx

The laryngopharynx lies between the base of the tongue and the entrance to the **esophagus** (see Figure 1–1). The **epiglottis** is directly anterior to the laryngopharynx. The **aryepiglottic folds** form the lateral borders of the laryngopharynx. The laryngopharynx is lined with nonciliated **stratified squamous epithelium** (see Figure 1–4A).

 ## THE LOWER AIRWAYS

THE LARYNX

The **larynx**, or voice box, is located between the base of the tongue and the upper end of the trachea (see Figure 1–1). The larynx is commonly described as a vestibule opening into the trachea from the pharynx. The larynx serves three functions: (1) it acts as a passageway of air between the pharynx and the trachea, (2) it works as a protective mechanism against the aspiration of solids and liquids, and (3) it generates sounds for speech.

Cartilages of the Larynx

The larynx consists of a framework of nine cartilages (Figure 1–7, page 12). Three are single cartilages: the **thyroid cartilage**, **cricoid cartilage**, and the **epiglottis**. Three are paired cartilages: the **arytenoid**, **corniculate**, and **cuneiform cartilages** (see Figure 1–7A, B). The cartilages of the larynx are held in position by ligaments, membranes, and **intrinsic** and **extrinsic muscles**. The interior of the larynx is lined with mucous membrane.

The **thyroid cartilage** (commonly called the Adam's apple) is the largest cartilage of the larynx. It is a double-winged structure that spreads over the anterior portion of the larynx. Along its superior border is a V-shaped notch, the **thyroid notch**. The upper portion of the thyroid cartilage is suspended from the horseshoe-shaped

Epiglottis

Hyoid bone

Thyrohyoid membrane

Corniculate cartilage

Arytenoid cartilage

Vocal process

Cricothyroid ligament

Vocal ligament

Cricoid cartilage

Trachea

Anterior view
A

LARYNGEAL CARTILAGES

Posterior view
B

Epiglottis

Aryepiglottic fold

Cuneiform tubercle
(cartilage)

Corniculate tubercle
(cartilage)

Aryepiglottic
muscle

Oblique
arytenoid muscle

Transverse
arytenoid muscle

Thyroarytenoid
muscle

Lateral
cricoaryteniod
muscle

Posterior
cricoarytenoid
muscle

Cricoid
cartilage

Cricothyroid muscle
(cut away)

Lateral view
C

Posterior view
D

INTRINSIC MUSCLES OF THE LARYNX

Figure 1–7. *Cartilages of the larynx.*

hyoid bone by the **thyrohyoid membrane**. Technically, the hyoid bone is not a part of the larynx.

The **epiglottis** is a broad, spoon-shaped fibrocartilaginous structure. Its base is attached to the medial surface of the thyroid cartilage, and it is free on its other borders. The epiglottis and the base of the tongue are connected by mucous membrane. The epiglottis prevents the aspiration of foods and liquids by covering the opening of the larynx during swallowing.

The **cricoid cartilage** is shaped like a signet ring. It is located inferior to the thyroid cartilage and forms a large portion of the posterior wall of the larynx. The inferior border of the cricoid cartilage is attached to the first C-shaped cartilage of the trachea (see Figure 1–7).

The paired **arytenoid cartilages** are shaped like a three-sided pyramid. The base of each arytenoid cartilage rests on the superior surface of the posterior portion of the cricoid cartilage. The apex of each arytenoid cartilage curves posteriorly and medially and flattens for articulation with the corniculate cartilages. At the base of each arytenoid cartilage is a projection called the **vocal process**. The **vocal ligaments**, which form the medial portion of the vocal folds, attach to the vocal process.

The paired **cuneiform cartilages** and **corniculate cartilages** are small accessory cartilages that are closely associated with the arytenoid cartilages. The cuneiform cartilages are embedded within the aryepiglottic folds that extend from the apices of the arytenoid cartilages to the epiglottis. They probably act to stiffen the folds. The two corniculate cartilages lie on top of the arytenoid cartilages.

Interior of the Larynx

The interior portion of the larynx is lined by a mucous membrane that forms two pairs of folds that protrude inward. The upper pair are called the **false vocal folds**, since they play no role in vocalization. The lower pair functions as the **true vocal folds** (vocal cords). The medial border of each vocal fold is composed of a strong band of elastic tissue called the **vocal ligament**. Anteriorly, the vocal cords attach to the posterior surface of the thyroid cartilage. Posteriorly, the vocal folds attach to the vocal process of the arytenoid cartilage. The arytenoid cartilages can rotate about a vertical axis through the cricoarytenoid joint, allowing the medial border to move anteriorly or posteriorly. This action, in turn, loosens or tightens the true vocal cords.

The space between the true vocal cords is termed the **rima glottidis** or, for ease of reference, the **glottis** (Figure 1–8, page 14). In the adult the glottis is the narrowest point in the larynx. In the infant the cricoid cartilage is the narrowest point.

Above the vocal cords, the laryngeal mucosa is composed of (nonciliated) **stratified squamous epithelium** (see Figure 1–4A). Below the vocal cords, the laryngeal mucosa is covered by **pseudostratified columnar epithelium** (see Figure 1–4B).

Laryngeal Musculature

The muscles of the larynx consist of the **extrinsic** and **intrinsic** muscle groups. The extrinsic muscles are subdivided into an **infrahyoid** and a **suprahyoid** group. The

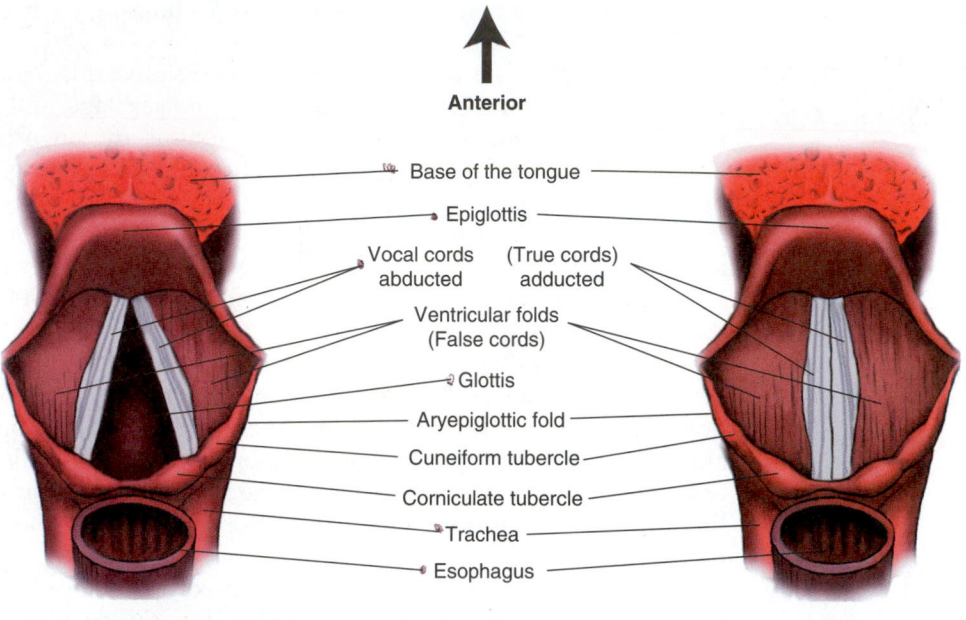

Anterior

Base of the tongue
Epiglottis
Vocal cords (True cords)
abducted adducted
Ventricular folds
(False cords)
Glottis
Aryepiglottic fold
Cuneiform tubercle
Corniculate tubercle
Trachea
Esophagus

Figure 1–8. *Superior view of vocal folds (cords).*

infrahyoid group consists of the **sternohyoid**, **sternothyroid**, **thyrohyoid**, and **omohyoid muscles** (Figure 1–9). These muscles pull the larynx and hyoid bone down to a lower position in the neck. The suprahyoid group consists of the **stylohyoid**, **mylohyoid**, **digastric**, **geniohyoid**, and **stylopharyngeus muscles**. These muscles pull the hyoid bone forward, upward, and backward (see Figure 1–9). The major **intrinsic muscles** that control the movement of the vocal folds are illustrated in Figure 1–7C, D. The action(s) of these muscles are described below.

Posterior Cricoarytenoid Muscles. These muscles pull inferiorly on the lateral angles of the arytenoids. This causes the vocal folds to move apart (*abduct*) and thus allows air to pass through (Figure 1–10A, page 16).

Lateral Cricoarytenoid Muscles. The action of these muscles is the opposite of the posterior cricoarytenoid muscles. These muscles pull laterally on the lateral angles of the arytenoids, causing the vocal folds to move together (*adduct*) (Figure 1–10B).

Transverse Arytenoid Muscles. These muscles pull the arytenoid cartilages together and thereby position the two vocal folds so that they vibrate as air passes between them during exhalation. Thus the sounds for speech or singing are generated (Figure 1–10C).

Thyroarytenoid Muscles. These muscles lie in the vocal folds lateral to the vocal ligaments. Contraction of the thyroarytenoid muscles pulls the arytenoid cartilages

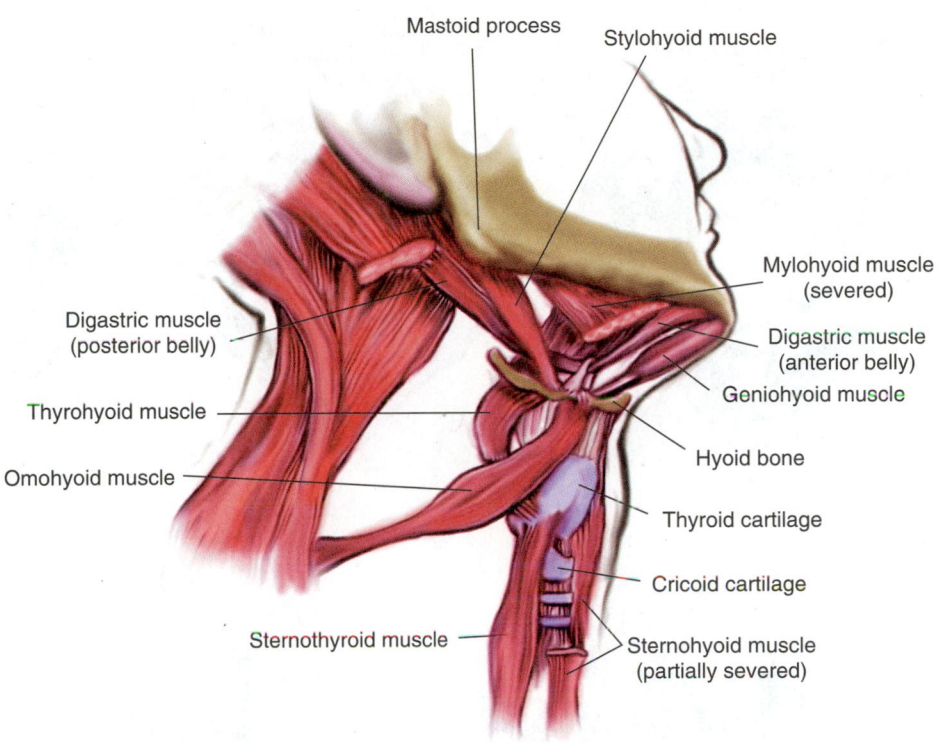

Figure 1–9. *Extrinsic laryngeal muscles.*

forward. This action loosens the vocal ligaments and allows a lower frequency of phonation (Figure 1–10D).

Cricothyroid Muscles. These muscles, which are located on the anterior surface of the larynx, can swing the entire thyroid cartilage anteriorly. This action provides an additional way to tense the vocal folds and thereby change the frequency of phonation (Figure 1–10E).

Ventilatory Function of the Larynx

A primary function of the larynx is to ensure a free flow of air to and from the lungs. During a quiet inspiration, the vocal folds move apart (abduct) and widen the glottis. During exhalation, the vocal folds move toward the midline slightly (adduct) but always maintain an open glottal airway.

A second vital function of the larynx is effort closure during exhalation, also known as **Valsalva's maneuver**. During this maneuver, there is a massive undifferentiated adduction of the laryngeal walls, including both the true and false vocal folds. As a result, the lumen of the larynx is tightly sealed, preventing air from escaping during physical work such as lifting, pushing, coughing, throat-clearing, vomiting, urination, defecation, and parturition.

Figure 1–10. *Intrinsic laryngeal muscles.*

THE TRACHEOBRONCHIAL TREE

After passing through the larynx, inspired air enters the tracheobronchial tree, which is a series of branching airways commonly referred to as *generations*, or *orders*. These airways become progressively narrower, shorter, and more numerous as they branch throughout the lungs (Figure 1–11). Table 1–1 lists the major subdivisions of the tracheobronchial tree.

In general, the airways exist in two major forms: (1) **cartilaginous airways** and (2) **noncartilaginous airways**. (The main structures of these airways are discussed in detail on page 25). The cartilaginous airways serve only to conduct air between the external environment and the sites of gas exchange. The noncartilaginous airways serve both as conductors of air and as sites of gas exchange. These will be discussed in detail below.

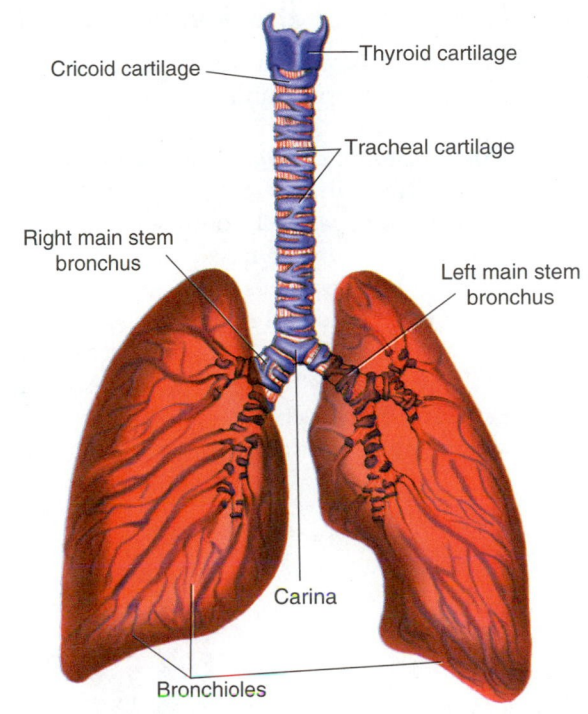

Figure 1–11. *Tracheobronchial tree.*

TABLE 1–1. **Major Structures and Corresponding Generations of the Tracheobronchial Tree**

	STRUCTURES OF THE LUNGS	GENERATIONS*	
Conducting Zone	Trachea	0	Cartilaginous airways
	Main stem bronchi	1	
	Lobar bronchi	2	
	Segmental bronchi	3	
	Subsegmental bronchi	4–9	
	Bronchioles	10–15	Noncartilaginous airways
	Terminal bronchioles	16–19	
Respiratory Zone	Respiratory bronchioles[†]	20–23	Sites of gas exchange
	Alveolar ducts[†]	24–27	
	Alveolar sacs[†]	28	

*NOTE: The precise number of generations between the subsegmental bronchi and the alveolar sacs is not known.
[†]These structures collectively are referred to as a primary lobule (see page 28) or lung parenchyma; they are also called terminal respiratory units and functional units.

Histology of the Tracheobronchial Tree

The tracheobronchial tree is composed of three major layers: an epithelial lining, the lamina propria, and a cartilaginous layer (Figure 1–12).

The Epithelial Lining.   The epithelial lining is predominantly composed of pseudostratified ciliated columnar epithelium interspersed with numerous mucous glands and separated from the lamina propria by a basement membrane (see Figure 1–12). Along the basement membrane of the epithelial lining are oval-shaped basal cells. These cells serve as a reserve supply of cells and replenish the superficial ciliated cells and mucous cells as needed.

The pseudostratified ciliated columnar epithelium extends from the trachea to the respiratory bronchioles. There are about 200 cilia per ciliated cell. The length of each cilium is about 5–7 μ (microns). As the bronchioles progressively become smaller, the columnar structure of the epithelium decreases in height and appears

Figure 1–12.   *Histology of the tracheobronchial tree.*

more cuboidal than columnar (see Figure 1–4C). The cilia progressively disappear in the terminal bronchioles and are completely absent in the respiratory bronchioles.

A mucus layer, commonly referred to as the **mucous blanket**, covers the epithelial lining of the tracheobronchial tree (Figure 1–13). In general, the mucous blanket is composed of 95 percent water, with the remaining 5 percent consisting of glycoproteins, carbohydrates, lipids, DNA, some cellular debris, and foreign particles. The mucus is produced by (1) the **goblet cells**, and (2) the **submucosal**, or **bronchial**, **glands** (see Figure 1–12). The goblet cells are located intermittently between the pseudostratified ciliated columnar cells and have been identified down to, and including, the terminal bronchioles. The submucosal glands, which produce most of the mucous blanket, extend deep into the lamina propria. These glands are innervated by the vagal parasympathetic nerve fibers (the tenth cranial nerve) and produce about 100 ml of bronchial secretions per day. Increased sympathetic activity decreases glandular secretions. The submucosal glands are particularly numerous in the medium-sized bronchi and disappear in the distal terminal bronchioles (see Figure 1–13).

The viscosity of the mucous blanket progressively increases from the epithelial lining to the inner luminal surface. The blanket has two distinct layers: (1) the **sol layer**, which is adjacent to the epithelial lining, and (2) the **gel layer**, which is the more viscous layer adjacent to the inner luminal surface. Under normal circumstances, the cilia move in a wavelike fashion through the less viscous sol layer and continually strike the innermost portion of the gel layer (approximately 1500 times per minute). This action propels the mucus layer, along with any foreign particles stuck to the gel layer, toward the larynx at an estimated average rate of

Figure 1–13. *Epithelial lining of the tracheobronchial tree.*

2 cm per minute. Precisely what causes the cilia to move is unknown. At the larynx, the cough mechanism moves secretions beyond the larynx and into the oropharynx. This process is commonly referred to as the **mucociliary transport mechanism** or the **mucociliary escalator**, and is an important part of the cleansing mechanism of the tracheobronchial tree. Clinically, there are a number of factors that are now known to slow the rate of the mucociliary transport. Some common factors are:

- Cigarette smoke
- Dehydration
- Positive pressure ventilation
- Endotracheal suctioning
- High inspired oxygen concentrations
- Hypoxia
- Atmospheric pollutants (e.g., sulfur dioxide, nitrogen dioxide, ozone)
- General anesthetics
- Parasympatholytics (e.g., atropine)

The Lamina Propria. The **lamina propria** is the submucosal layer of the tracheobronchial tree. Within the lamina propria there is a loose, fibrous tissue that contains tiny blood vessels, lymphatic vessels, and branches of the vagus nerve. Also found within the lamina propria are two sets of smooth muscle fibers. These sets of muscles wrap around the tracheobronchial tree in fairly close spirals, one clockwise and the other counterclockwise. The smooth muscle fibers extend down to, and including, the alveolar ducts (see the section on sites of gas exchange in this chapter). The outer portion of the lamina propria is surrounded by a thin connective tissue called the **peribronchial sheath** (see Figure 1–16, page 23).

Immune Response. **Mast cells** play an important role in the immunologic mechanism. They are also found in the lamina propria—near the branches of the vagus nerve and blood vessels and scattered throughout the smooth muscle bundles, in the intra-alveolar septa, and as one of the cell constituents of the submucosal glands (Figure 1–14). Outside of the lungs, mast cells are found in loose connective tissue of skin and intestinal submucosa.

When they are activated, numerous substances are released from the mast cells which can significantly alter the diameter of the bronchial airways. Because of this fact, a basic understanding of how the mast cells function in the immunologic system is essential to the respiratory care practitioner.

There are two major immune responses: **cellular immunity** and **humoral immunity**. The *cellular immune response* involves the sensitized lymphocytes that are responsible for tissue rejection in transplants. This immune response is also termed a type IV, or delayed, type of hypersensitivity.

The *humoral immune response* involves the circulating antibodies that are involved in allergic responses such as allergic asthma. Antibodies (also called immunoglobulins) are serum globulins, or proteins, that defend against invading environmental antigens such as pollen, ragweed, animal dander, and feathers. Although five different immunoglobulins (IgG, IgA, IgM, IgD, and IgE) have been

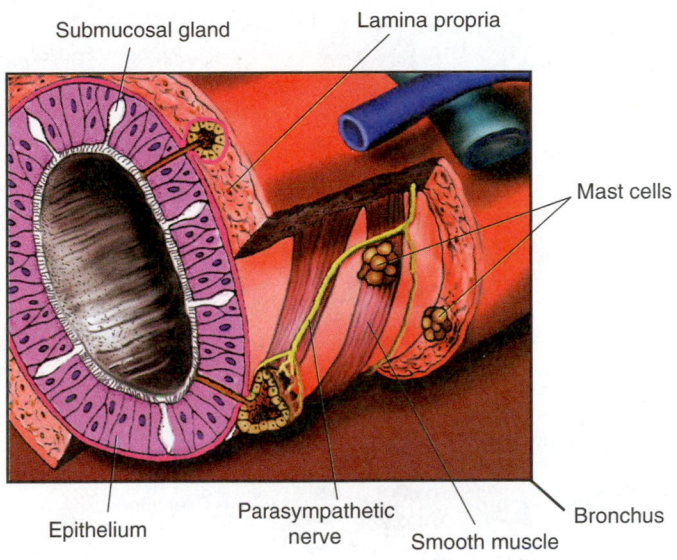

Submucosal gland   Lamina propria

Mast cells

Epithelium   Parasympathetic nerve   Smooth muscle   Bronchus

Figure 1–14. *Mast cells of the lamina propria.*

identified, the IgE (reaginic) antibody is basic to the allergic response. The mechanism of the IgE antibody-antigen reaction is as follows:

1. When a susceptible individual is exposed to a certain antigen, the lymphoid tissues release specific IgE antibodies. The newly formed IgE antibodies travel through the blood stream and attach to surface receptors on the mast cells. It is estimated that there are between 100,000 and 500,000 IgE receptor sites on the surface of each mast cell. Once the IgE antibodies attach to the mast cell, the individual (or more specifically, the mast cell) is said to be sensitive to the specific antigen (Figure 1–15A, page 22).

2. Each mast cell also has about 1000 secretory granules that contain several chemical mediators of inflammation (see below). Continued exposure, or re-exposure, to the same antigen creates an IgE antibody-antigen reaction on the surface of the mast cell, which works to destroy or inactivate the antigen. This response, however, causes the mast cell to degranulate (break down) and to release the following chemical mediators (Figure 1–15B):
   a. Histamine
   b. Heparin
   c. Slow-reacting substance of anaphylaxis (SRS-A)
   d. Platelet-activating factor (PAF)
   e. Eosinophilic chemotactic factor of anaphylaxis (ECF-A)

3. The release of these chemical mediators causes increased vascular permeability, smooth muscle contraction, increased mucus secretion, and vasodilation with edema.

Such a reaction in the lungs can be extremely dangerous and is seen in individuals during an allergic asthmatic episode. The production of IgE antibodies

Figure 1–15. *Immunologic mechanisms.*

may be 20 times greater than normal in some asthmatic patients (the normal IgE antibody level in the serum is about 200 ng/ml). During an asthmatic attack, the patient demonstrates bronchial edema, bronchospasms and wheezing, increased mucus production, mucus plugging, air trapping, and lung hyperinflation (Figure 1–15C).

The Cartilaginous Layer. The cartilaginous layer, which is the outermost layer of the tracheobronchial tree, progressively diminishes in size as the airways extend into the lungs. Cartilage is completely absent in bronchioles less than 1 millimeter (mm) in diameter (see Figure 1–12).

The Cartilaginous Airways

As shown in Table 1–1, the cartilaginous airways consist of the trachea, main stem bronchi, lobar bronchi, segmental bronchi, and subsegmental bronchi. Collectively, the cartilaginous airways are referred to as the conducting zone.

Trachea. The adult trachea is about 11 to 13 centimeters (cm) long and 1.5 to 2.5 centimeters in diameter (Figure 1–16). It extends vertically from the cricoid cartilage of the larynx to about the level of the second costal cartilage, or fifth thoracic vertebra. At this point, the trachea divides into the right and left main stem bronchi. The bifurcation of the trachea is known as the carina. Approximately 15 to 20 C-shaped cartilages support the trachea. These cartilages are incomplete posteriorly where the trachea and the esophagus share a fibroelastic membrane (Figure 1–17, page 24).

Main Stem Bronchi. The right main stem bronchus branches off the trachea at about a 25-degree angle; the left main stem bronchus forms an angle of 40 to 60

Figure 1–16. *Trachea.*

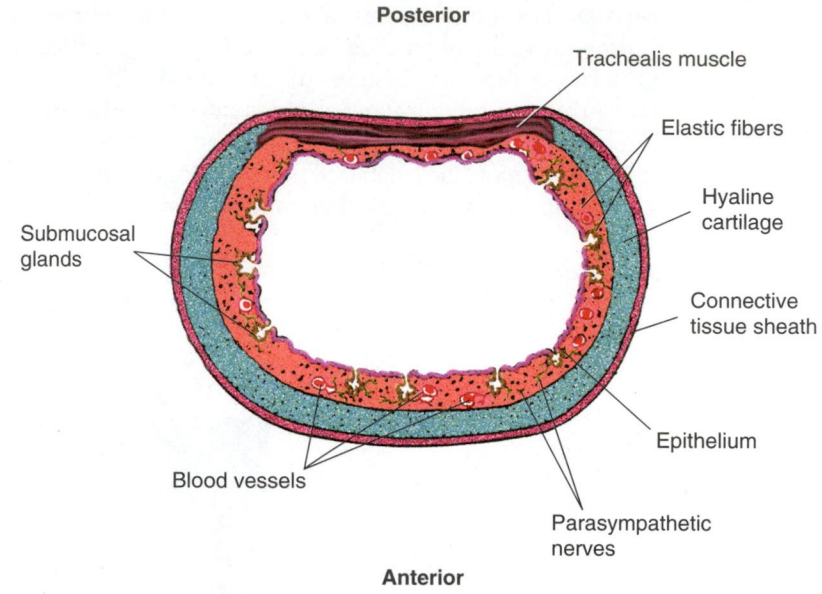

Posterior

Trachealis muscle

Elastic fibers

Hyaline cartilage

Connective tissue sheath

Submucosal glands

Epithelium

Blood vessels

Parasympathetic nerves

Anterior

Figure 1–17. *Cross-section of trachea.*

degrees with the trachea. The right main stem bronchus is wider, more vertical, and about 5 cm shorter than the left main stem bronchus. Similar to the trachea, the main stem bronchi are supported by C-shaped cartilages. In the newborn, both the right and left main stem bronchi form about a 55-degree angle with the trachea. The main stem bronchi are the tracheobronchial tree's first generation.

Lobar Bronchi. The right main stem bronchus divides into the upper, middle, and lower lobar bronchi. The left main stem bronchus branches into the upper and lower lobar bronchi. The lobar bronchi are the tracheobronchial tree's second generation. The C-shaped cartilages that support the trachea and the main stem bronchi progressively form cartilaginous plates around the lobar bronchi.

Segmental Bronchi. A third generation of bronchi branch off the lobar bronchi to form the segmental bronchi. There are ten segmental bronchi in the right lung and eight in the left lung. Each segmental bronchus is named according to its location within a particular lung lobe.

Subsegmental Bronchi. The tracheobronchial tree continues to subdivide between the fourth and approximately the ninth generation into progressively smaller airways called subsegmental bronchi. These bronchi range in diameter from 1 to 4 mm. Peribronchial connective tissue containing nerves, lymphatics, and bronchial arteries surrounds the subsegmental bronchi to about the 1-mm diameter level. After this point, the connective tissue sheaths disappear.

The Noncartilaginous Airways

The noncartilaginous airways are composed of the **bronchioles** and the **terminal bronchioles**.

Bronchioles. When the bronchi decrease to less than 1 mm in diameter and are no longer surrounded by connective tissue sheaths, they are called bronchioles. The bronchioles are found between the tenth and fifteenth generations. At this level, cartilage is absent and the lamina propria is directly connected with the lung parenchyma (see lung parenchyma in the section on sites of gas exchange in this chapter). The bronchioles are surrounded by spiral muscle fibers and the epithelial cells are more cuboidal in shape (see Figure 1–12). The rigidity of the bronchioles is very low when compared with the cartilaginous airways. Because of this, the airway patency at this level may be substantially altered by intra-alveolar and intrapleural pressures and by alterations in the size of the lungs. This lack of airway support often plays a major role in respiratory disease.

Terminal Bronchioles. The conducting tubes of the tracheobronchial tree end with the terminal bronchioles between the sixteenth and nineteenth generations. The average diameter of the terminal bronchioles is about 0.5 mm. At this point, the cilia and the mucous glands progressively disappear, the epithelium flattens and becomes cuboidal in shape (see Figures 1–4C and 1–12).

As the walls of the terminal bronchioles progressively become thinner, small channels, called the **canals of Lambert**, begin to appear between the inner luminal surface of the terminal bronchioles and the adjacent alveoli that surround them (Figure 1–18, page 26). Although specific information as to their function is lacking, it is believed that these tiny pathways may be important secondary avenues for collateral ventilation in patients with certain respiratory disorders (e.g., chronic obstructive pulmonary disease).

Also unique to the terminal bronchioles is the presence of **Clara cells**. These cells have thick protoplasmic extensions that bulge into the lumen of the terminal bronchioles. The precise function of the Clara cells is not known. They may have secretory functions that contribute to the extracellular liquid lining the bronchioles and alveoli. They may also contain enzymes that work to detoxify inhaled toxic substances.

The anatomic structures beyond the terminal bronchioles are the normal sites of gas exchange and, although directly connected, are not considered part of the tracheobronchial tree.

Bronchial Cross-Sectional Area

The total cross-sectional area of the tracheobronchial tree steadily increases from the trachea to the terminal bronchioles. The total cross-sectional area increases significantly beyond the terminal bronchioles because of the many branches that occur at this level. The anatomic structures distal to the terminal bronchioles are, collectively, referred to as the **respiratory zone** (Figure 1–19, page 27).

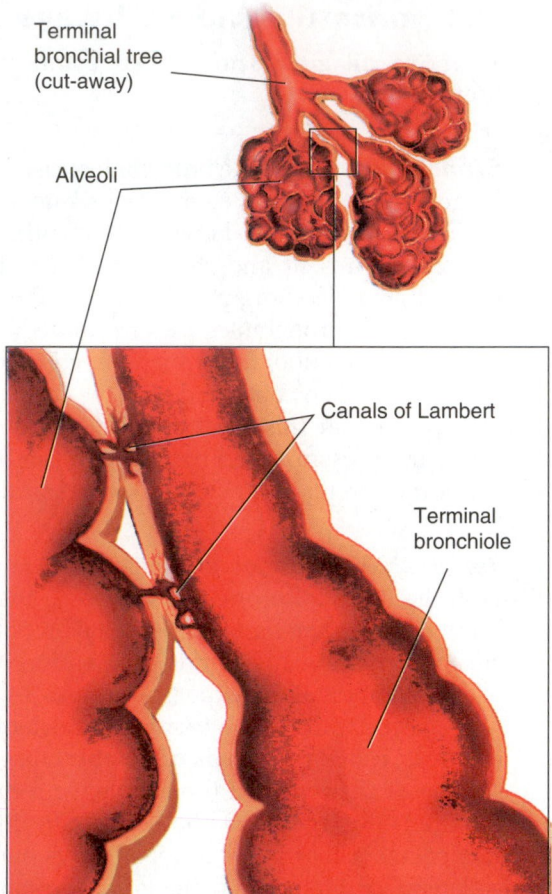

Terminal
bronchial tree
(cut-away)

Alveoli

Canals of Lambert

Terminal
bronchiole

Figure 1–18.   *Canals of Lambert.*

Air flows down the tracheobronchial tree as a mass to about the level of the terminal bronchioles, similar to water flowing through a tube. Because the cross-sectional area becomes so great beyond this point, however, the forward motion essentially stops and the natural molecular movement of gas becomes the dominant mechanism of ventilation.

BRONCHIAL BLOOD SUPPLY

The bronchial arteries nourish the tracheobronchial tree. The arteries arise from the aorta and follow the tracheobronchial tree as far as the terminal bronchioles. Beyond the terminal bronchioles, the bronchial arteries lose their identity and merge with the pulmonary arteries and capillaries, which are part of the pulmonary vascular system. The normal bronchial arterial blood flow is about 1 percent of the cardiac output. In addition to the tracheobronchial tree, the bronchial arteries nourish the mediastinal lymph nodes, the pulmonary nerves, some muscular pulmonary arteries and veins, a portion of the esophagus, and of the visceral pleura.

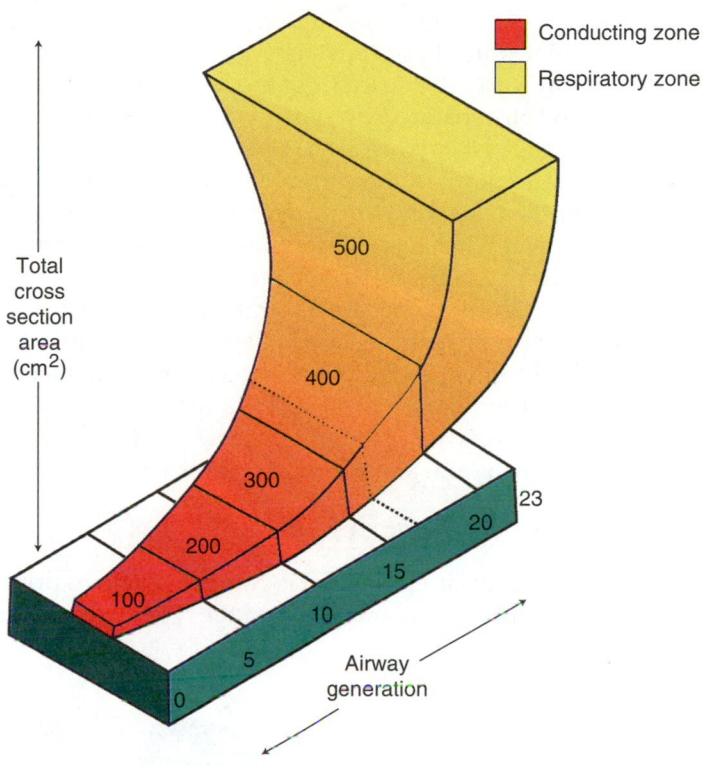

Figure 1–19. *Cross-section of bronchial area. Note the rapid increase in the total cross-sectional area of the airways in the respiratory zone.*

About one-third of the bronchial venous blood returns to the right atrium by way of the **azygos**, **hemiazygos**, and **intercostal veins**. Most of this blood comes from the first two or three generations of the tracheobronchial tree. The remaining two-thirds of the bronchial venous blood drains into the pulmonary circulation, via **bronchopulmonary anastomoses**, and then flows to the left atrium by way of the pulmonary veins. In effect, the bronchial venous blood, which is low in oxygen and high in carbon dioxide, mixes with blood that has just passed through the alveolar-capillary system, which is high in oxygen and low in carbon dioxide. The mixing of venous blood and freshly oxygenated blood is known as **venous admixture**. (The effects of venous admixture are discussed in greater detail in Chapter Seven.)

 ## THE SITES OF GAS EXCHANGE

The anatomic structures distal to the terminal bronchioles are the functional units of gas exchange. They are composed of about three generations of **respiratory bronchioles**, followed by about three generations of **alveolar ducts**, and finally, ending in 15 to 20 grapelike clusters, the **alveolar sacs** (Figure 1–20). The respiratory bronchioles are characterized by alveoli budding from their walls. The walls of the alveolar ducts that arise from the respiratory bronchioles are completely composed of alveoli separated by septal walls that contain smooth muscle fibers. Most gas exchange takes place at the alveolar-capillary membrane (Figure 1–21). In the lungs of the adult male, there are approximately 300 million alveoli between 75 μ and 300 μ in diameter, and small pulmonary capillaries cover about 85 to 95 percent of the alveoli. This anatomic arrangement provides an average surface area of 70 square meters (about the size of a tennis court) available for gas exchange.

Collectively, the respiratory bronchioles, alveolar ducts, and alveolar clusters that originate from a single terminal bronchiole are referred to as a **primary lobule**. Each primary lobule is about 3.5 mm in diameter and contains about 2000 alveoli. It is estimated that there are approximately 130,000 primary lobules in the lung. Synonyms for primary lobule include **acinus**, **terminal respiratory unit**, **lung parenchyma**, and **functional units** (see Table 1–1).

ALVEOLAR EPITHELIUM

The alveolar epithelium is composed of two principal cell types: the **type I cell**, or **squamous pneumocyte**, and the **type II cell**, or **granular pneumocyte**.

Figure 1–20. *Schematic drawing of the anatomic structures distal to the terminal bronchioles; collectively, these are referred to as the primary lobule.*

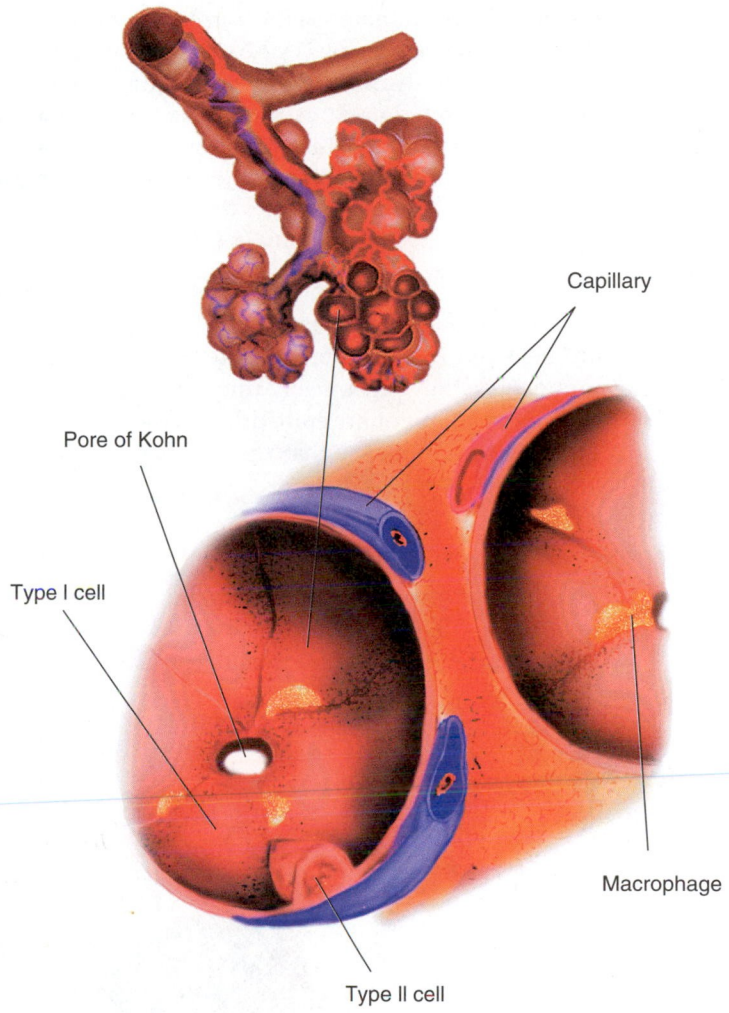

Capillary

Pore of Kohn

Type I cell

Macrophage

Type II cell

Figure 1–21. *Alveolar-capillary network.*

Type I cells are primarily composed of a cytoplasmic ground substance. They are broad, thin cells that form about 95 percent of the alveolar surface. They are between 0.1 μ and 0.5 μ thick and are the major sites of alveolar gas exchange.

Type II cells form the remaining 5 percent of the total alveolar surface. They have microvilli and are cuboidal in shape. They are believed to be the primary source of **pulmonary surfactant**. Surfactant molecules are situated at the air–liquid interface of the alveoli and play a major role in decreasing the surface tension of the fluid that lines the alveoli (see Figure 1–21).

PORES OF KOHN

The **pores of Kohn** are small holes in the walls of the interalveolar septa (see Figure 1–21). They are between 3 μ and 13 μ in diameter and permit gas to move between adjacent alveoli. The formation of the pores may include one or more of the following processes: (1) the desquamation (i.e., shedding or peeling) of epithelial cells due to disease, (2) the normal degeneration of tissue cells as a result of age, and (3) the movement of macrophages, which may leave holes in the alveolar walls. The formation of alveolar pores is accelerated by diseases involving the lung parenchyma, and the number and size of the pores increase progressively with age.

ALVEOLAR MACROPHAGES

Alveolar macrophages, or type III alveolar cells, play a major role in removing bacteria and other foreign particles that are deposited within the acini. Macrophages are believed to originate from stem cell precursors in the bone marrow. Then, as monocytes, they presumably migrate through the blood stream to the lungs, where they move about or are embedded in the extracellular lining of the alveolar surface. There is also evidence that the alveolar macrophages reproduce within the lung (see Figure 1–21).

INTERSTITIUM

The alveolar-capillary clusters are surrounded, supported, and shaped by the **interstitium** (Figure 1–22). The interstitium is a gel-like substance composed of hyaluronic acid molecules that are held together by a weblike network of collagen

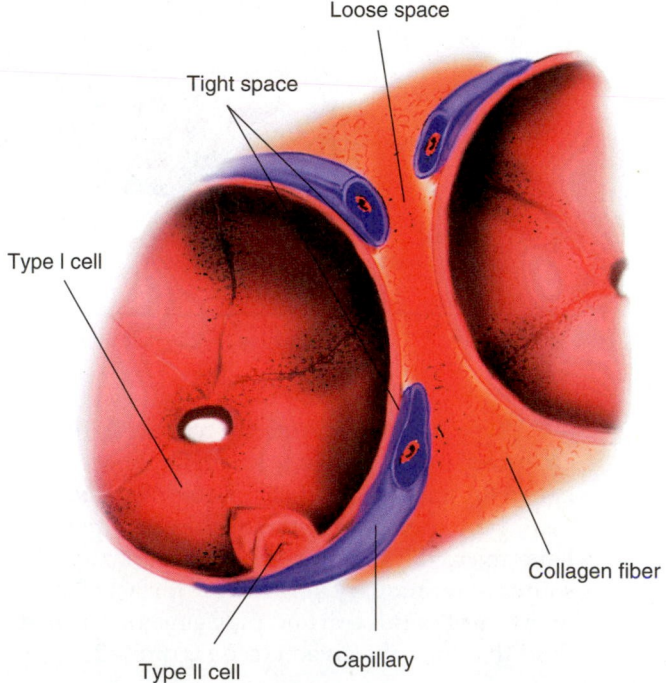

Figure 1–22.   *Interstitium. Most gas exchange occurs in the tight space area. The area around the bronchioles, respiratory bronchioles, alveolar ducts, and alveolar sacs is called the loose space.*

fibers. The interstitium has two major compartments: the **tight space** and the **loose space**. The tight space is the area between the alveolar epithelium and the endothelium of the pulmonary capillaries—the area where most gas exchange occurs. The loose space is primarily the area that surrounds the bronchioles, respiratory bronchioles, alveolar ducts, and alveolar sacs. Lymphatic vessels and neural fibers are found in this area. Water content in this area can increase more than 30 percent before a significant pressure change develops.

The collagen in the interstitium is believed to limit alveolar distensibility. Expansion of a lung unit beyond the limits of the interstitial collagen can (1) occlude the pulmonary capillaries or (2) damage the structural framework of the collagen fibers and, subsequently, the wall of the alveoli.

PULMONARY VASCULAR SYSTEM

The pulmonary vascular system can be viewed as an independent vascular network with the sole purpose of delivering blood to and from the lungs for gas exchange. In addition to gas exchange, the pulmonary vascular system provides nutritional substances to the anatomic structures distal to the terminal bronchioles. Similar to the systemic vascular system, the pulmonary vascular system is composed of **arteries**, **arterioles**, **capillaries**, **venules**, and **veins**.

ARTERIES

The right ventricle of the heart pumps deoxygenated blood into the **pulmonary artery**. Just beneath the aorta the pulmonary artery divides into the right and left branches (Figure 1–23, page 32). The branches then penetrate their respective lung through the hilum, which is that part of the lung where the main stem bronchi, vessels, and nerves enter. In general, the pulmonary artery follows the tracheobronchial tree in a posterolateral relation, branching or dividing as the tracheobronchial tree does.

The arteries have three layers of tissue in their walls (Figure 1–24, page 33). The inner layer is called the **tunica intima** and is composed of endothelium and a thin layer of connective and elastic tissue. The middle layer is called the **tunica media** and consists primarily of elastic connective tissue in large arteries and smooth muscle in medium-sized to small arteries. The tunica media is the thickest layer in the arteries. The outermost layer is called the **tunica adventitia** and is composed of connective tissue. This layer also contains small vessels that nourish all three tissue layers. Because of the different layers, the arteries are relatively stiff vessels that are well suited for carrying blood under high pressures in the systemic system.

ARTERIOLES

The walls of the arterioles consist of an endothelial layer, an elastic layer, and a layer of smooth muscle fibers (see Figure 1–24). The elastic and smooth muscle fibers gradually disappear just before entering the alveolar-capillary system. The pulmonary arterioles supply nutrients to the respiratory bronchioles, alveolar

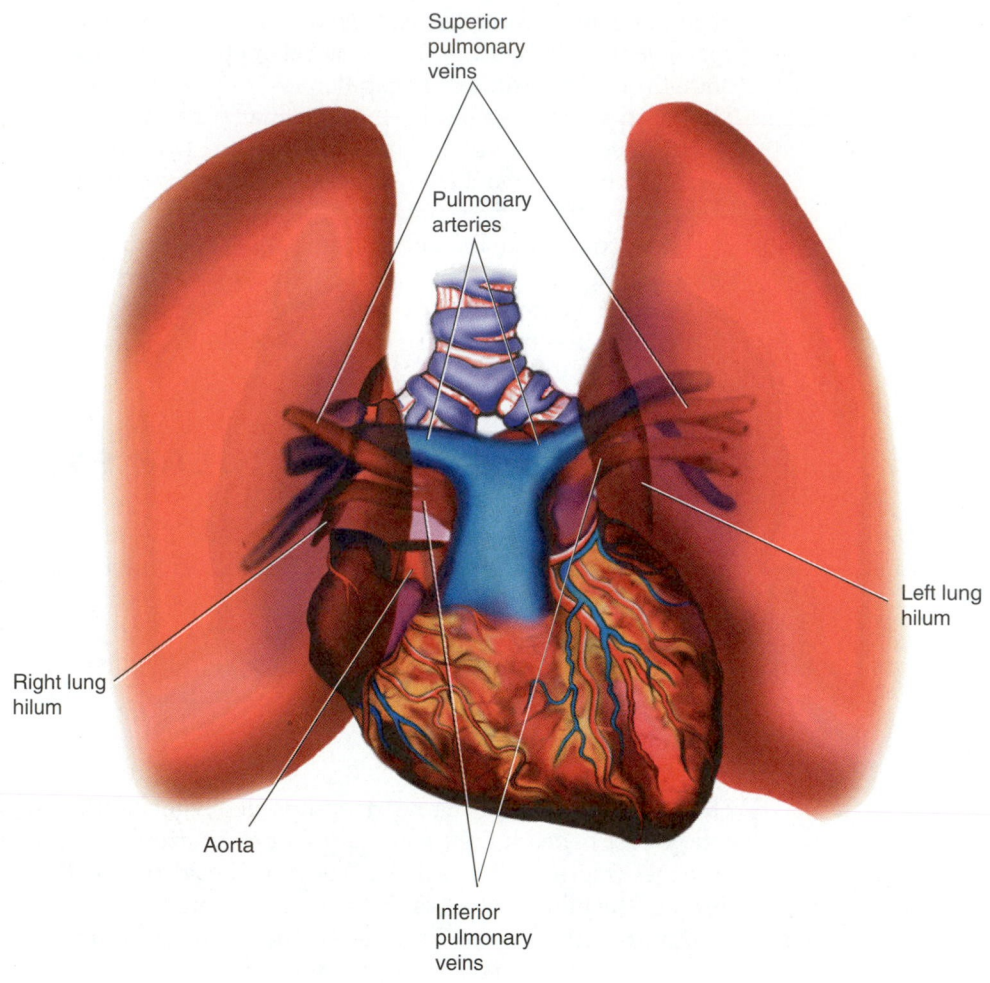

Figure 1–23.   *Major pulmonary vessels.*

ducts, and alveoli. By virtue of their smooth muscle fibers, the arterioles play an important role in the distribution and regulation of blood and are called the **resistance vessels**.

CAPILLARIES

The pulmonary arterioles give rise to a complex network of capillaries that surround the alveoli. The capillaries are composed of an endothelial layer (a single layer of squamous epithelial cells) (see Figure 1–24). The capillaries are essentially an extension of the inner lining of the larger vessels. The walls of the pulmonary capillaries are less than 0.1 μ thick and the external diameter of each vessel is about 10 μ. The capillaries are where gas exchange occurs. The pulmonary capillary endothelium also has a selective permeability to substances such as water, electrolytes, and sugars.

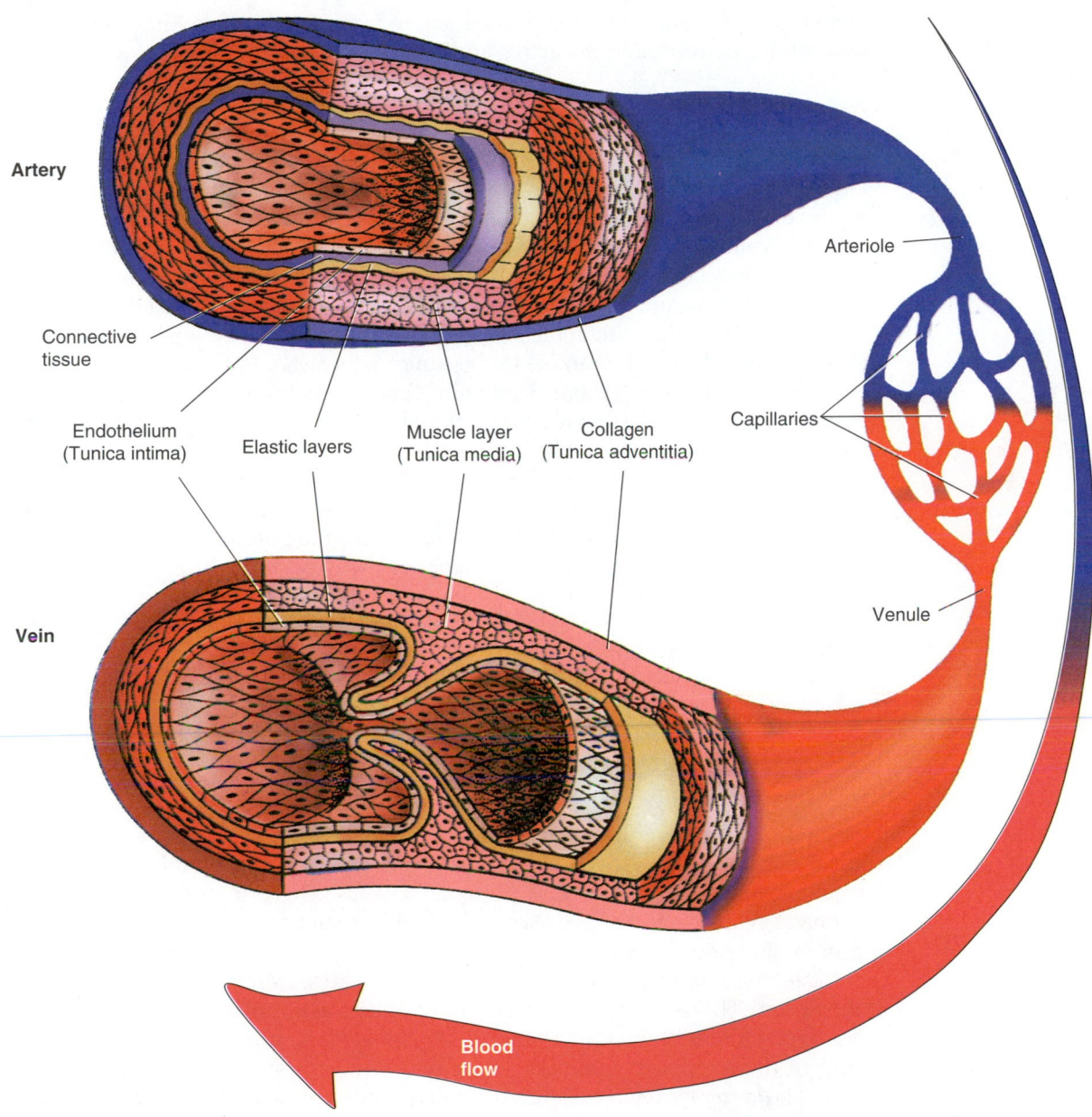

Figure 1–24. *Schematic drawing of the components of the major blood vessels.*

In addition to gas and fluid exchange, the pulmonary capillaries play an important biochemical role in the production and destruction of a broad range of biologically active substances. For example, serotonin, norepinephrine, and some prostaglandins are destroyed by the pulmonary capillaries. Some prostaglandins are produced and synthesized by the pulmonary capillaries, and some circulating inactive peptides are converted to their active form; for example, the inactive angiotensin I is converted to the active angiotensin II.

VENULES AND VEINS

After blood moves through the pulmonary capillaries, it enters the pulmonary venules. The venules are actually tiny veins continuous with the capillaries. The venules empty into the veins, which carry blood back to the heart. Similar to the arteries, the veins usually have three layers of tissue in their walls (see Figure 1–24).

The veins differ from the arteries, however, in that the middle layer is poorly developed. As a result, the veins have thinner walls and contain less smooth muscle and less elastic tissue than the arteries. There are only two layers in the smaller veins, lacking a layer comparable to the tunica adventitia. In the systemic circulation, many medium- and large-sized veins (particularly those in the legs) contain one-way, flaplike valves that aid blood flow back to the heart. The valves open as long as the flow is toward the heart, but close if flow moves away from the heart.

The veins also differ from the arteries in that they are capable of collecting a large amount of blood with very little pressure change. Because of this unique feature, the veins are called **capacitance vessels**. Unlike the pulmonary arteries, which generally parallel the airways, the veins move away from the bronchi and take a more direct route out of the lungs. Ultimately, the veins in each lung merge into two large veins and exit through the lung hilum. The four pulmonary veins then empty into the left atrium of the heart (see Figure 1–23).

THE LYMPHATIC SYSTEM

Lymphatic vessels are found superficially around the lungs just beneath the visceral pleura and in the dense connective tissue wrapping of the bronchioles, bronchi, pulmonary arteries, and pulmonary veins. The primary function of the lymphatic vessels is to remove excess fluid and protein molecules that leak out of the pulmonary capillaries.

Deep within the lungs, the lymphatic vessels arise from the loose space of the interstitium. The vessels follow the bronchial airways, pulmonary arteries, and veins to the hilum of the lung (Figure 1–25). Single-leaf, funnel-shaped valves are found in the lymphatic channels. These one-way valves direct fluid toward the hilum. The larger lymphatic channels are surrounded by smooth muscle bands that actively produce peristaltic movements regulated by the autonomic nervous system. Both the smooth muscle activity and the normal, cyclic pressure changes generated in the thoracic cavity move lymphatic fluid toward the hilum. The vessels end in the pulmonary and bronchopulmonary **lymph nodes** located just inside and outside the lung parenchyma (Figure 1–26, page 36).

The lymph nodes are organized collections of lymphatic tissue interspersed along the course of the lymphatic stream. Lymph nodes produce lymphocytes and monocytes. The nodes act as filters, keeping particulate matter and bacteria from gaining entrance to the bloodstream.

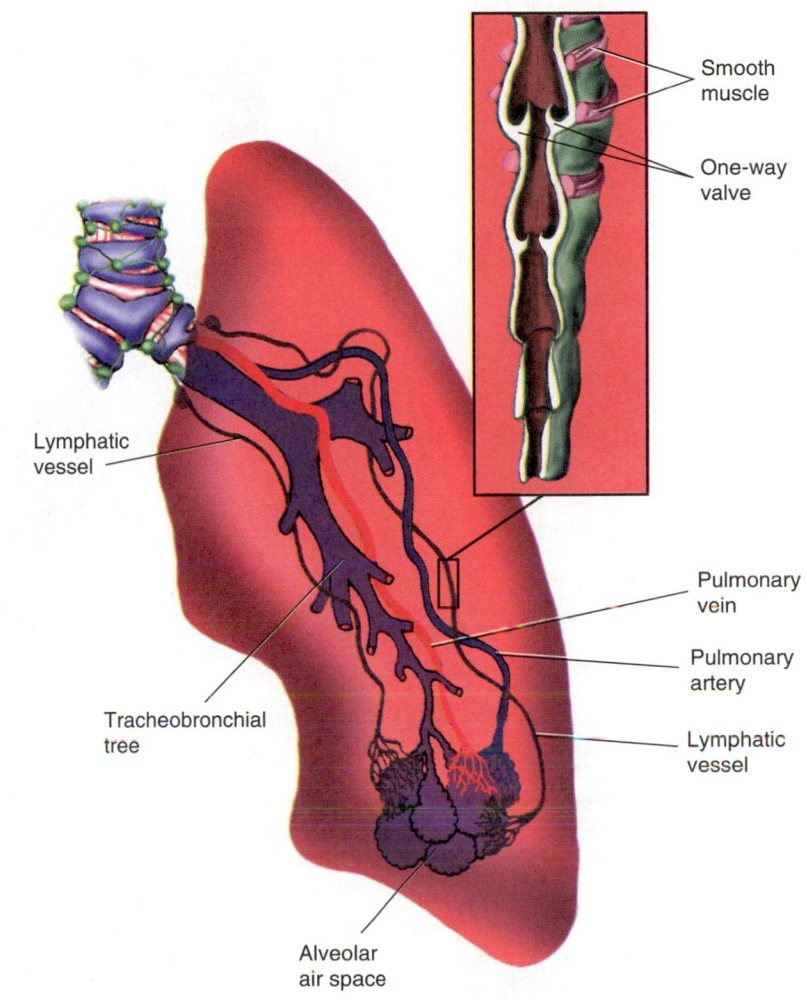

Figure 1–25. *Lymphatic vessels of the bronchial airways, pulmonary arteries, and veins.*

There are no lymphatic vessels in the walls of the alveoli. Some alveoli, however, are strategically located immediately adjacent to peribronchovascular lymphatic vessels. These vessels are called **juxta-alveolar lymphatics** and are thought to play an active role in the removal of excess fluid and other foreign material that gain entrance into the interstitial space of the lung parenchyma.

Superficially, there are more lymphatic vessels on the surface of the lower lung lobes than on that of the upper or middle lobes. The lymphatic channels on the left lower lung lobe are more numerous and larger in diameter than the lymphatic vessels on the surface of the right lower lung lobe (Figure 1–27, page 36). This anatomic difference provides a possible explanation why patients with **bilateral effusion** (i.e., the escape of fluid from the blood vessels from both lungs) commonly have more fluid in the lower right lung than in the lower left.

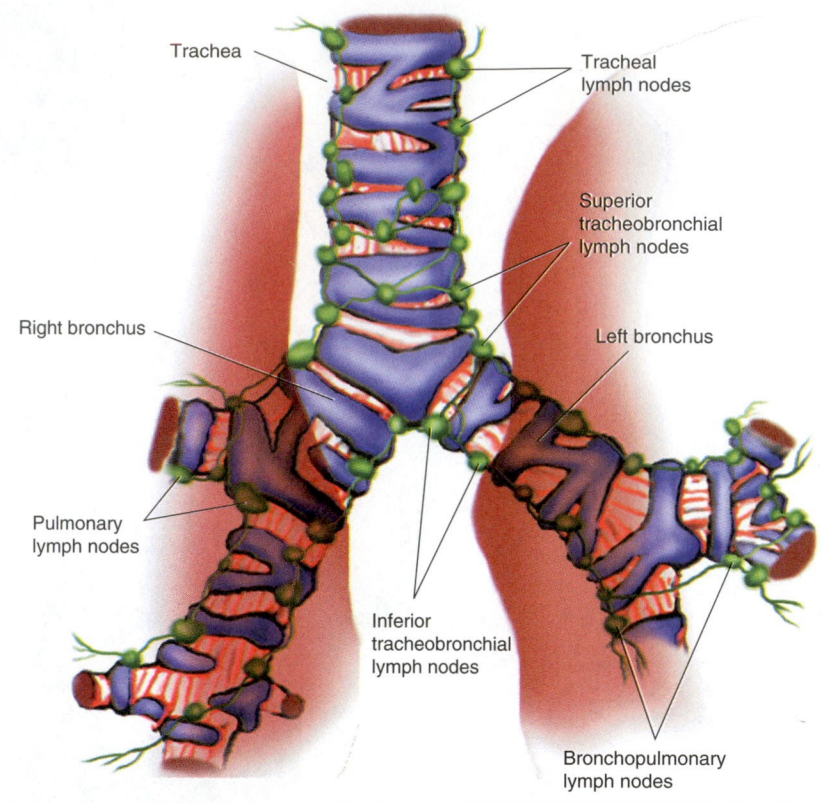

Figure 1–26. *Lymph nodes associated with the trachea and the right and left main stem bronchi.*

Figure 1–27. *Lymphatic vessels of the visceral pleura of the lungs.*

NEURAL CONTROL OF THE LUNGS

The balance, or tone, of the bronchial and arteriolar smooth muscle of the lungs is controlled by the autonomic nervous system. The autonomic nervous system is the part of the nervous system that regulates involuntary vital functions, including the activity of the cardiac muscle, the smooth muscle, and glands. It has two divisions: (1) the sympathetic nervous system, which accelerates the heart rate, constricts blood vessels, relaxes bronchial smooth muscles, and raises blood pressure; and (2) the parasympathetic nervous system, which slows the heart rate, constricts bronchial smooth muscles, and increases intestinal peristalsis and gland activity. Table 1–2 lists some effects of the two divisions of the autonomic nervous system.

The neural fibers of the sympathetic and parasympathetic nervous systems control the smooth muscle tone in the following way.

When the sympathetic nervous system is activated, neural transmitters, such as epinephrine and norepinephrine, are released. These agents stimulate (1) the beta$_2$ receptors in the bronchial smooth muscles, causing relaxation of the airway musculature, and (2) the alpha receptors of the smooth muscles of the arterioles, causing the pulmonary vascular system to constrict. When the parasympathetic nervous system is activated, the neutral transmitter acetylcholine is released, causing constriction of the bronchial smooth muscle.

Inactivity of either the sympathetic or the parasympathetic nervous system allows the action of the other to dominate the bronchial smooth muscle response. For example, if a beta$_2$-blocking agent such as propranolol is administered to a patient, the parasympathetic nervous system becomes dominant and bronchial constriction ensues. In contrast, if a patient receives a parasympathetic blocking agent such as atropine, the sympathetic nervous system becomes dominant and bronchial relaxation occurs.

TABLE 1–2.   **Some Effects of Autonomic Nervous System Activity**

EFFECTOR SITE	SYMPATHETIC NERVOUS SYSTEM	PARASYMPATHETIC NERVOUS SYSTEM
Heart	Increases rate	Decreases rate
	Increases strength of contraction	Decreases strength of contraction
Bronchial smooth muscle	Relaxation	Constriction
Bronchial glands	Decreases secretions	Increases secretions
Salivary glands	Decreases secretions	Increases secretions
Stomach	Decreases motility	Increases motility
Intestines	Decreases motility	Increases motility
Eye	Widens pupils	Constricts pupils

THE LUNGS

The apex of each lung is somewhat pointed and the base is broad and concave to accommodate the convex diaphragm (Figures 1–28 and 1–29). As shown in Figure 1–30, the apices of the lungs rise to about the level of the first rib. The base extends anteriorly to about the level of the sixth rib (xiphoid process level), and posteriorly to about the level of the eleventh rib (two ribs below the inferior angle of the scapula). The **mediastinal border** of each lung is concave to fit the heart and other mediastinal structures. At the center of the mediastinal border is the **hilum**, where the right and left main stem bronchi, blood vessels, lymph vessels, and various nerves enter and exit the lungs.

The **right lung** is larger and heavier than the left. It is divided into the **upper**, **middle**, and **lower lobes** by the **oblique** and the **horizontal fissures**. The oblique fissure extends from the costal to the mediastinal borders of the lung and separates the upper and middle lobes from the lower lobe. The horizontal fissure extends horizontally from the oblique fissure to about the level of the fourth costal cartilage and separates the middle from the upper lobe.

The **left lung** is divided into only two lobes—the **upper** and the **lower**. These two lobes are separated by the **oblique fissure**, which extends from the costal to the mediastinal borders of the lung.

All lobes are further subdivided into **bronchopulmonary segments**. In Figure 1–31 (page 40), the segments are numbered to demonstrate their relationship.

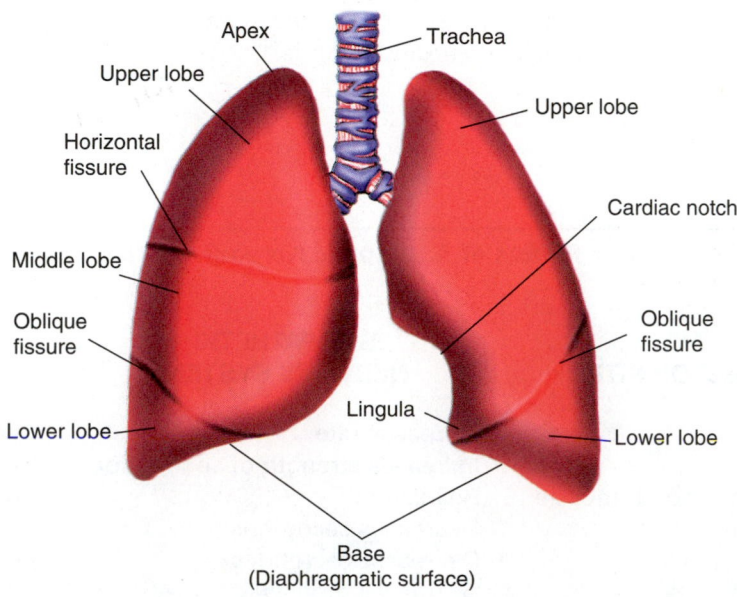

Figure 1–28. *Anterior view of the lungs.*

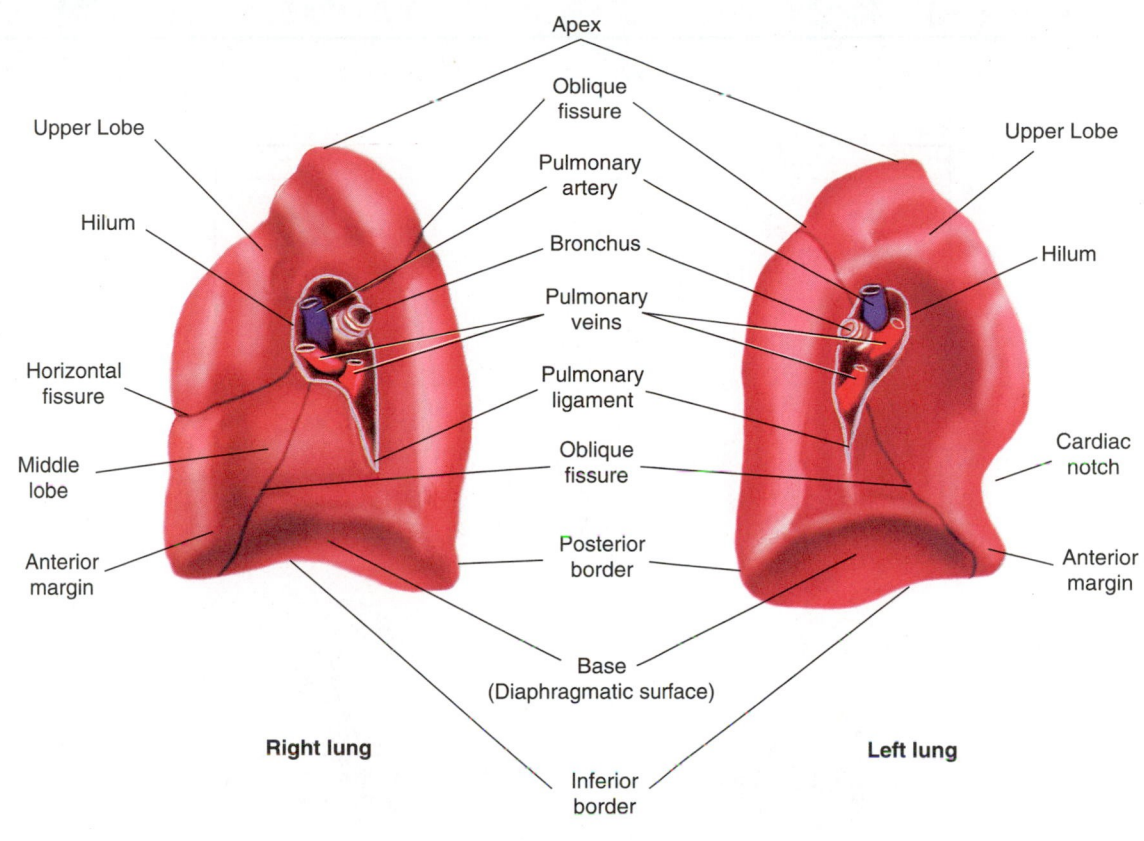

Figure 1–29. *Medial view of the lungs.*

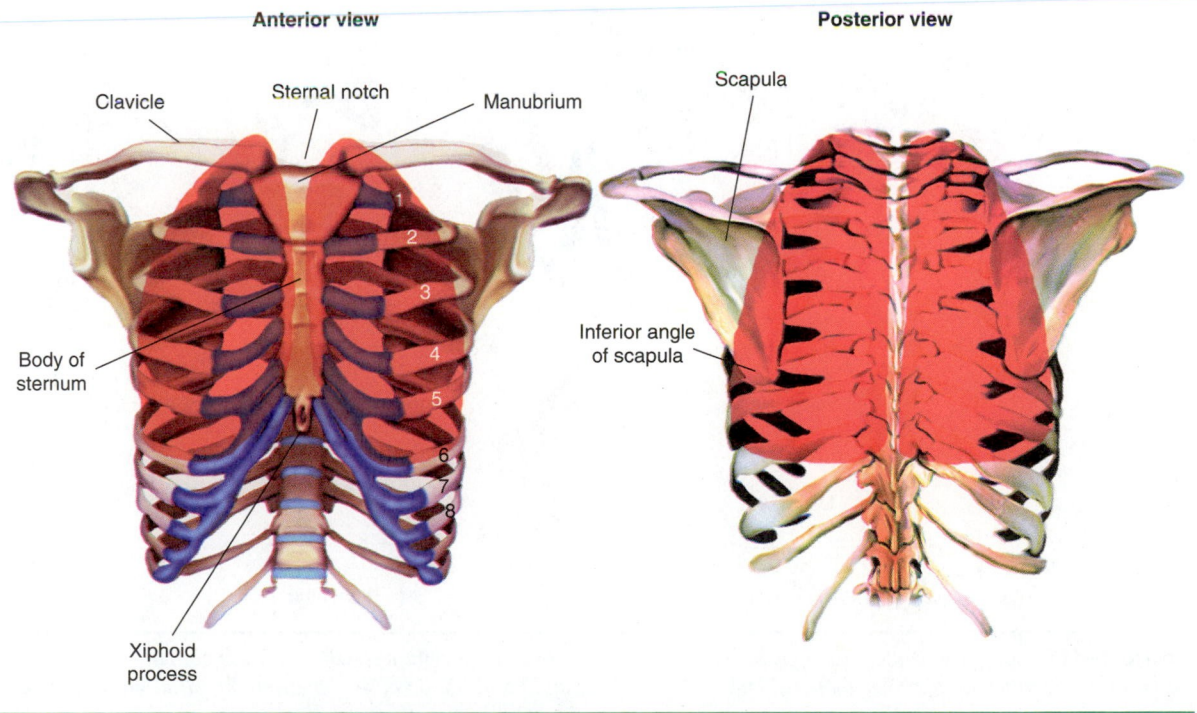

Figure 1–30. *Anatomic relationship of the lungs and the thorax.*

	Right lung		Left lung	
Upper lobe			**Upper lobe**	
Apical	1		**Upper division**	
Posterior		2	Apical/Posterior	1 & 2
Anterior		3	Anterior	3
Middle lobe			**Lower division (lingular)**	
Lateral	4		Superior lingula	4
Medial	5		Inferior lingula	5
Lower lobe			**Lower lobe**	
Superior		6	Superior	6
Medial basal		7	Anterior medial	7 & 8
Anterior basal		8	Lateral basal	9
Lateral basal		9	Posterior basal	10
Posterior basal		10		

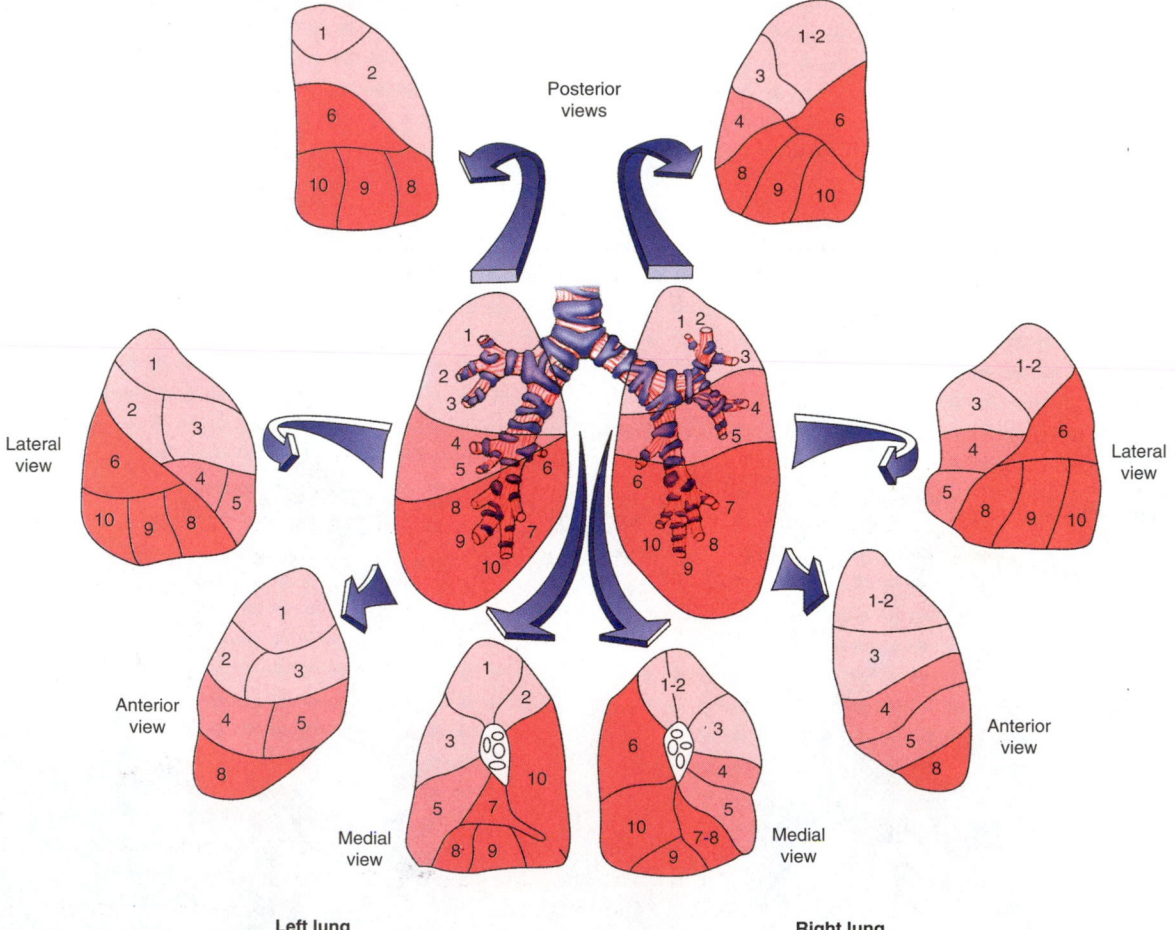

Figure 1–31. *Lung segments. Although the segment subdivisions of the right and left lungs are similar, there are some slight anatomic differences, which are noted by combined names and numbers. Because of these slight variations, some workers consider that, technically, there are only eight segments in the left lung and that the apical-posterior segment is number 1 and the anteromedial is number 6.*

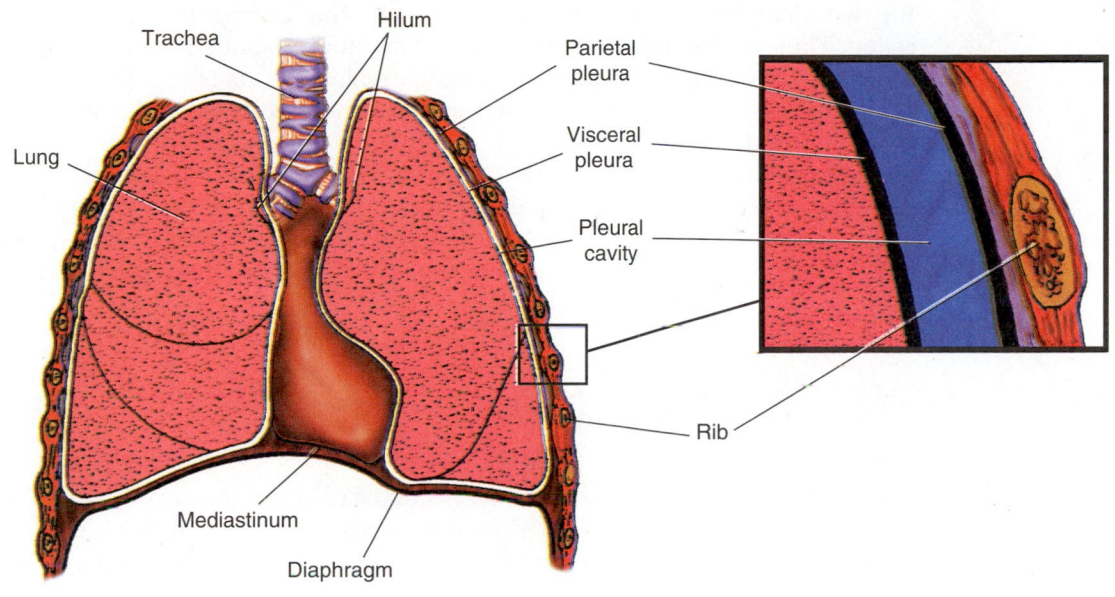

Figure 1–32. *Major structures around the lungs.*

THE MEDIASTINUM

The **mediastinum** is a cavity that contains organs and tissues in the center of the thoracic cage between the right and left lungs (Figure 1–32). It is bordered anteriorly by the sternum and posteriorly by the thoracic vertebrae. The mediastinum contains the trachea, the heart, the major blood vessels (commonly known as the great vessels) that enter and exit from the heart, various nerves, portions of the esophagus, the thymus gland, and lymph nodes. If the mediastinum is compressed or distorted, it can severely compromise the cardiopulmonary system.

THE PLEURAL MEMBRANES

Two moist, slick-surfaced membranes, called the **visceral** and **parietal pleurae**, are closely associated with the lungs. The visceral pleura is firmly attached to the outer surface of each lung and extends into each of the interlobar fissures. The parietal pleura lines the inside of the thoracic walls, the thoracic surface of the diaphragm, and the lateral portion of the mediastinum. The potential space between the visceral and parietal pleurae is called the **pleural cavity** (see Figure 1–32).

    The visceral and parietal pleurae are held together by a thin film of serous fluid—somewhat like two flat, moistened pieces of glass. This fluid layer allows the two pleural membranes to glide over each other during inspiration and expiration. Thus, during inspiration the pleural membranes hold the lung tissue to the inner surface of the thorax and diaphragm, causing the lungs to expand.

Because the lungs have a natural tendency to collapse and the chest wall has a natural tendency to expand, a negative or subatmospheric pressure (negative intrapleural pressure) normally exists between the parietal and visceral pleurae. Should air or gas be introduced into the pleural cavity (e.g., as a result of a chest puncture wound), the intrapleural pressure rises to atmospheric pressure and causes the pleural membranes to separate. This condition is called a **pneumothorax**.

THE THORAX

The **thorax** houses and protects the organs of the cardiopulmonary system. Twelve **thoracic vertebrae** form the posterior midline border of the thoracic cage. The **sternum** forms the anterior border of the chest. The sternum is composed of the **manubrium sterni**, the **body**, and the **xiphoid process** (Figure 1–33).

The twelve pairs of ribs form the lateral boundary of the thorax. The ribs attach directly to the vertebral column posteriorly and indirectly by way of the costal

Figure 1–33. *The thorax.*

Figure 1–34. *The intercostal space.*

cartilage anteriorly to the sternum. The first seven ribs are referred to as **true ribs**, since they are attached directly to the sternum by way of their costal cartilage. Because the cartilage of the eighth, ninth, and tenth ribs attaches to the cartilage of the ribs above, they are referred to as **false ribs**. Ribs eleven and twelve float freely anteriorly and are called **floating ribs**. There are eleven intercostal spaces between the ribs; these spaces contain blood vessels, intercostal nerves, and the external and internal intercostal muscles (Figure 1–34).

THE DIAPHRAGM

The **diaphragm** is the major muscle of ventilation (Figure 1–35, page 44). It is a dome-shaped musculofibrous partition located between the thoracic cavity and the abdominal cavity. Although the diaphragm is generally referred to as one muscle, it is actually composed of two separate muscles known as the **right** and **left**

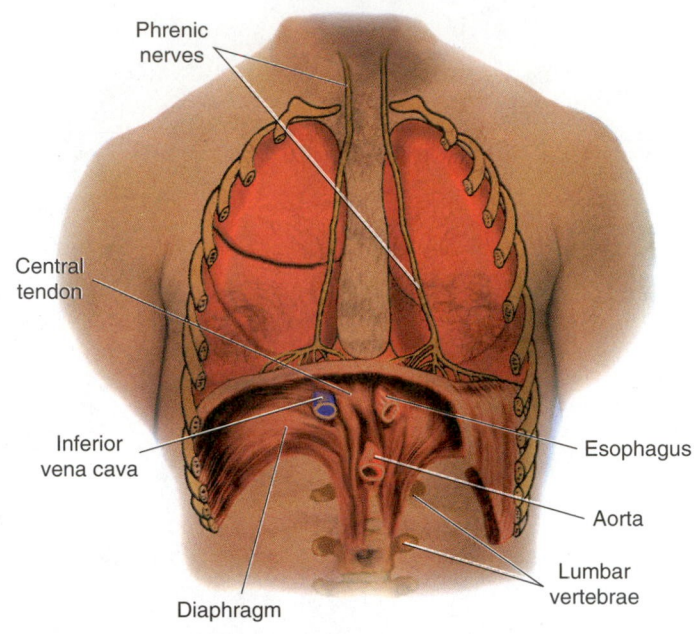

Figure 1–35.   *The diaphragm.*

hemidiaphragms. Each hemidiaphragm arises from the lumbar vertebrae, the costal margin, and the xiphoid process. The two muscles then merge together at the midline into a broad connective sheet called the **central tendon**. The diaphragm is pierced by the esophagus, the aorta, several nerves, and the inferior vena cava. Terminal branches of the **phrenic nerves**, which leave the spinal cord between the third and fifth cervical segments, supply the primary motor innervation to each hemidiaphragm. The **lower thoracic nerves** also contribute to the motor innervation of each hemidiaphragm.

When stimulated to contract, the diaphragm moves downward and the lower ribs move upward and outward. This action increases the volume of the thoracic cavity, which, in turn, lowers the intrapleural and intra-alveolar pressures in the thoracic cavity. As a result, gas from the atmosphere flows into the lungs. During expiration, the diaphragm relaxes and domes upward into the thoracic cavity. This action increases the intra-alveolar and intrapleural pressures, causing gas to flow out of the lungs.

THE ACCESSORY MUSCLES OF VENTILATION

During normal ventilation by a healthy person, the diaphragm alone can manage the task of moving gas in and out of the lungs. During vigorous exercise, however, and during the advanced stages of chronic obstructive pulmonary disease, the accessory muscles of inspiration and expiration are activated to assist the diaphragm.

THE ACCESSORY MUSCLES OF INSPIRATION

The accessory muscles of inspiration are those muscles that are recruited to assist the diaphragm in creating a subatmospheric pressure in the lungs to enable adequate inspiration. Following are the major accessory muscles of inspiration:

- Scalene muscles
- Sternocleidomastoid muscles
- Pectoralis major muscles
- Trapezius muscles
- External intercostal muscles

Scalene Muscles

The **scalene muscles** are three separate muscles that function as a unit. They are known as the **anterior**, the **medial**, and the **posterior** scalene muscles. They originate on the transverse processes of the second to the sixth cervical vertebrae and insert into the first and second ribs (Figure 1–36). The primary function of these muscles is to flex the neck. When used as accessory muscles for inspiration, they elevate the first and second ribs. This action works to decrease the intrapleural pressure.

Figure 1–36. *Scalenus muscles.*

Sternocleidomastoid Muscles

The sternocleidomastoid muscles are located on each side of the neck (Figure 1–37). They originate from the sternum and the clavicle and insert into the mastoid process and occipital bone of the skull. Normally the sternocleidomastoid muscle pulls from its sternoclavicular origin and rotates the head to the opposite side and turns it upward. When the sternocleidomastoid muscle functions as an accessory muscle of inspiration, the head and neck are fixed by other muscles and the sternocleidomastoid pulls from its insertion on the skull and elevates the sternum. This action increases the anteroposterior diameter of the chest.

Pectoralis Major Muscles

The pectoralis major muscles are powerful, fan-shaped muscles located on each side of the upper chest. They originate from the clavicle and the sternum and insert into the upper part of the humerus.

Normally, the pectoralis majors pull from their sternoclavicular origin and bring the upper arm to the body in a hugging motion (Figure 1–38). When functioning as accessory muscles of inspiration, they pull from the humeral insertion and elevate the chest, resulting in an increased anteroposterior diameter. It is common to observe patients with chronic obstructive pulmonary disease bracing their arms against something stationary and using their pectoralis majors to increase the diameter of their chests (Figure 1–39).

Figure 1–37. *Sternocleidomastoid muscle.*

Pectoralis
major

Figure 1–38.   *Pectoralis major muscles.*

Trapezius Muscles

The **trapezius muscles** are large, flat, triangular muscles that are situated superficially in the upper back and the back of the neck. They originate from the occipital bone, the ligamentum nuchae, and the spinous processes of the seventh cervical vertebra and all the thoracic vertebrae. They insert into the spine of the scapula, the acromion process, and the lateral third of the clavicle (Figure 1–40, page 48).

Normally, the trapezius muscles rotate the scapula, raise the shoulders, and abduct and flex the arms. Their action is typified in shrugging of the shoulders (Figure 1–41, page 48). When used as accessory muscles of inspiration, the trapezius muscles help to elevate the thoracic cage.

Figure 1–39.   *How an individual may appear when using the pectoralis major muscles for inspiration.*

Figure 1–40. *Trapezius muscles.*

Figure 1–41. *Shrugging of the shoulders typifies the action of the trapezius muscles.*

External Intercostal Muscles

The external intercostal muscles arise from the lower border of each rib (the upper limit of an intercostal space), and insert into the upper border of the rib below. Anteriorly, the fibers run downward and medially. Posteriorly, the fibers run downward and laterally (Figure 1–42). The external intercostal muscles contract during inspiration and pull the ribs upward and outward, increasing both the lateral and anteroposterior diameters of the thorax (an antagonist action to the internal intercostal muscles). This action increases lung volume and prevents intercostal space retractions during an excessively forceful inspiration.

THE ACCESSORY MUSCLES OF EXPIRATION

The accessory muscles of expiration are those muscles that are recruited to assist in exhalation when airway resistance becomes significantly elevated. When these muscles contract, they increase the intrapleural pressure and offset the increased airway resistance. Following are the major accessory muscles of exhalation:

- Rectus abdominis muscles
- External abdominis obliquus muscles
- Internal abdominis obliquus muscles
- Transversus abdominis muscles
- Internal intercostal muscles

Figure 1–42. *Internal and external intercostal muscles.*

Rectus Abdominis Muscles

The rectus abdominis muscles are a pair of muscles that extend the entire length of the abdomen. Each muscle forms a vertical mass about four inches wide and is separated from the other by the linea alba. The muscles arise from the iliac crest and pubic symphysis and insert into the xiphoid process and the fifth, sixth, and seventh ribs.

When contracted, the rectus abdominis muscles assist in compressing the abdominal contents. This compression, in turn, pushes the diaphragm into the thoracic cage (Figure 1–43A), thereby assisting in exhalation.

External Abdominis Oblique Muscles

The external abdominis obliquus muscles are broad, thin, muscles positioned on the anterolateral sides of the abdomen. They are the longest and the most superficial of all the anterolateral abdominal muscles. They arise by eight digitations from the lower eight ribs and the abdominal aponeurosis and insert into the iliac crest and the linea alba.

When contracted, the external abdominis obliquus muscles assist in compressing the abdominal contents, which, in turn, push the diaphragm into the thoracic cage (Figure 1–43B), thereby assisting in exhalation.

Internal Abdominis Oblique Muscles

Smaller and thinner than the external abdominis obliques, the internal abdominis obliquus muscles are located in the lateral and ventral parts of the abdominal wall directly under the external abdominis obliquus muscles. They arise from the in-

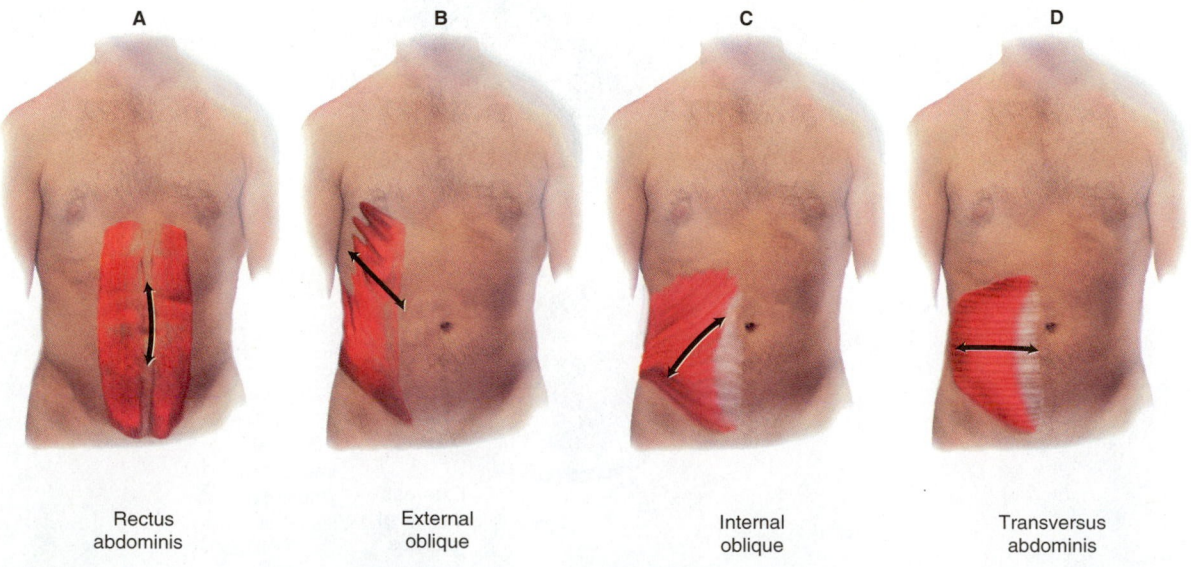

A	B	C	D
Rectus abdominis	External oblique	Internal oblique	Transversus abdominis

Figure 1–43. *Accessory muscles of expiration.*

guinal ligament, the iliac crest, and the lower portion of the lumbar aponeurosis. They insert into the last four ribs and into the linea alba.

The internal abdominis obliquus muscles also assist in exhalation by compressing the abdominal contents and in pushing the diaphragm into the thoracic cage (Figure 1–43C).

Transversus Abdominis Muscles

The transversus abdominis muscles are found immediately under the internal abdominis obliquus muscles. These muscles arise from the inguinal ligament, the iliac crest, the thoracolumbar fascia, and the lower six ribs, and insert into the linea alba. When activated, they also help to constrict the abdominal contents (Figure 1–43D).

When all four pairs of accessory muscles of exhalation contract, the abdominal pressure increases and drives the diaphragm into the thoracic cage. As the diaphragm moves into the thoracic cage during exhalation, the intrapleural pressure increases, enhancing the amount of gas flow (Figure 1–44).

Internal Intercostal Muscles

The internal intercostal muscles run between the ribs immediately beneath the external intercostal muscles. The muscles arise from the inferior border of each rib and insert into the superior border of the rib below. Anteriorly, the fibers run in a downward and lateral direction. Posteriorly, the fibers run downward and in a

Bronchial
gas flow

Diaphragmatic
pressure

Figure 1–44. *The collective action of the accessory muscles of expiration causes the intrapleural pressure to increase, the chest to move outward, and bronchial gas flow to increase.*

medial direction (see Figure 1–42). The internal intercostal muscles contract during expiration and pull the ribs downward and inward, decreasing both the lateral and anteroposterior diameters of the thorax (an antagonist action to the external intercostal muscles). This action decreases lung volume and offsets intercostal bulging during excessive expiration.

REVIEW QUESTIONS

1. Which of the following line the anterior one-third of the nasal cavity?
   a. Stratified squamous epithelium
   b. Simple cuboidal epithelium
   c. Type I cells
   d. Pseudostratified ciliated columnar epithelium
   e. Simple squamous epithelium
2. Which of the following form(s) the nasal septum?
   I. Frontal process of the maxilla bone
   II. Ethmoid bone
   III. Nasal bones
   IV. Vomer
      a. I only
      b. III only
      c. IV only
      d. I and III only
      e. II and IV only
3. Which of the following prevents the aspiration of foods and liquids?
   a. Epiglottis
   b. Cricoid cartilage
   c. Arytenoid cartilages
   d. Thyroid cartilages
   e. Corniculate cartilages
4. The canals of Lambert are found in the
   a. trachea
   b. terminal bronchioles
   c. alveoli
   d. main stem bronchi
   e. alveolar ducts
5. The eustachian tubes are found in the
   a. nasopharynx
   b. oropharynx
   c. laryngopharynx
   d. oral cavity
   e. tracheobronchial tree
6. The inferior portion of the larynx is composed of the
   a. arytenoid cartilage

b. thyroid cartilage

c. hyoid bone

d. glottis

e. cricoid cartilage

7. Which of the following has the greatest cross-sectional area?

a. Terminal bronchioles

b. Main stem bronchi

c. Lobar bronchi

d. Trachea

e. Segmental bronchi

8. The left main stem bronchus angles off from the carina at about

a. 5–10 degrees from the carina

b. 10–20 degrees from the carina

c. 20–30 degrees from the carina

d. 30–40 degrees from the carina

e. 40–60 degrees from the carina

9. Ninety-five percent of the alveolar surface is composed of which of the following?

I. Type I cells

II. Granular pneumocytes

III. Type II cells

IV. Squamous pneumocytes

a. I only

b. II only

c. III only

d. I and IV only

e. II and IV only

10. Which of the following is/are released when the parasympathetic nerve fibers are stimulated?

I. Norepinephrine

II. Atropine

III. Epinephrine

IV. Acetylcholine

a. II only

b. IV only

c. I and III only

d. I, II, and III only

e. I, II, III and IV

11. Which of the following is/are released when the sympathetic nerve fibers are stimulated?

I. Norepinephrine

II. Propranolol

III. Acetylcholine

IV. Epinephrine

a. I only

b. II only

    c. I and IV only

    d. II, III, and IV only

    e. I, II, III and IV

12. Pseudostratified ciliated columnar epithelium lines which of the following?

    I. Oropharynx

    II. Trachea

    III. Nasopharynx

    IV. Oral cavity

    V. Laryngopharynx

       a. I only

       b. II only

       c. IV only

       d. II and III only

       e. I, II, III, and V only

13. Which of the following is/are accessory muscles of inspiration?

    I. Trapezius muscles

    II. Internal abdominis obliquus muscles

    III. Scalene muscles

    IV. Transversus abdominis muscles

       a. I only

       b. II only

       c. I and III only

       d. II and IV only

       e. II, III, and IV only

14. The horizontal fissure separates the

    a. middle and upper lobes of the right lung

    b. upper and lower lobes of the left lung

    c. middle and lower lobes of the right lung

    d. oblique fissure of the left lung

    e. oblique fissure of the right lung

15. Which of the following supply the motor innervation of each hemidiaphragm?

    I. Vagus nerve (tenth cranial nerve)

    II. Phrenic nerve

    III. Lower thoracic nerves

    IV. Glossopharyngeal nerve (ninth cranial nerve)

       a. I only

       b. II only

       c. IV only

       d. I and IV only

       e. II and III only

16. The lung segment called the superior lingula is found in the

    a. left lung, lower division of the upper lobe

    b. right lung, lower lobe

    c. left lung, upper division of the upper lobe

    d. right lung, upper lobe

    e. left lung, lower lobe

17. Cartilage is found in which of the following structures of the tracheobron-chial tree?
    I. Bronchioles
    II. Respiratory bronchioles
    III. Segmental bronchi
    IV. Terminal bronchioles
    a. I only
    b. III only
    c. IV only
    d. I and IV only
    e. I, II, and IV only

18. The bronchial arteries nourish the tracheobronchial tree down to, and in-cluding, which of the following?
    a. Respiratory bronchioles
    b. Subsegmental bronchi
    c. Alveolar ducts
    d. Terminal bronchioles
    e. Segmental bronchi

19. Which of the following elevates the soft palate?
    a. Palatoglossal muscle
    b. Levator veli palatine muscle
    c. Transverse arytenoid muscle
    d. Stylopharyngeus muscles
    e. Palatopharyngeal muscle

20. Which of the following are called the resistance vessels?
    a. Arterioles
    b. Veins
    c. Capillaries
    d. Venules
    e. Arteries

CHAPTER TWO

VENTILATION

By the end of this chapter, the student should be able to:

1. Define ventilation.
2. Differentiate between the following pressure differences across the lungs:
   —Driving pressure
   —Transairway pressure
   —Transpulmonary pressure
   —Transthoracic pressure
3. Describe the role of the diaphragm in ventilation.
4. Explain how the excursion of the diaphragm affects the intrapleural pressure, intra-alveolar pressure, and bronchial gas flow during
   —inspiration
   —end-inspiration
   —expiration
   —end-expiration
5. Define the term static.
6. Define lung compliance.
7. Calculate lung compliance.
8. Explain how Hooke's law can be applied to the elastic properties of the lungs.
9. Define surface tension.
10. Describe the physical principles of Laplace's law.
11. Describe how Laplace's law can be applied to the alveolar fluid lining.
12. Explain how pulmonary surfactant offsets alveolar surface tension.
13. List respiratory disorders that cause a deficiency of pulmonary surfactant.
14. Define the term dynamic.
15. Describe how Poiseuille's law arranged for flow relates to the radius of the bronchial airways.
16. Describe how Poiseuille's law arranged for pressure relates to the radius of the bronchial airways.
17. Describe how Poiseuille's law can be rearranged to simple proportionalities.
18. Define airway resistance and explain how it relates to
    —laminar flow
    —turbulent flow
19. Calculate airway resistance.
20. Define time constants and explain how they relate to alveolar units with
    —increased airway resistance
    —decreased compliance
21. Define dynamic compliance and explain how it relates to
    —increased airway resistance
    —frequency dependence
22. Describe how the following relates to the normal ventilatory pattern:
    —Tidal volume (V_T)
    —Ventilatory rate
    —I : E ratio

(continues)

23. Differentiate between alveolar ventilation and deadspace ventilation, and include an explanation of the following:
    —Anatomic dead space
    —Alveolar dead space
    —Physiologic dead space
24. Describe how the following affect the total alveolar ventilation:
    —Depth of breathing
    —Rate of breathing
25. Calculate an individual's total alveolar ventilation in one minute (minute ventilation) when given the following information:
    —Alveolar ventilation
    —Deadspace ventilation
    —Breaths per minute
26. Describe how the normal intrapleural pressure differences cause regional differences in normal lung ventilation.
27. Describe how the following alter the ventilatory pattern (i.e., the respiratory rate and tidal volume):
    —Decreased lung compliance
    —Increased airway resistance
28. Define the following specific ventilatory patterns:
    —Apnea
    —Eupnea
    —Biot's breathing
    —Hyperpnea
    —Hyperventilation
    —Hypoventilation
    —Tachypnea
    —Cheyne-Stokes breathing
    —Kussmaul breathing
    —Orthopnea
    —Dyspnea
29. Complete the review questions at the end of this chapter.

The term **ventilation** is defined as the process that exchanges gases between the external environment and the alveoli. It is the mechanism by which oxygen is carried from the atmosphere to the alveoli and by which carbon dioxide (delivered to the lungs in mixed venous blood) is carried from the alveoli to the atmosphere.

To understand the process of ventilation, the respiratory care practitioner must understand (1) how the excursion of the diaphragm changes the intra-alveolar and intrapleural pressures, (2) the static characteristics of the lungs, (3) the dynamic characteristics of the lungs, and (4) the characteristics of normal and abnormal ventilatory patterns.

PRESSURE DIFFERENCES ACROSS THE LUNGS

Understanding the following pressure differences across the lungs is an essential building block in the study of ventilation.

Driving pressure is the pressure difference between two points in a tube or vessel; it is the force moving gas or fluid through the tube or vessel. For example, if the gas pressure at the beginning of a tube is 20 mm Hg, and the pressure at the end of the same tube is 5 mm Hg, the driving pressure is 15 mm Hg. In other words, the force required to move the gas through the tube is 15 mm Hg.

Transairway pressure (P_{ta}) is the barometric pressure difference between the mouth pressure (P_m) and the alveolar pressure (P_{alv}).

$$P_{ta} = P_m - P_{alv}$$

For example, if the P_{alv} is 757 mm Hg and the P_m is 760 mm Hg during inspiration, the P_{ta} is 3 mm Hg (Figure 2–1A).

$$P_{ta} = P_m - P_{alv}$$
$$= 760 \text{ mm Hg} - 757 \text{ mm Hg}$$
$$= 3 \text{ mm Hg}$$

Or, if the P_{alv} is 763 mm Hg and the P_m is 760 mm Hg during expiration, the P_{ta} is −3 mm Hg. Gas in this example, however, is moving in the opposite direction (Figure 2–1B). In essence, the P_{ta} represents the driving pressure (the pressure difference between the mouth and the alveolus) that forces gas in or out of the lungs.

Transpulmonary pressure (P_{tp}) is the difference between the alveolar pressure (P_{alv}) and the pleural pressure (P_{pl}).

$$P_{tp} = P_{alv} - P_{pl}$$

For example, if the P_{pl} is 755 mm Hg and the P_{alv} is 760 mm Hg (e.g., inspiration), the P_{tp} is 5 mm Hg (Figure 2–2A).

$$P_{tp} = P_{alv} - P_{pl}$$
$$= 760 \text{ mm Hg} - 755 \text{ mm Hg}$$
$$= 5 \text{ mm Hg}$$

Figure 2–1. *Transairway pressure: The difference between the pressure at the mouth (P_m) and the alveolar pressure (P_{alv}). Even though gas is moving in opposite directions in A and B, the transairway pressure is 3 mm Hg in both examples. Note: In this illustration, the pressure of the mouth (P_m) is equal to the barometric pressure (P_B).*

Figure 2–2. *Transpulmonary pressure: The difference between the alveolar pressure (P_{alv}) and the pleural pressure (P_{pl}). This illustration assumes a barometric pressure (P_B) of 761 mm Hg.*

Or, if the P_{alv} is 763 mm Hg and the P_{pl} is 758 mm Hg (e.g., expiration), the P_{tp} is 5 mm Hg (Figure 2–2B).

Transthoracic pressure (P_{tt}) is the difference between the alveolar pressure (P_{alv}) and the body surface pressure (P_{bs}).

$$P_{tt} = P_{alv} - P_{bs}$$

For example, if the P_{alv} is 757 mm Hg and the P_{bs} is 760 mm Hg (e.g., inspiration), the P_{tt} is −3 mm Hg (Figure 2–3A).

$$P_{tt} = P_{alv} - P_{bs}$$

$$= 757 \text{ mm Hg} - 760 \text{ mm Hg}$$

$$= -3 \text{ mm Hg}$$

Or, if the P_{alv} is 763 mm Hg and the P_{bs} is 760 mm Hg (e.g., expiration), the P_{tt} is 3 mm Hg (Figure 2–3B).

Figure 2–3. *Transthoracic pressure: The difference between the alveolar pressure (P_{alv}) and the body surface pressure (P_{bs}). Note: In this illustration, the body surface pressure (P_{bs}) is equal to the barometric pressure (P_B).*

Technically, there is no real difference between the transairway pressure (P_{ta}) and the transthoracic pressure (P_{tt}). The P_{tt} is merely another way to view the pressure differences across the lungs.

ROLE OF THE DIAPHRAGM IN VENTILATION

The flow of gas in and out of the lungs is caused by the transpulmonary and transairway pressure changes that occur in response to the action of the diaphragm (Figure 2–4). When stimulated to contract during inspiration, diaphragmatic leaves move downward, causing the thoracic volume to increase and the intrapleural and intra-alveolar pressures to decrease (see Boyle's law, Chapter Three). Because the intra-alveolar pressure is less than the barometric pressure during this period, gas from the atmosphere moves down the tracheobronchial tree until the intra-alveolar pressure and the barometric pressure are in equilibrium. This equilibrium point is known as **end-inspiration** (pre-expiration).

During expiration, each diaphragmatic leaf relaxes and moves upward, causing the thoracic volume to decrease and the intrapleural and intra-alveolar pressures to increase. During this period, the intra-alveolar pressure is greater than the barometric pressure and gas flows out of the lungs until the intra-alveolar pressure and the barometric pressure are once again in equilibrium (Figure 2–5). This equilibrium point is known as **end-expiration** (pre-inspiration). The intrapleural pres-

Figure 2–4. *The diaphragm.*

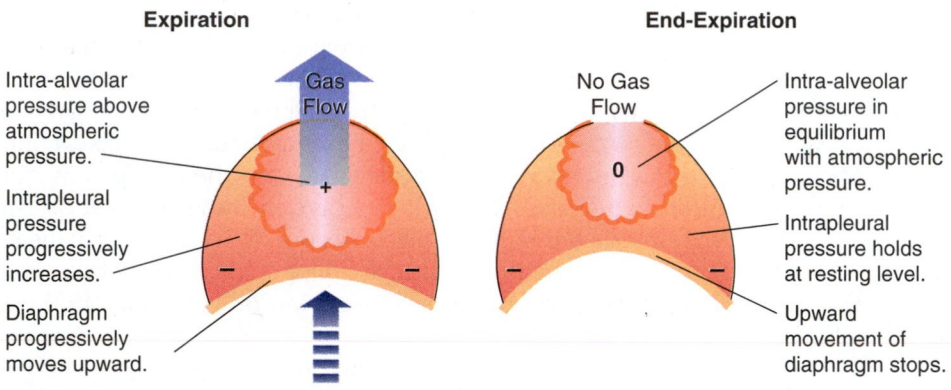

Figure 2–5.   *How the excursion of the diaphragm affects the intrapleural pressure, intra-alveolar pressure, and bronchial gas flow during inspiration and expiration.*

sure during normal inspiration and expiration is always less than the barometric pressure.

At rest, the normal excursion (movement) of the diaphragm is about 1.5 cm, and the normal intrapleural pressure change is about 3 to 6 cm H_2O pressure (2 to 4 mm Hg). During a deep inspiration, however, the diaphragm may move as much as 6 to 10 cm, a fact which can cause the average intrapleural pressure to drop as low as 50 cm H_2O subatmospheric. During a forced expiration, the intrapleural pressure may climb between 70 and 100 cm H_2O above atmospheric.

STATIC CHARACTERISTICS OF THE LUNGS

The term **static** refers to the study of matter at rest and the forces bringing about or maintaining equilibrium. Normally, the lungs have a natural tendency to recoil inward, or to collapse. In contrast, the chest wall has a natural tendency to move outward, or to expand. Because of these two opposing forces, the lungs are at their resting volume (**functional residual capacity**) when the inward recoil force of the lungs is equal to the outward, or expanding, force of the chest wall. In other words, the functional residual capacity is the volume remaining in the lungs when the recoil pressure of the lungs and the outward pressure generated by the chest wall cancel each other out.

There are two major static forces in the lungs that cause an inflated lung to recoil inward: (1) the elastic properties of the lung tissue itself and (2) the surface tension produced by the layer of fluid that lines the inside of the alveoli.

ELASTIC PROPERTIES OF THE LUNG

How readily the elastic force of the lungs accepts a volume of inspired air is known as **lung compliance** (C_L). C_L is defined as the change in lung volume (ΔV) per unit pressure change (ΔP). Mathematically, C_L is expressed in liters per centimeters of water pressure (L/cm H_2O). In other words, compliance determines how much air, in liters (L), the lungs will accommodate for each centimeter of water pressure change (cm H_2O) (e.g., each transpulmonary pressure change).

For example, if an individual generates a negative intrapleural pressure change of 5 cm H_2O during inspiration, and the lungs accept a new volume of .75 L of gas, the C_L of the lungs would be expressed as .15 L/cm H_2O:

$$C_L = \frac{\Delta V \, (L)}{\Delta P \, (cm \, H_2O)}$$

$$= \frac{.75 \, L \, of \, gas}{5 \, cm \, H_2O}$$

$$= .15 \, L/cm \, H_2O \, (or, \, 150 \, ml/cm \, H_2O)$$

It is irrelevant whether the change in driving pressure is in the form of a positive or negative pressure. In other words, a negative 5 cm H_2O pressure generated in the intrapleural space around the lungs will produce the same volume change as a positive 5 cm H_2O pressure generated at the airway (e.g., by means of a mechanical ventilator) (Figure 2–6).

At rest, the average C_L for each breath is about 0.1 L/cm H_2O. In other words, approximately 100 ml of air is delivered into the lungs per 1 cm H_2O pressure change (see Figure 2–6). When lung compliance is increased, the lungs accept a greater volume of gas per unit of pressure change. When C_L is decreased, the lungs accept a smaller volume of gas per unit of pressure change. This relationship is also illustrated by the volume-pressure curve in Figure 2–7 (page 65).

Finally, it should be noted that C_L—both in the normal and abnormal lung—progressively decreases as the alveoli approach their total filling capacity. This occurs because the elastic force of the alveoli steadily increases as the lungs expand, which, in turn, reduces the ability of the lungs to accept an additional volume of gas (see Figure 2–7).

Hooke's Law

Hooke's law provides another way to conceptualize the meaning of compliance by describing the physical properties of an elastic substance. **Elastance** is the natural

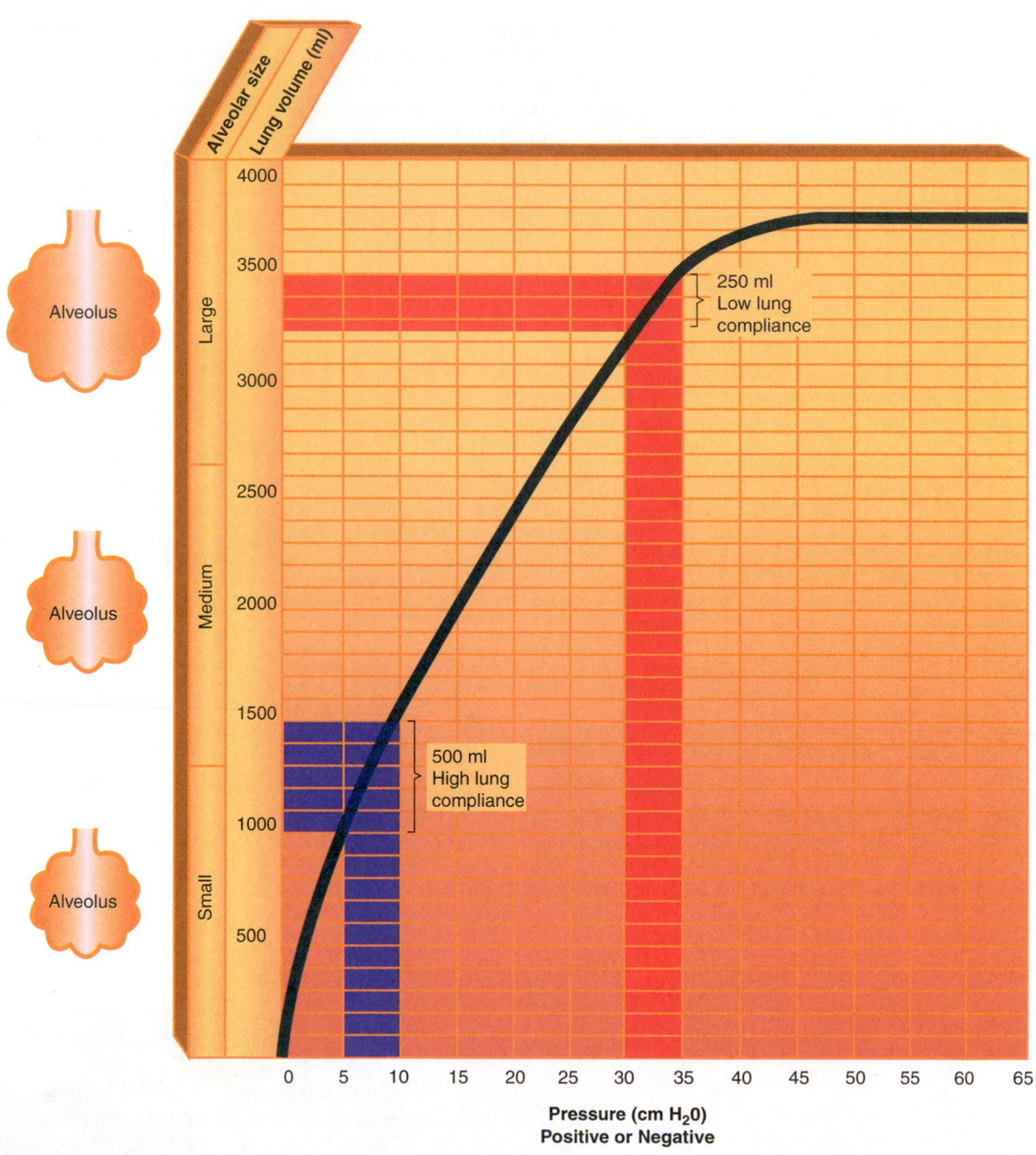

Figure 2–6. *Normal volume-pressure curve. The curve shows that lung compliance progressively decreases as the lungs expand in response to more volume. For example, note the greater volume change between 5 and 10 cm H_2O (small/medium alveoli) than between 30 and 35 cm H_2O (large alveoli).*

Figure 2–7. *How changes in lung compliance affect the volume-pressure curve. When lung compliance decreases, the volume-pressure curve shifts to the right. When lung compliance increases, the volume-pressure curve shifts to the left.*

ability of matter to respond directly to force and to return to its original resting position or shape after the external force no longer exists. In pulmonary physiology, elastance is defined as the change in pressure per change in volume:

$$\text{Elastance} = \frac{\Delta P}{\Delta V}$$

Elastance is the reciprocal (opposite) of compliance. Thus, lungs with high compliance (greater ease of filling) have low elastance; lungs with low compliance (lower ease of filling) have high elastance.

Hooke's law states that when a truly elastic body, like a spring, is acted on by 1 unit of force, the elastic body will stretch 1 unit of length, and when acted on by 2 units of force it will stretch 2 units of length, and so forth. This phenomenon is only true, however, within the elastic body's normal functional range. That is, when the force goes beyond the elastic limit of the substance, the ability of length to directly increase in response to force ceases. Should the force continue to rise, the elastic substance will ultimately break (Figure 2–8, page 66).

When Hooke's law is applied to the elastic properties of the lungs, *volume* is substituted for *length*, and *pressure* is substituted for *force*. Thus, over the normal physiologic range of the lungs, volume varies directly with pressure. The lungs behave in a manner similar to the spring, and once the elastic limit of the lung unit is reached, little or no volume change occurs in response to pressure changes. Should the change in pressure continue to rise, the lung unit will rupture (Figure 2–9, page 67).

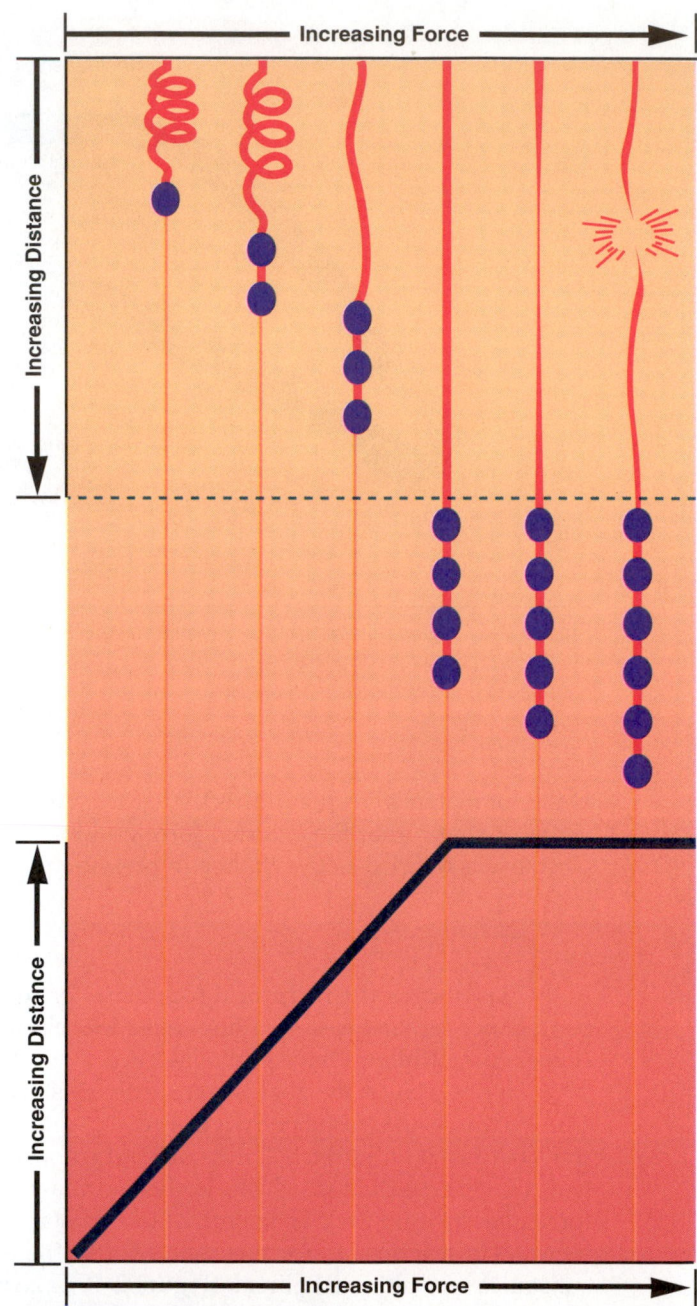

Figure 2–8. *Hooke's law. When a truly elastic body—such as the spring in this illustration—is acted on by 1 unit of force, the elastic body will stretch 1 unit of length; when acted on by 2 units of force, it will stretch 2 units of length; and so forth. When the force goes beyond the elastic limit of the substance, however, the ability of length to increase in response to force quickly ceases.*

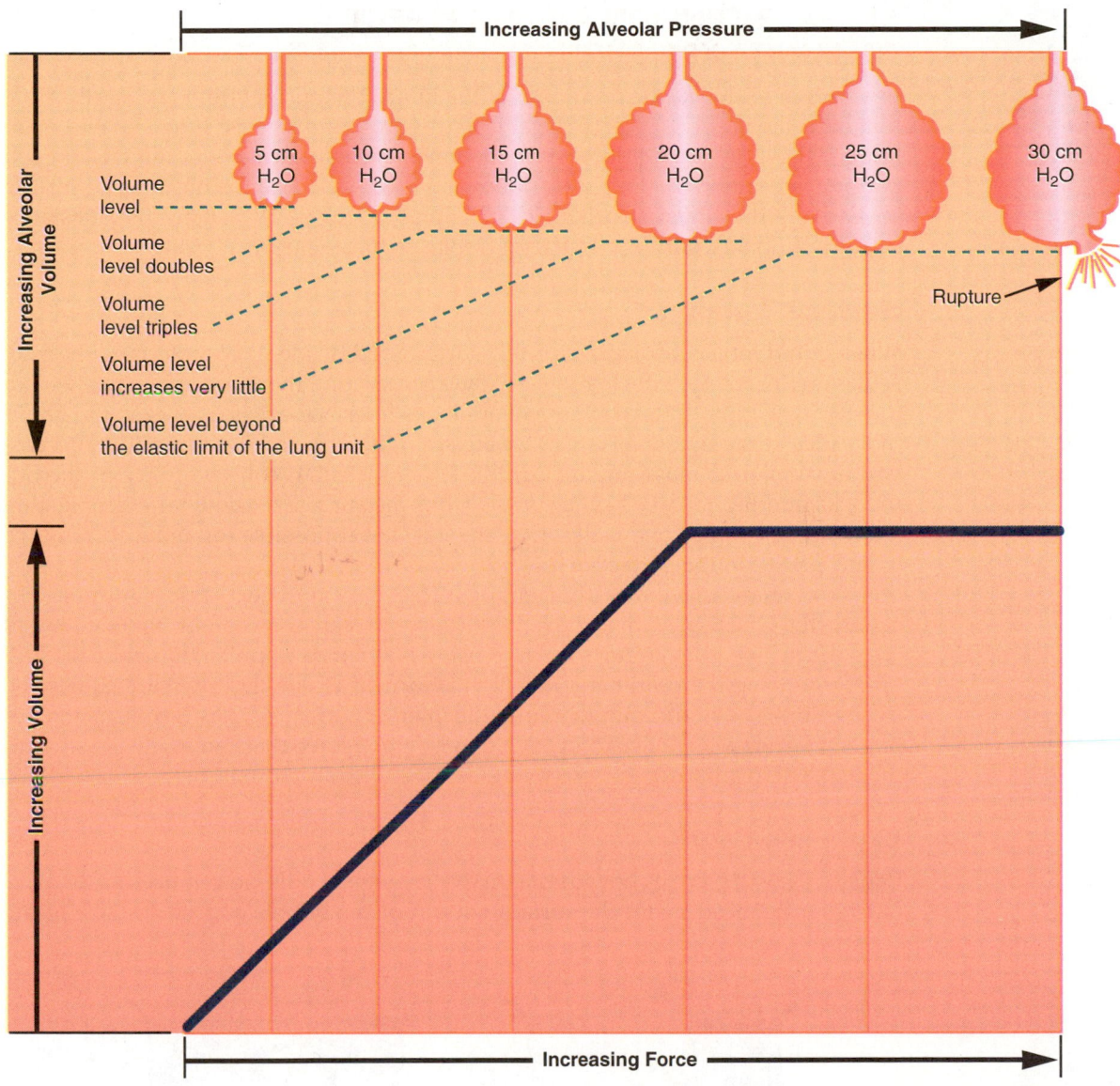

Figure 2–9. *Hooke's law applied to the elastic properties of the lungs. Over the normal physiologic range of the lungs, volume changes vary directly with pressure changes. Once the elastic limit is reached, however, little or no volume change occurs in response to pressure changes.*

Clinically, this phenomenon explains a hazard associated with mechanical ventilation. That is, if the pressure during mechanical ventilation (positive pressure breath) causes the lung unit to expand beyond its elastic capability, the lung unit could rupture, allowing alveolar gas to move into the intrapleural space, and thus causing the lungs to collapse. This condition is called a **pneumothorax**.

SURFACE TENSION AND ITS EFFECT ON LUNG EXPANSION

In addition to the elastic properties of the lungs, the normal fluid (primarily H_2O) that lines the inner surface of the alveoli can profoundly resist lung expansion. To understand how the liquid coating the intra-alveolar surface can hinder lung expansion, an understanding of the following is essential: (1) the meaning of surface tension, (2) the physical principles of Laplace's law, and (3) how the substance called pulmonary surfactant offsets alveolar surface tension.

Surface Tension

When liquid molecules are completely surrounded by identical molecules, the molecules are mutually attracted toward one another and, therefore, move freely in all directions (Figure 2–10A). When a liquid–gas interface exists, however, the liquid molecules at the liquid–gas interface are strongly attracted to the liquid molecules within the liquid mass (Figure 2–10B). This molecular, cohesive force at the liquid–gas interface is called *surface tension*. It is the surface tension, for example, that maintains the shape of a water droplet, or makes it possible for an insect to move or stay afloat on the surface of a pond.

The quantitative measurement of surface tension is expressed in dynes per centimeter. One dyne/cm is the force necessary to cause a tear 1 centimeter long in the surface layer of a liquid, similar to using two hands to pull a thin piece of cloth apart until a split 1 centimeter in length is formed (1 cm H_2O pressure equals 980 dynes/cm). The liquid film that lines the interior surface of the alveoli has the potential to exert a force in excess of 70 dynes/cm, a force that can easily cause complete alveolar collapse.

Laplace's Law

Laplace's law describes how the *distending pressure* of a liquid bubble (not an alveolus) is influenced by (1) the surface tension of the bubble and (2) the size of the

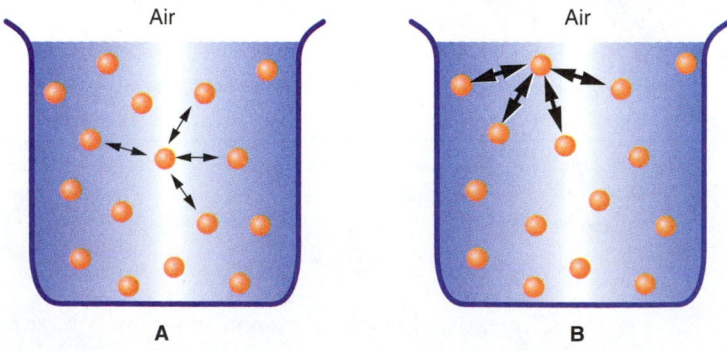

Figure 2–10. *In model A, the liquid molecules in the middle of the container are mutually attracted toward each other and, therefore, move freely in all directions. In model B, the liquid molecules near the surface (liquid–gas interface) are strongly attracted to the liquid molecules within the liquid mass. This molecular force at the liquid–gas interface is called surface tension.*

bubble itself. When Laplace's law is applied to a sphere with one liquid–gas interface (e.g., a bubble completely submerged in a liquid), the equation is written as follows:

$$P = \frac{2\,ST}{r}$$

where P is the pressure difference (dynes/cm^2), ST is surface tension (dynes/cm), and r is the radius of the liquid sphere (cm); the factor 2 is required when the law is applied to a liquid sphere with one liquid–gas interface.

When the law is applied to a bubble with two liquid–gas interfaces (e.g., a soap bubble blown on the end of a tube has a liquid–gas interface both on the inside and on the outside of the bubble), the numerator contains the factor 4 rather than 2:

$$P = \frac{4\,ST}{r}$$

The mathematical arrangement of Laplace's law shows that the *distending pressure* of a liquid sphere is (1) directly proportional to the surface tension of the liquid and (2) inversely proportional to the radius (size) of the sphere.

In other words, the numerator of Laplace's law shows that (a) as the surface tension of a liquid bubble increases, the distending pressure necessary to hold the bubble open increases, or (b) the opposite—when the surface tension of a liquid bubble decreases, the distending pressure of the bubble decreases (Figure 2–11). The denominator of Laplace's law shows that (a) when the size (radius) of a liquid bubble increases, the distending pressure necessary to hold the bubble open decreases, or (b) the opposite—when the size of the bubble decreases, the distending pressure of the bubble increases (Figure 2–12, page 70). Because of this interesting physical phenomenon, when two different size bubbles—having the same

Figure 2–11. *Bubbles A and B are the same size. The surface tension (ST) of bubble A is 10 dynes/cm and requires a distending pressure (P) of 5 cm H$_2$O to maintain its size. The surface tension of bubble B is 20 dynes/cm H$_2$O (twice the surface tension of bubble A) and requires a distending pressure of 10 cm H$_2$O (twice that of bubble A) to maintain its size (r = radius).*

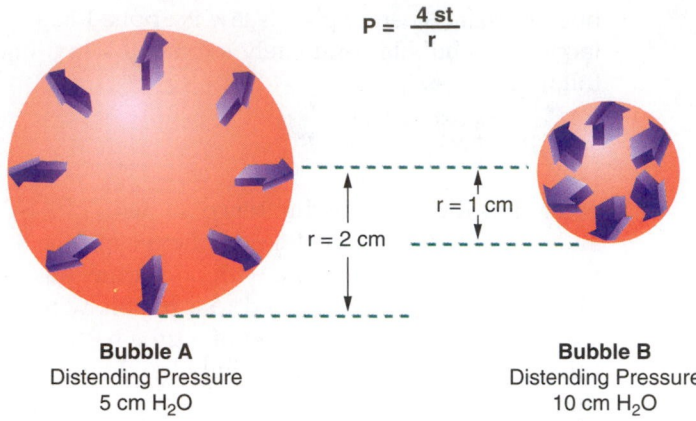

$$P = \frac{4\ st}{r}$$

r = 1 cm

r = 2 cm

Bubble A
Distending Pressure
5 cm H_2O

Bubble B
Distending Pressure
10 cm H_2O

Figure 2–12. *The surface tension (ST) of bubbles A and B is identical. The radius (r) of bubble A is 2 cm, and it requires a distending pressure (P) of 5 cm H_2O to maintain its size. The radius of bubble B is 1 cm (one-half that of bubble A), and it requires a distending pressure of 10 cm H_2O (twice that of bubble A) to maintain its size.*

surface tension—are in direct communication, the greater pressure in the smaller bubble will cause the smaller bubble to empty into the larger bubble (Figure 2–13).

During the formation of a new bubble (e.g., a soap bubble blown on the end of a tube), the principles of Laplace's law do not come into effect until the distending pressure of the liquid sphere goes beyond what is called the *critical opening pres-*

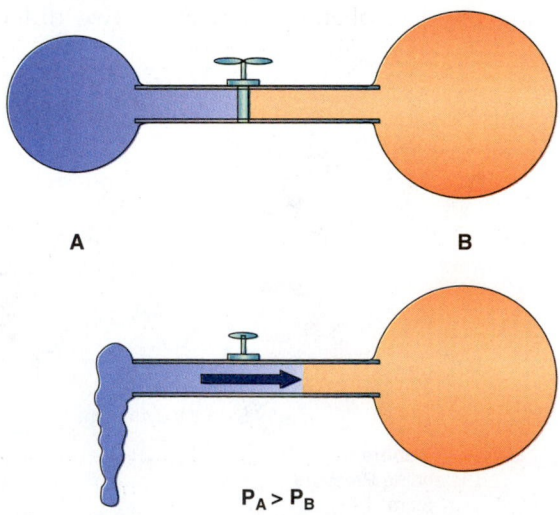

A   B

$P_A > P_B$

Figure 2–13. *Bubbles A and B have the same surface tension. When the two bubbles are in direct communication, the higher pressure in the smaller bubble (A) causes it to empty into the large bubble (B).*

sure. As shown in Figure 2–14, the critical opening pressure is the high pressure (with little volume change) that is initially required to overcome the liquid molecular force during the formation of a new bubble—similar to the high pressure first required to blow up a new balloon. Figure 2–14 also shows that, prior to the critical opening pressure, the distending pressure must progressively increase to enlarge the size of the bubble. In other words, the distending pressure is *directly proportional* to the radius of the bubble (the opposite of what Laplace's law states).

Once the critical opening pressure is reached, however, the distending pressure progressively decreases as the bubble increases in size—the distending pressure, as described by Laplace's law, is *inversely proportional* to the radius of the bubble. The distending pressure will continue to decrease until the bubble enlarges to its breaking point and ruptures. It is interesting to note that just before the bubble breaks, the distending pressure is at its lowest level (see Figure 2–14).

Conversely: Laplace's law shows that as an inflated bubble decreases in size, the distending pressure proportionally increases until the pressure reaches what is called the *critical closing pressure* (actually the same pressure as the critical opening pressure). When the size of the bubble decreases beyond this point, the liquid molecular force of the bubble becomes greater than the distending pressure and the bubble collapses (see Figure 2–14).

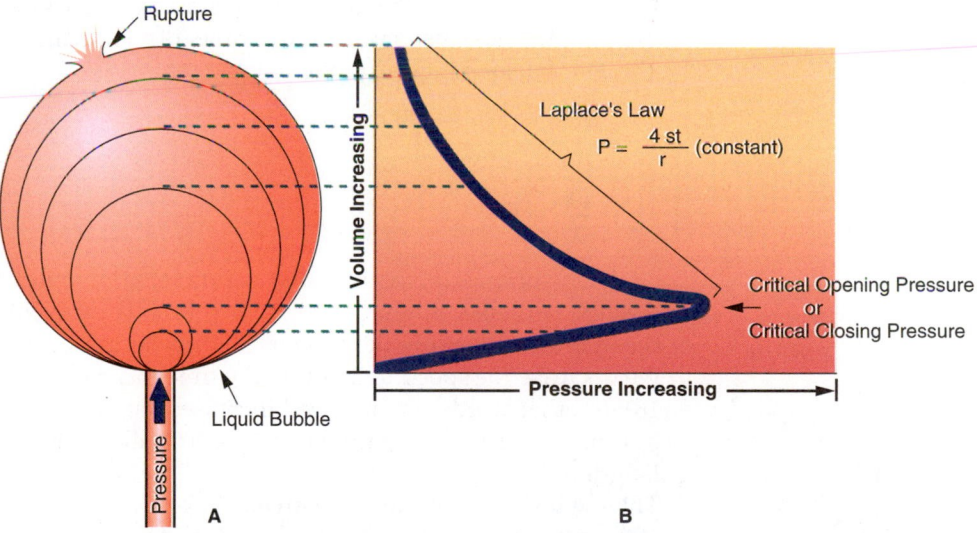

Figure 2–14. *A) Model showing the formation of a new liquid bubble at the end of a tube. B) Graph showing the distending pressure required to maintain the bubble's size (volume) at various stages. Initially, a very high pressure, with little volume change, is required to inflate the bubble. Once the critical opening pressure (same as critical closing pressure) is reached, however, the distending pressure progressively decreases as the size of the bubble increases. Thus, between the critical opening pressure and the point at which the bubble ruptures, the bubble behaves according to Laplace's law. In essence, Laplace's law applies to the normal functional size range of the bubble.*

It should be emphasized that *Laplace's law does not state that the surface tension varies with the size of the bubble.* To the contrary, the law shows that as a liquid bubble changes in size, it is the *distending pressure*, not the *surface tension*, that varies inversely with the radius. In fact, as the radius of the sphere increases, the surface tension remains the same until the size of the bubble goes beyond its natural elastic limit and ruptures.

The fact that the surface tension remains the same while the radius of a liquid sphere changes can be illustrated mathematically by rearranging Laplace's law as follows:

a. Since surface tension is a property of the fluid and is constant for any specific fluid, Laplace's law can be restated as:

$$P = \frac{k}{r}$$

where k is a constant (in this case, the constant k equals surface tension) and P (pressure) is inversely proportional to r (radius).

b. The equation $P = k \div r$ can be rearranged as follows:

$$Pr = k$$

The formula now shows that the variable quantities (Pr) are inversely proportional and that their product is a constant (k). Thus, as one variable increases, the other must decrease to maintain a constant product (k).

To demonstrate this concept, consider taking a 400-mile automobile trip. With the formula distance = rate × time (d = rt), which represent product (d) and variable quantities (rt), we have:

$$400 = rt \ (d = 400 \text{ miles})$$

or

$$\frac{400}{r} = t$$

On such a trip, assume that we travel at 50 miles per hour (mph) and that the trip takes 8 hours (400 ÷ 50 = 8). If we travel by train and increase the speed to 100 mph, the time of the trip decreases to 4 hours. If, however, we decrease the speed to 25 mph, the time increases to 16 hours (400 ÷ 25 = 16). In other words, as the speed increases the time decreases and vice versa, but the product (d) remains a constant 400 miles, which is determined by the length of the trip.

c. Thus, when two variables are inversely proportional, such as rt = 400 or t = 400 ÷ r, the time increases as the rate decreases, and time decreases as the rate increases (Figure 2–15). Note the similarity of the graph in Figure 2–15 to the portion of the graph that represents Laplace's law in Figure 2–14B.

Laplace's Law Applied to the Alveolar Fluid Lining

Since the liquid film that lines the alveolus resembles a bubble or sphere, according to Laplace's law, when the alveolar fluid is permitted to behave according to its

$$Time = \frac{Distance}{Rate} \quad (constant\ 400\ mi)$$

or

$$Distance = Rate \times Time$$

Figure 2–15. *Rate and time are inversely proportional (as rate increases, time decreases; and as rate decreases, time increases).*

natural tendency, a high transpulmonary pressure must be generated to keep the small alveoli open (see Figure 2–14). Fortunately, in the healthy lung the natural tendency for the smaller alveoli to collapse is offset by a fascinating substance called **pulmonary surfactant**.

How Pulmonary Surfactant Offsets Alveolar Surface Tension

Pulmonary surfactant is a phospholipid (dipalmitoyl phosphatidyl choline) produced by the alveolar Type II cells (see Figure 1–21, page 29). The surfactant molecule has both a hydrophobic (water-insoluble) end and a hydrophilic (water-soluble) end. This unique hydrophobic/hydrophilic characteristic causes the surfactant molecule to position itself at the alveolar gas–liquid interface so that the hydrophilic end is in the liquid phase and the hydrophobic end is in the gas phase. The interruption of the alveolar fluid caused by the surfactant hydrophilic/hydrophobic ends has the ability to profoundly lower the alveolar surface tension as described below.

The presence of pulmonary surfactant at the alveolar gas–liquid interface causes surface tension to decrease in proportion to the ratio of surfactant to alveolar surface area. That is, when the alveolus decreases in size (decreased volume), the proportion of surfactant to alveolar surface area increases. This mechanism, in turn, increases the physiologic effect of the pulmonary surfactant and causes the alveolar surface tension to decrease (Figure 2–16A, page 74).

On the other hand, as the alveolus increases in size (increased volume), the relative amount of surfactant to alveolar surface area decreases (since the number of surfactant molecules does not change when the size of the alveolus changes).

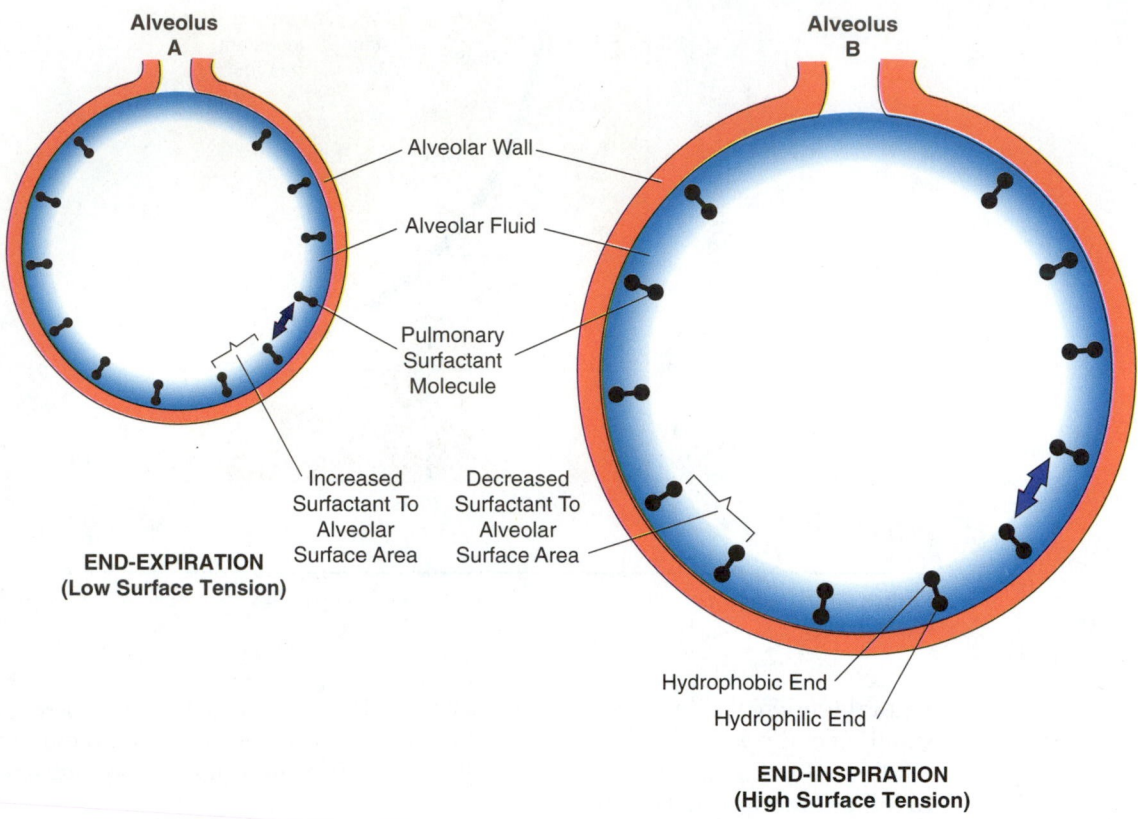

Figure 2–16. *In the normal lung, the surface tension is low in the small alveolus (A) because the ratio of surfactant to alveolar surface is high. As the alveolus enlarges (B), the surface tension steadily increases because the ratio of surfactant to alveolar surface decreases.*

This mechanism, in turn, decreases the physiologic effect of pulmonary surfactant and causes the alveolar surface tension to increase (Figure 2–16B). In fact, as the alveolus enlarges, the surface tension will progressively increase to the value it would naturally have in the absence of pulmonary surfactant. Clinically, however, the fact that surface tension increases as the alveolus enlarges is not significant—since, as Laplace's law demonstrates, the distending pressure required to maintain a bubble size progressively decreases as the size of the bubble increases (see Figure 2–14).

It is estimated that the surface tension of the average alveolus varies from 1 to 5 dynes/cm (when the alveolus is very small) to about 50 dynes/cm (when the alveolus is fully distended) (Figure 2–17). Because pulmonary surfactant has the ability to reduce the surface tension of the small alveoli (the numerator in Laplace's law), the high distending pressure that would otherwise be required to offset the critical closing pressure of the small alveoli is virtually eliminated.

In the absence of pulmonary surfactant, however, the alveolar surface tension increases to the force it would naturally have (50 dynes/cm), and the distending

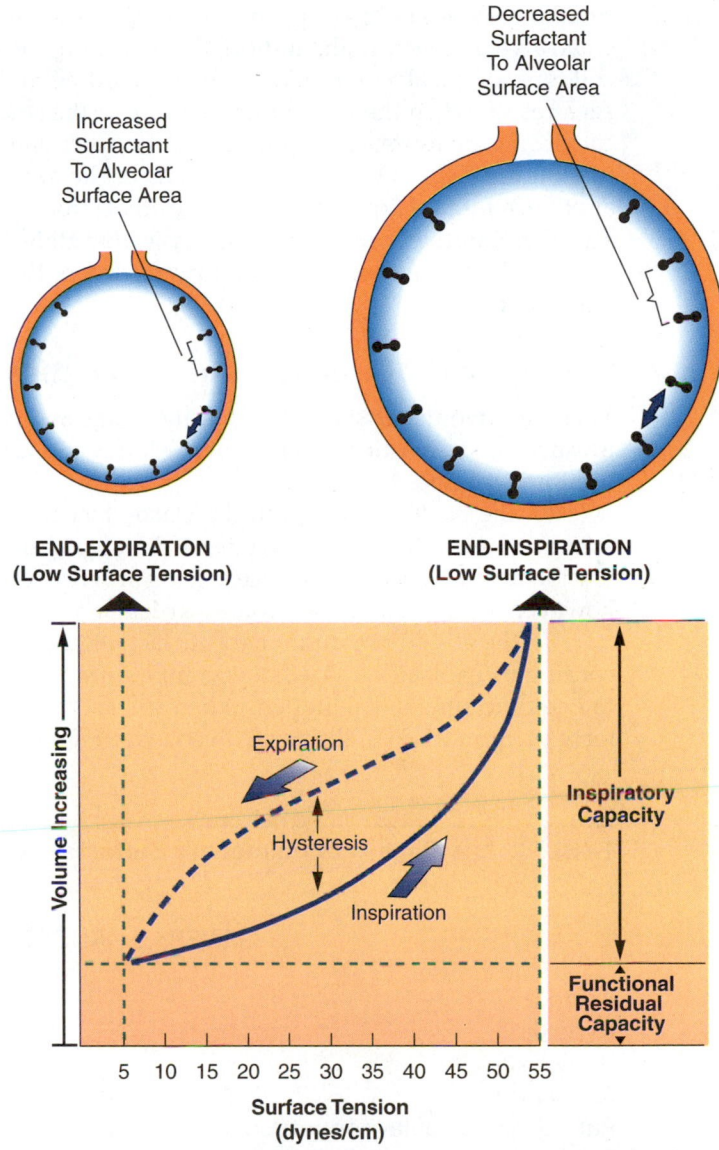

Figure 2–17. *In the normal lung, the surface tension force progressively increases as the alveolar size increases. Similarly, as the alveolar size decreases, the surface tension force progressively decreases. Note that, because of the alveolar surface tension, the actual physical change of the alveolus lags behind the pressure applied to it. When such a phenomenon occurs in the field of physics (i.e., a physical manifestation lagging behind a force), a* hysteresis *is said to exist. When this lung characteristic is plotted on a volume-pressure curve, the alveolus is shown to deflate along a different curve than that inscribed during inspiration and the curve has a looplike appearance. The hysteresis loop shows graphically that at any given pressure the alveolar volume is less during inspiration than it is during expiration. This alveolar hysteresis is virtually eliminated when the lungs are inflated experimentally with saline; such an experimental procedure removes the alveolar liquid–gas interface and, therefore, the alveolar surface tension. Inspiratory capacity is the volume of air that can be inhaled after a normal exhalation. Functional residual capacity is the volume of air remaining in the lungs after a normal exhalation.*

pressure necessary to overcome the recoil forces of the liquid film that coats the small alveoli is very high. In short, the distending pressure required to offset the recoil force of the alveolar fluid behaves according to the principles of Laplace's law. As a result, when the distending pressure of the small alveoli falls below the critical closing pressure, the liquid molecular force snaps the alveolar walls together (see Figure 2–14). Once the liquid walls of the alveolus come in contact with one another, a mutual liquid bond develops that strongly resists the re-expansion of the alveolus. Complete alveolar collapse is called **atelectasis**.

Table 2–1 lists some respiratory disorders that cause pulmonary surfactant deficiency.

Summary of the Static Characteristics of the Lungs

There are two major static forces in the lungs that cause an inflated lung to recoil inward: (1) the elastic properties of the lungs and (2) the surface tension of the liquid film that lines the alveolus.

In the healthy lung, both the elastic tension and the degree of surface tension are low in the small alveoli. As the alveoli increase in size, both the elastic tension and the degree of surface tension progressively increase. The elastic tension, however, is the predominant force, particularly in the large alveoli (Figure 2–18).

In the absence of pulmonary surfactant, the alveolar fluid lining behaves according to Laplace's law—that is, a high intrapleural pressure must be generated to keep the small alveoli open. When such a condition exists, the surface tension force predominates in the small alveoli (see Figure 2–18).

TABLE 2–1. **Causes of Pulmonary Surfactant Deficiency**

GENERAL CAUSES

Acidosis
Hypoxia
Hyperoxia
Atelectasis
Pulmonary vascular congestion

SPECIFIC CAUSES

Adult respiratory distress syndrome (ARDS)
Infant respiratory distress syndrome (IRDS)
Pulmonary edema
Pulmonary embolism
Pneumonia
Excessive pulmonary lavage or hydration
Drowning
Extracorporeal oxygenation

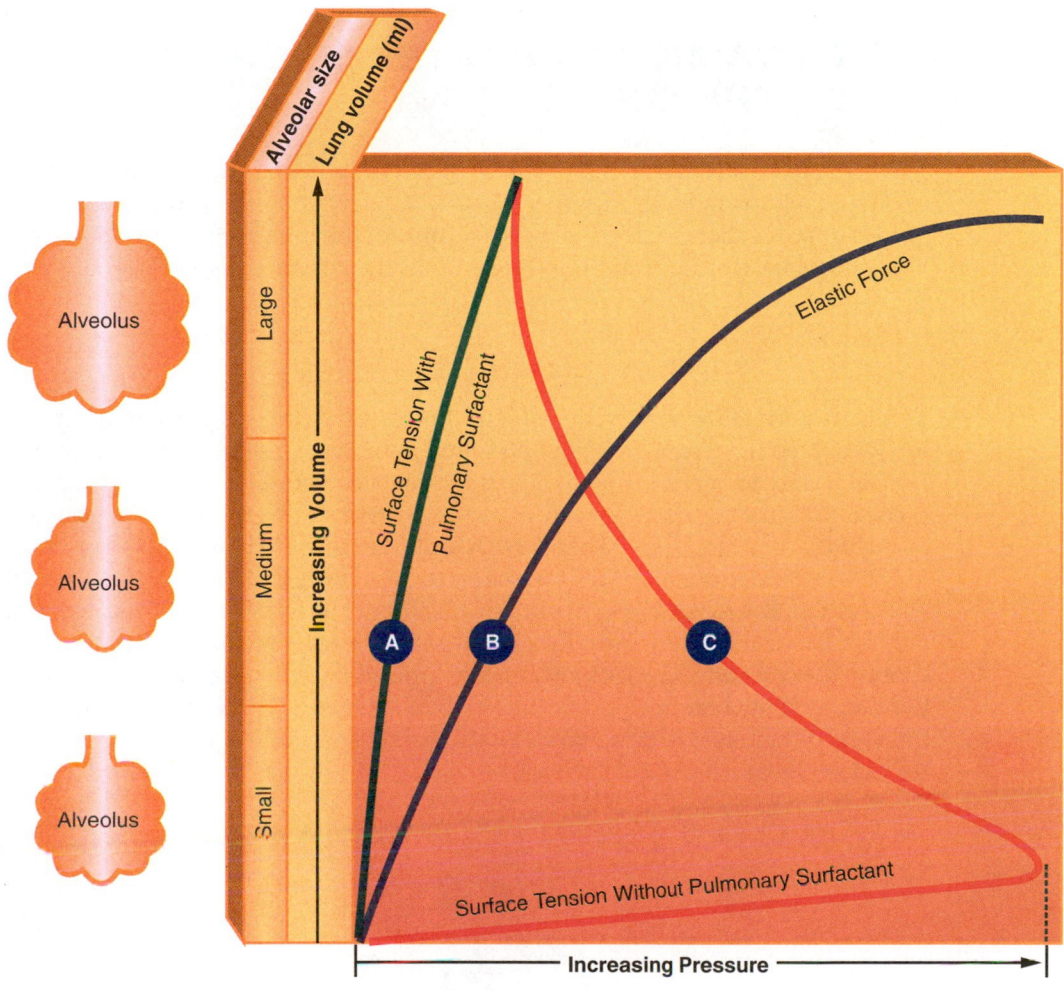

Figure 2–18. *In the normal lung, both the surface tension force (A) and the elastic force (B) progressively increase as the alveolus enlarges. The elastic force is the predominant force in both the small and the large alveoli. In the absence of pulmonary surfactant, the surface tension force (C) predominates in the small alveoli. The elastic force (B) still predominates in the large alveoli. Note that, as the alveolus enlarges, the pressure required to offset the "abnormal" surface tension force (C) ultimately decreases to the same pressure required to offset the "normal" surface tension force (B). Thus, it can be seen that when there is a deficiency of pulmonary surfactant, the surface tension of the small alveoli creates a high recoil force. If a high pressure is not generated to offset this surface tension force, the alveoli will collapse.*

DYNAMIC CHARACTERISTICS OF THE LUNGS

The term **dynamic** refers to the study of forces in action. In the lungs, dynamic refers to the movement of gas in and out of the lungs and the pressure changes required to move the gas. The dynamic features of the lung are best explained by (1) Poiseuille's law for flow and pressure and (2) the airway resistance equation.

POISEUILLE'S LAW FOR FLOW AND PRESSURE APPLIED TO THE BRONCHIAL AIRWAYS

During a normal inspiration, intrapleural pressure decreases from its normal resting level (about -3 to -6 cm H_2O pressure), which causes the bronchial airways to lengthen and to increase in diameter (*passive dilation*). During expiration, intrapleural pressure increases (or returns to its normal resting state), which causes the bronchial airways to decrease in length and in diameter (*passive constriction*) (Figure 2–19). Under normal circumstances, such anatomic changes of the bronchial airways are not remarkable. In certain respiratory disorders (e.g., emphysema or chronic bronchitis), however, bronchial gas flow and intrapleural pressure may change significantly, particularly during expiration, when passive constriction of the tracheobronchial tree occurs. The reason for this is best explained in the relationship of factors described in Poiseuille's law. Poiseuille's law can be arranged for either flow or pressure.

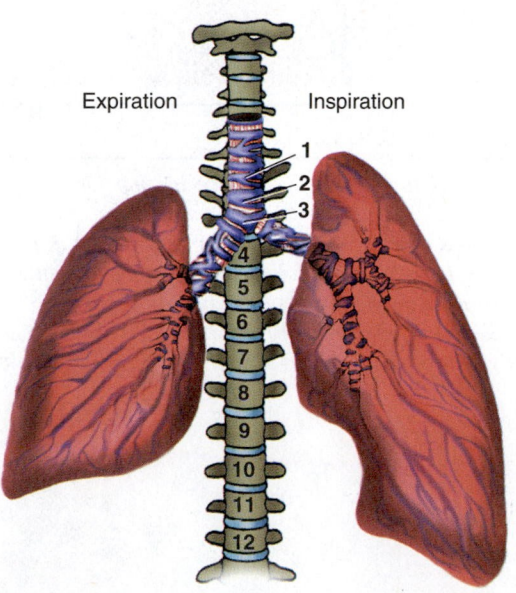

Figure 2–19. *During inspiration, the bronchial airways lengthen and increase in diameter. During expiration, the bronchial airways decrease in length and diameter.*

Poiseuille's Law Arranged for Flow

When Poiseuille's law is arranged for flow, it is written as follows:

$$\dot{V} = \frac{\Delta P r^4 \pi}{8l\eta}$$

where η = the viscosity of a gas (or fluid), Δ (Delta) P = the change of pressure from one end of the tube to the other, r = the radius of the tube, l = the length of the tube, $\dot{V}$ = the gas (or fluid) flowing through the tube; $\pi \div 8$ = constants, which will be excluded from the discussion.

The equation states that flow is directly proportional to P and r^4 and inversely proportional to l and η. In other words, flow will decrease in response to a decreased P and tube radius, and flow will increase in response to a decreased tube length and fluid viscosity. Conversely, flow will increase in response to an increased P and tube radius and decrease in response to an increased tube length and fluid viscosity.

It should be emphasized that flow is profoundly affected by the radius of the tube. As Poiseuille's law illustrates, $\dot{V}$ is a function of the fourth power of the radius (r^4). In other words, assuming that pressure (P) remains constant, decreasing the radius of a tube by one-half reduces the gas flow to 1/16 of its original flow.

For example, if the radius of a bronchial tube through which gas flows at a rate of 16 ml per second (ml/sec) is reduced to one-half its original size because of mucosal swelling, the flow rate through the bronchial tube would decrease to 1 ml/sec (1/16 the original flow rate) (Figure 2–20).

Similarly, decreasing a tube radius by 16 percent decreases gas flow to one-half its original rate. For instance, if the radius of a bronchial tube through which

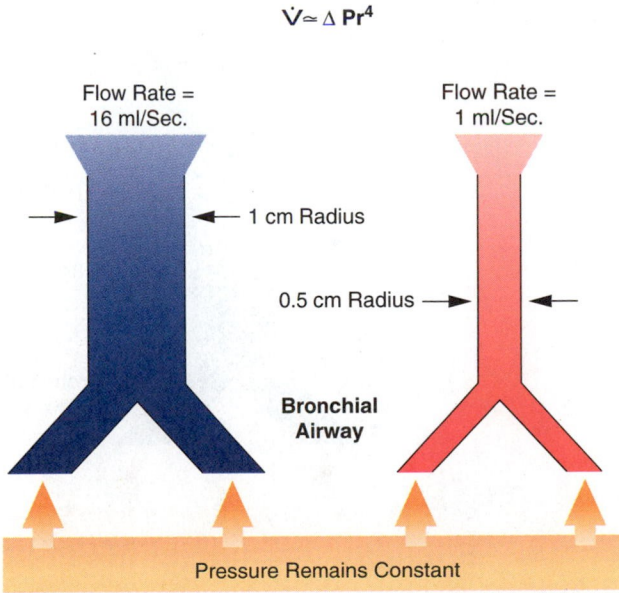

Figure 2–20. *Poiseuille's law for flow applied to a bronchial airway with its radius reduced 50 percent.*

gas flows at a rate of 16 ml/sec is decreased by 16 percent (because of mucosal swelling, for example), the flow rate through the bronchial tube would decrease to 8 ml/sec (one-half the original flow rate) (Figure 2–21).

Poiseuille's Law Arranged for Pressure

When Poiseuille's law is arranged for pressure, it is written as follows:

$$P = \frac{\dot{V}8l\eta}{r^4\pi}$$

The equation now states that pressure is directly proportional to $\dot{V}$, l, and η and inversely proportional to r^4. In other words, pressure will increase in response to a decreased tube radius and decrease in response to a decreased flow rate, tube length, or viscosity. The opposite is also true: pressure will decrease in response to an increased tube radius, and increase in response to an increased flow rate, tube length, or viscosity.

Pressure is a function of the radius to the fourth power and therefore is profoundly affected by the radius of a tube. In other words, if flow ($\dot{V}$) remains constant, decreasing a tube radius to one-half of its previous size requires an increase in pressure to 16 times its original level.

For example, if the radius of a bronchial tube with a driving pressure of 1 cm H_2O is reduced to one-half its original size because of mucosal swelling, the driving pressure through the bronchial tube would have to increase to 16 cm H_2O ($16 \times 1 = 16$) to maintain the same flow rate (Figure 2–22).

Figure 2–21. *Poiseuille's law for flow applied to a bronchial airway with its radius reduced 16 percent.*

$$P \approx \frac{\dot{V}}{r^4}$$

Flow Rate Remains Constant

1 cm Radius

0.5 cm Radius

**Bronchial
Airway**

1 cm H$_2$O
Driving Pressure

16 cm H$_2$O
Driving Pressure

Figure 2–22. *Poiseuille's law for pressure applied to a bronchial airway with its radius reduced 50 percent.*

Similarly, decreasing the bronchial tube radius by 16 percent increases the pressure to twice its original level. For instance, if the radius of a bronchial tube with a driving pressure of 10 cm H$_2$O is decreased by 16 percent because of mucosal swelling, the driving pressure through the bronchial tube would have to increase to 20 cm H$_2$O (twice its original pressure) to maintain the same flow (Figure 2–23, page 82).

Poiseuille's Law Rearranged to Simple Proportionalities

When Poiseuille's law is applied to the tracheobronchial tree during spontaneous breathing, the two equations can be rewritten as simple proportionalities:

$$\dot{V} \approx Pr^4$$

$$P \approx \frac{\dot{V}}{r^4}$$

Based on the proportionality for flow, it can be stated that since gas flow varies directly with r^4 of the bronchial airway, flow must diminish during exhalation because the radius of the bronchial airways decreases. Stated differently, assuming that the pressure remains constant as the radius (r) of the bronchial airways decreases, gas flow ($\dot{V}$) also decreases. During normal spontaneous breathing, however, the gas flow reduction during exhalation is negligible.

In terms of the proportionality for pressure (P $\approx$ $\dot{V} \div r^4$), if gas flow is to remain constant during exhalation, the transthoracic pressure must vary inversely

$$P \simeq \frac{\dot{V}}{r^4}$$

Flow Rate Remains Constant

1 cm Radius

.84 cm Radius

Bronchial Airway

10 cm H$_2$O
Driving Pressure

20 cm H$_2$O
Driving Pressure

Figure 2–23. *Poiseuille's law for pressure applied to a bronchial airway with its radius reduced 16 percent.*

with the fourth power of the radius of the airway. In other words, as the radius of the bronchial airways decreases during exhalation, the driving pressure must increase to maintain a constant gas flow.*

During normal spontaneous breathing, the need to increase the transairway pressure during exhalation in order to maintain a certain gas flow is not significant. However, in certain respiratory disorders (e.g., emphysema and bronchitis), gas flow reductions and transthoracic pressure increases may be substantial as a result of the bronchial narrowing that develops in such disorders.

AIRWAY RESISTANCE

Airway resistance (R_{aw}) is defined as the pressure difference between the mouth and the alveoli (*transairway pressure*) divided by flow rate. In other words, the rate at which a certain volume of gas flows through the bronchial airways is a function of the pressure gradient and the resistance created by the airways to the flow of gas. Mathematically, R_{aw} is measured in centimeters of water per liter per second (L/sec), according to the following equation:

$$R_{aw} = \frac{\Delta P \text{ (cm H}_2\text{O)}}{\dot{V}\text{(L/sec)}}$$

*See Mathematical Discussion of Poiseuille's Law in Appendix III.

For example, if an individual produces a flow rate of 4 L/sec during inspiration by generating a transairway pressure of 4 cm H_2O, R_{aw} would equal 1 cm H_2O/L/sec:

$$R_{aw} = \frac{\Delta P}{\dot{V}}$$

$$= \frac{4 \text{ cm } H_2O}{4 \text{ L/sec}}$$

$$= 1 \text{ cm } H_2O/\text{L/sec}$$

Normally, the R_{aw} in the tracheobronchial tree is about 1.0 to 2.0 cm H_2O/L/sec in adults. However, in chronic obstructive pulmonary diseases (e.g., emphysema or asthma), R_{aw} may be very high. It is also much higher in newborn infants than in normal adults (see Chapter Eleven).

The movement of gas through a tube (or bronchial airway) can be classified as (1) laminar flow, or (2) turbulent flow (Figure 2–24).

Laminar Flow

Laminar gas flow refers to a gas flow that is streamlined. The gas molecules move through the tube in a pattern parallel to the sides of the tube. This flow pattern occurs at low flow rates and at low pressure gradients.

Turbulent Flow

Turbulent gas flow refers to gas molecules that move through a tube in a random manner. Gas flow encounters resistance from both the sides of the tube and from

Figure 2–24. *Types of gas flow.*

the collision with other gas molecules. This flow pattern occurs at high flow rates and at high pressure gradients.

TIME CONSTANTS

A product of airway resistance (R_{aw}) and lung compliance (C_L) is a phenomenon called **time constant**. Time constant is defined as the time (in seconds) necessary to inflate a particular lung region to 60 percent of its potential filling capacity. For example, lung regions that have either an increased R_{aw} or an increased C_L require more time to inflate. These alveoli are said to have a *long time constant*. In contrast, lung regions that have either a decreased R_{aw} or a decreased C_L require less time to inflate. These alveoli are said to have a *short time constant*.

Mathematically, the time constant (T_C) is arranged as follows:

$$T_C \text{ (sec)} = \underbrace{\frac{\Delta P \text{ (cm H}_2\text{O)}}{\dot{V} \text{ (L/sec)}}}_{(R_{aw})} \times \underbrace{\frac{\Delta V \text{ (L)}}{\Delta P \text{ (cm H}_2\text{O)}}}_{(C_L)}$$

$$= \frac{\text{cm H}_2\text{O} \times \text{L}}{\text{L/sec} \times \text{cm H}_2\text{O}}$$

This equation shows that as R_{aw} increases, the value for pressure (P, in cm H_2O) in the numerator increases. Or, when C_L decreases, the value for volume (V) in liters (L) in the numerator decreases.

Thus, assuming that all other variables remain constant, if the R_{aw} of a specific lung region doubles, the time constant will also double (i.e., the lung unit will take twice as long to inflate). In contrast, if the C_L is reduced by half, the time constant will also be reduced by half—and, it is important to note, the potential filling capacity of the lung region is also reduced by half. To help illustrate this concept, consider the time constants illustrated in Figure 2–25.

In Figure 2–25A, two alveolar units have identical R_{aw} and C_L. Thus, the two alveoli require the same amount of time to inflate—they have the same time constants. Figure 2–25B shows two alveolar units with the same R_{aw} but with two different C_L. Because the C_L in Unit B is one-half the C_L of Unit A, Unit B (low compliance) receives one-half the volume of Unit A (high compliance). It is important to realize that (1) Unit B has a shorter time constant than Unit A, and (2) Unit B receives only one-half the volume received by Unit A.

In Figure 2–25C, the two alveolar units have the same compliance, but two different R_{aw}. Because the R_{aw} leading to Unit B is two times greater than the R_{aw} leading to Unit A, Unit B (high R_{aw}) requires twice the time to fill to the same volume as Unit A (low R_{aw}). It is important to note that the two alveolar units do not have the same time constant—the time constant for Unit B is two times longer than that of Unit A. Thus, it is also important to note that as the breathing frequency increases, the time necessary to fill Unit B may not be adequate. Clinically, how readily a lung region fills during a period of gas flow is called **dynamic compliance**.

DYNAMIC COMPLIANCE

The measurement called dynamic compliance is a product of the time constants. Dynamic compliance is defined as the change in the volume of the lungs divided

Figure 2–25. *Time constants for hypothetical alveoli with differing lung compliances (C_L), supplied by airways with differencing resistances (R_{aw}).*

by the change in the transpulmonary pressure (obtained via a partially swallowed esophageal pressure balloon) during the time required for one breath. Dynamic compliance is distinctively different from the static lung compliance (C_L) defined earlier in this chapter as the change in lung volume (ΔV) per unit pressure change (ΔP) (see Figure 2–6). In short, static compliance is determined during a period of no gas flow; whereas dynamic compliance is measured during a period of gas flow.

In the healthy lung, the dynamic compliance is about equal to static compliance at all breathing frequencies (the ratio of dynamic compliance to static compliance is 1 : 1) (Figure 2–26, page 86).

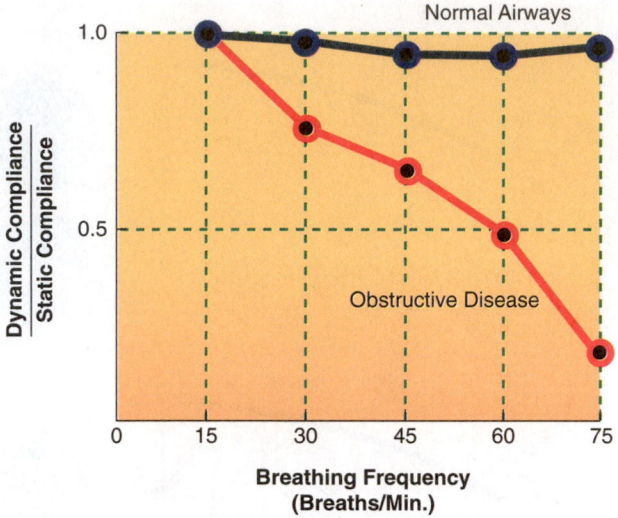

Figure 2–26. *Dynamic compliance/static compliance ratio at different breathing frequencies. In normal subjects there is essentially no ratio change. In individuals with obstructive disorders, however, the ratio decreases dramatically as the respiratory rate increases.*

In patients with partially obstructed airways, however, the ratio of dynamic compliance to static compliance falls significantly as the breathing frequency rises (see Figure 2–26). In other words, the alveoli distal to the obstruction do not have enough time to fill to their potential filling capacity as the breathing frequency increases. The compliance of such alveoli is said to be frequency dependent.

VENTILATORY PATTERNS

THE NORMAL VENTILATORY PATTERN

The ventilatory pattern consists of (1) the tidal volume (V_T), (2) the ventilatory rate, and (3) the time relationship between inhalation and exhalation (I : E ratio).

Tidal volume is defined as the volume of air that normally moves into and out of the lungs in one quiet breath. Normally, V_T is about 7 to 9 ml/kg (3 to 4 ml/lb) of ideal body weight. The normal adult ventilatory rate is about 15 breaths per minute. The I : E ratio is usually about 1 : 2. That is, the time required to inhale a normal breath is about one-half the time required to exhale the same breath.

Technically, though, the time required to inhale and exhale while at rest is about equal (a 1 : 1 ratio) in terms of "true" gas flow. The reason exhalation is considered twice as long as inhalation in the I : E ratio is that the ratio includes the normal pause, during which there is no gas flow, that typically occurs at end-expiration as part of the exhalation phase (Figure 2–27).

This normal pause that occurs at end-exhalation is usually about equal, in terms of time, to either the inspiratory or expiratory phase. Thus, when an indi-

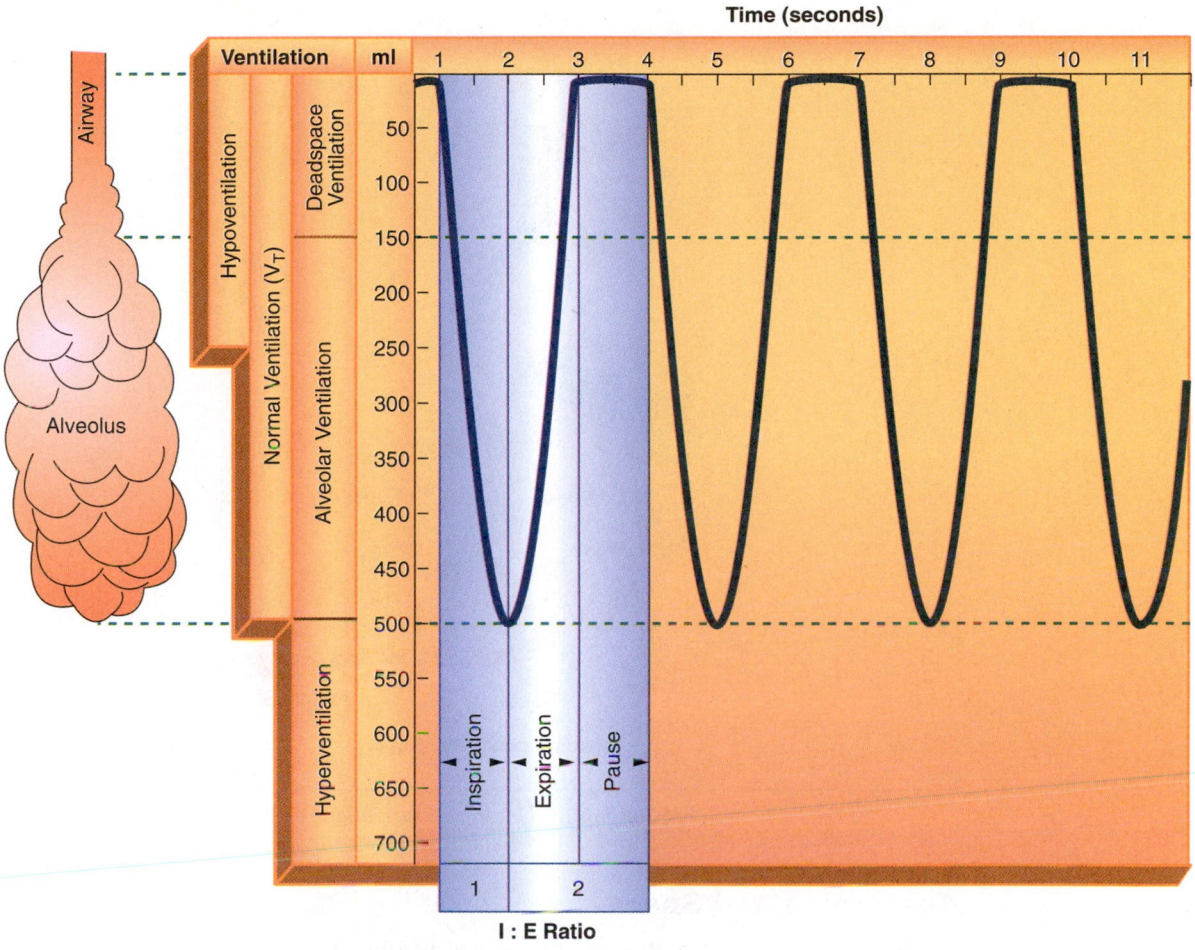

Figure 2–27. *Normal, spontaneous breathing (eupnea). The I : E ratio is typically 1 : 2.*

vidual is at rest, the time required for a normal ventilatory cycle consists of approximately three equal phases: (1) the inspiratory phase, (2) the expiratory phase, and (3) the pause phase at end-expiration (see Figure 2–27).

ALVEOLAR VENTILATION VERSUS DEADSPACE VENTILATION

Only the inspired air that reaches the alveoli is physiologically effective in terms of gas exchange. This portion of the inspired gas is referred to as alveolar ventilation. The volume of inspired air that does not reach the alveoli is not physiologically effective. This portion of gas is referred to as deadspace ventilation (Figure 2–28, page 88). There are three types of dead space: (1) anatomic dead space, (2) alveolar dead space, and (3) physiologic dead space.

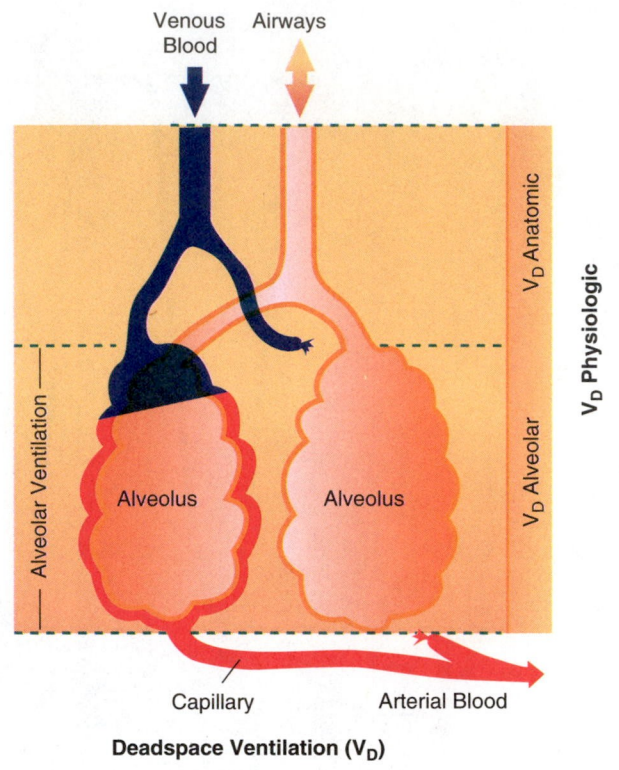

Deadspace Ventilation (V$_D$)

Figure 2–28. *Deadspace ventilation (V$_D$).*

Anatomic Dead Space

Anatomic dead space is the volume of gas in the conducting airways: the nose, mouth, pharynx, larynx, and lower airways down to, but not including, the respiratory bronchioles. The volume of anatomic dead space is approximately equal to 1 ml/lb (2.2 ml/kg) of normal body weight. Thus, if an individual weighs 150 pounds, approximately 150 ml of inspired gas would be anatomic dead space gas (or physiologically ineffective).

Because of the anatomic dead space, moreover, the gas that does enter the alveoli during each inspiration (alveolar ventilation) is actually a combination of (1) anatomic deadspace gas (non-fresh gas) and (2) gas from the atmosphere (fresh gas). To visualize this, consider the inspiration and expiration of 450 ml (V$_T$) in an individual with an anatomic dead space of 150 ml (Figure 2–29).

Inspiration. As shown in Figure 2–29A, 150 ml of gas fill the anatomic dead space at pre-inspiration. This gas was the last 150 ml of gas to leave the alveoli during the previous exhalation. Thus, as shown in Figure 2–29B, the first 150 ml of gas to enter the alveoli during inspiration are from the anatomic dead space (non-fresh gas). The next 300 ml of gas to enter the alveoli are from the atmosphere (fresh gas). The last 150 ml of fresh gas inhaled fill the anatomic dead space (see Figure 2–29B).

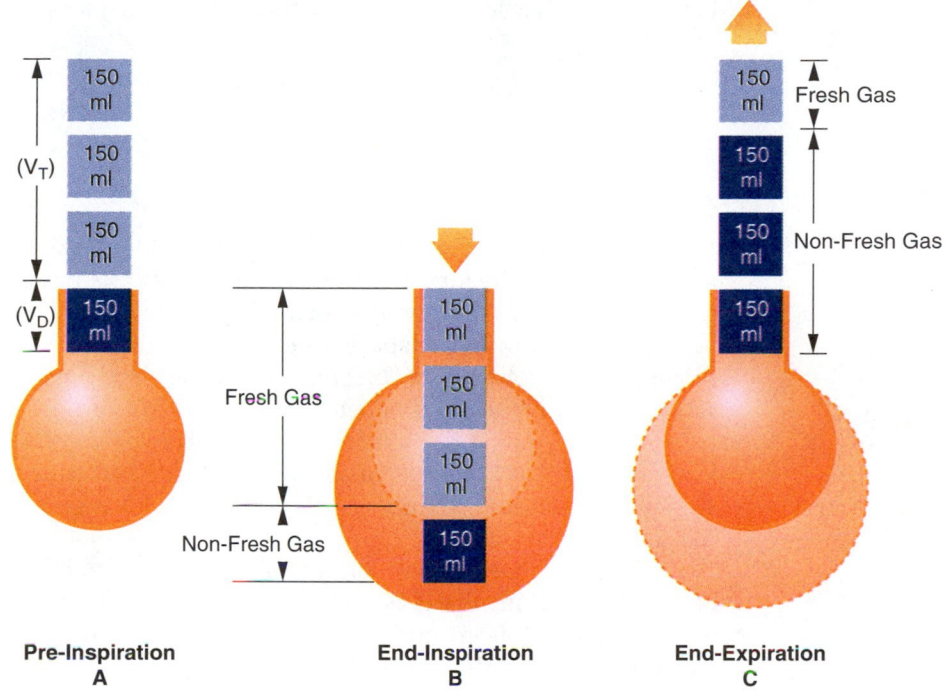

Figure 2–29. *Alveolar ventilation versus deadspace ventilation during one ventilatory cycle. (See text for explanation.)*

Thus, of the 450 ml of gas that enter the alveoli, 150 ml come from the conducting airways (non-fresh gas) and 300 ml come from the atmosphere (fresh gas).

Expiration. As shown in Figure 2–29C, 450 ml of gas are forced out of the alveoli during expiration. The first 150 ml of gas exhaled are from the anatomic dead space. This gas was the last 150 ml that entered the conducting airways during the previous inspiration (see Figure 2–29B). The next 300 ml of gas exhaled come from the alveoli. The last 150 ml of gas to leave the alveoli fill the anatomic dead space. During the next inspiration, the last 150 ml of gas exhaled from the alveoli will, again, reenter the alveoli, thus diluting the oxygen concentration of any atmospheric gas that enters the alveoli (see Figure 2–29A).

Therefore minute alveolar ventilation (V_A) is equal to the tidal volume (V_T) minus the deadspace ventilation (V_D) multiplied by the breaths per minute (frequency):

$$\dot{V}_A = (V_T - V_D) \times \text{breaths/min}$$

For example, if:

$$V_T = 450 \text{ ml}$$

$$V_D = 150 \text{ ml}$$

Breaths/min = 12

then minute alveolar ventilation would be computed as follows:

$$\dot{V}_A = V_T - V_D \times breaths/min$$

$$= 450 \text{ ml} - 150 \text{ ml} \times 12$$

$$= 300 \times 12$$

$$= 3600 \text{ ml}$$

Finally, an individual's breathing pattern (depth and rate of breathing) can profoundly alter the total alveolar ventilation. For example, Table 2–2 shows three different subjects, each having a total minute ventilation (MV) of 6000 ml and each having an anatomic deadspace volume of 150 ml. Each subject, however, has a different tidal volume and breathing frequency. Subject A has a tidal volume of 150 ml and a breathing frequency of 40 breaths/min. Even though gas rapidly moves in and out of the lungs, the actual alveolar ventilation is zero. Subject A is merely moving 150 ml of gas in and out of the anatomic dead space at a rate of 40 times per minute. Clinically, this subject would become unconscious in a few minutes.

Subject B has a tidal volume of 500 ml and a breathing frequency of 12 breaths/min. This subject has an alveolar ventilation of 4200 ml. Subject C has a tidal volume of 1000 ml and a frequency of 6 breaths/min. This subject has an alveolar ventilation of 5100 ml.

The important deduction to be drawn from Table 2–2 is that *an increased depth of breathing is far more effective than an equivalent increase in breathing rate in increasing an individual's total alveolar ventilation.* Or, conversely, a decreased depth of breathing can lead to a significant and, perhaps, a critical reduction of alveolar ventilation. This is because the anatomic deadspace volume represents a fixed volume (normally about one-third), and the fixed volume will make up a larger portion of a decreasing tidal volume. This fraction increases as the tidal volume decreases until, as demonstrated by subject A, it represents the entire tidal volume. On the other hand, any increase in the tidal volume beyond the anatomic dead space goes entirely toward increasing alveolar ventilation.

TABLE 2–2. **Effect of Breathing Depth and Frequency on Alveolar Ventilation**

SUBJECT	BREATHING DEPTH (V_T) (ml)	BREATHING FREQUENCY (BREATHS/MIN)	TOTAL MV* (ml/MIN)	V_D† (ml/MIN)	V_A‡ (ml/MIN)
A	150	40	6000	$150 \times 40 = 6000$	0
B	500	12	6000	$150 \times 12 = 1800$	4200
C	1000	6	6000	$150 \times 6 = 900$	5100

*Total pulmonary ventilation, or minute ventilation (MV), is the product of breathing depth, or tidal volume (V_T), times breathing frequency, or breaths per minute.
†Total deadspace ventilation (V_D) is the product of anatomic deadspace volume (150 ml in each subject) times breathing frequency.
‡V_A = alveolar ventilation.

Alveolar Dead Space

Alveolar dead space occurs when an alveolus is ventilated but not perfused with pulmonary blood. Thus, the air that enters the alveolus is not physiologically effective in terms of gas exchange, since there is no pulmonary capillary blood flow. The amount of alveolar dead space is unpredictable.

Physiologic Dead Space

Physiologic dead space is the sum of the anatomic dead space and alveolar dead space. Since neither of these two forms of dead space is physiologically effective in terms of gas exchange, the two forms are combined and are referred to as physiologic dead space.

HOW NORMAL INTRAPLEURAL PRESSURE DIFFERENCES CAUSE REGIONAL DIFFERENCES IN NORMAL LUNG VENTILATION

As discussed earlier, the diaphragm moves air in and out of the lungs by changing the intrapleural and intra-alveolar pressures. Ordinarily, the intrapleural pressure is always below atmospheric pressure during both inspiration and expiration (see Figure 2–5).

The intrapleural pressure, however, is not evenly distributed within the thorax. In the normal individual in the upright position, there is a natural intrapleural pressure gradient from the upper lung region to the lower. The negative intrapleural pressure at the apex of the lung is normally greater (from −7 to −10 cm H_2O pressure) than at the base (from −2 to −3 cm H_2O pressure). This gradient is gravity dependent and is thought to be due to the normal weight distribution of the lungs above and below the hilum. In other words, because the lung is suspended from the hilum, and because the lung base weighs more than the apex (primarily due to the increased blood flow in the lung base), the lung base requires more pressure for support than the lung apex. This causes the negative intrapleural pressure around the lung base to be less.

Because of the greater negative intrapleural pressure in the upper lung regions, the alveoli in those regions are expanded more than the alveoli in the lower regions. In fact, many of the alveoli in the upper lung regions may be close to, or at, their total filling capacity. This means, therefore, that the compliance of the alveoli in the upper lung regions is normally less than the compliance of the alveoli in the lower lung regions in the normal person in the upright position. As a result, during inspiration the alveoli in the upper lung regions are unable to accommodate as much gas as the alveoli in the lower lung regions. Thus, in the normal individual in the upright position, ventilation is usually much greater and more effective in the lower lung regions (Figure 2–30, page 92).

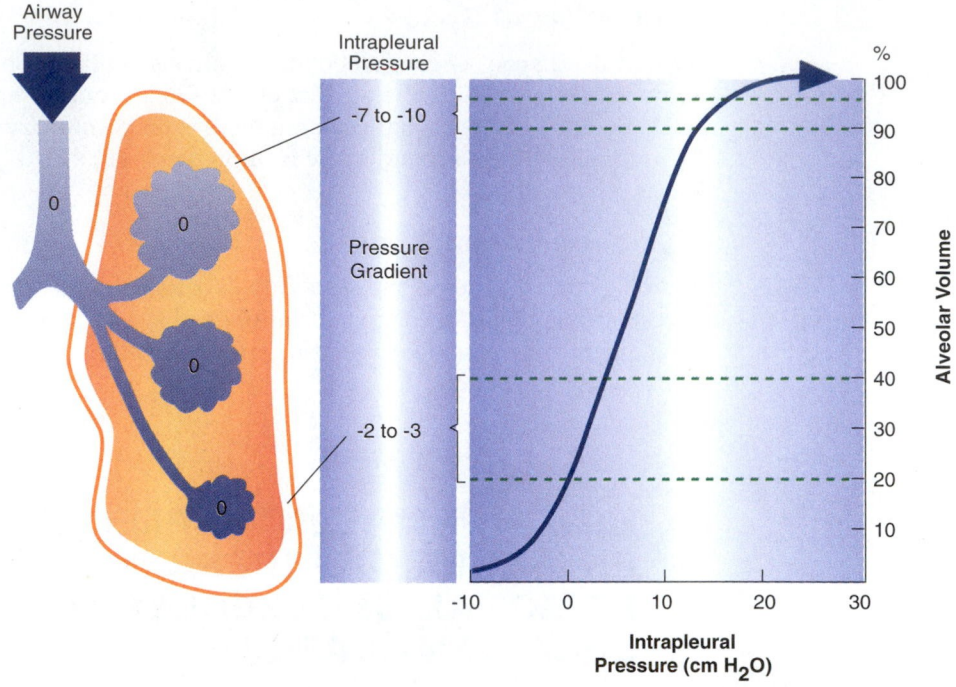

Figure 2–30. *Intrapleural pressure gradient in the upright position. The negative intrapleural pressure is normally greater in the upper lung regions as compared to the lower lung regions. Because of this, the alveoli in the upper lung regions expand more than the alveoli in the lower lung regions. This condition causes alveolar compliance to be lower in the upper lung regions, and ventilation to be greater in the lower lung regions.*

THE EFFECT OF AIRWAY RESISTANCE AND LUNG COMPLIANCE ON VENTILATORY PATTERNS

As already mentioned, the respiratory rate and tidal volume presented by an individual is known as the *ventilatory pattern*. The normal ventilatory pattern is a respiratory rate of about 15 breaths per minute and a tidal volume of about 500 ml. Although the precise mechanism is not clear, it is well documented that these ventilatory patterns frequently develop in response to changes in lung compliance and airway resistance.

When lung compliance decreases, the patient's ventilatory rate generally increases while, at the same time, the tidal volume decreases. When airway resistance increases, the patient's ventilatory frequency usually decreases while, at the same time, the tidal volume increases (Figure 2–31).

The ventilatory pattern adopted by the patient is thought to be based on minimum work requirements rather than ventilatory efficiency. In physics, work is defined as the force applied multiplied by the distance moved (work = force × dis-

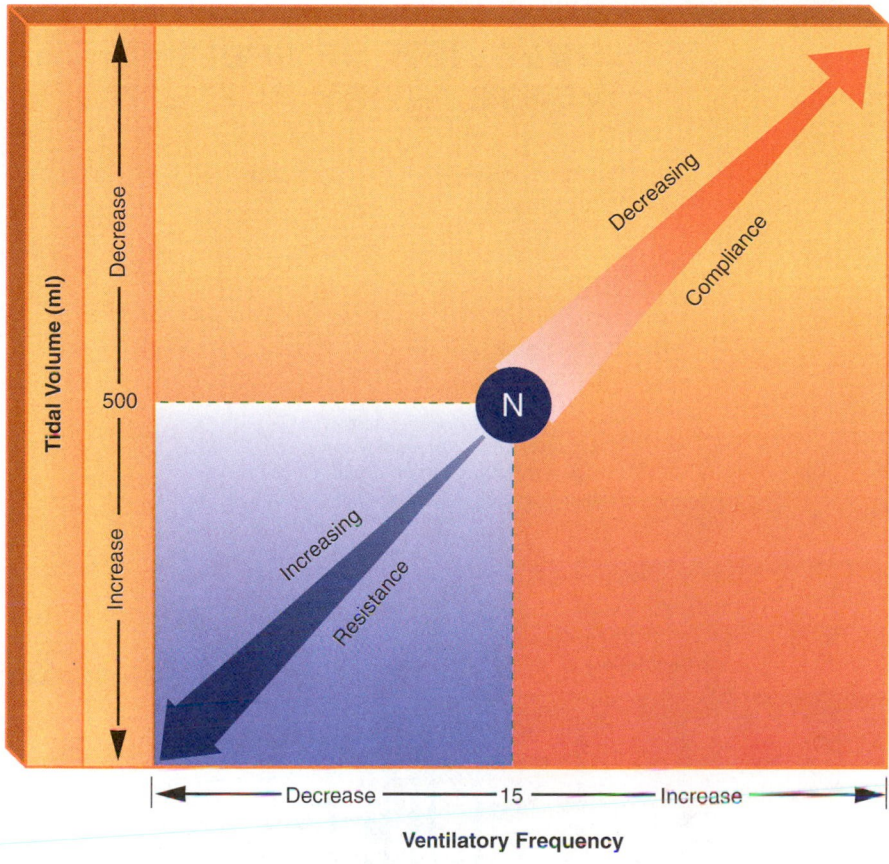

Figure 2–31. *The effects of increased airway resistance and decreased lung compliance on ventilatory frequency and tidal volume.*

tance). In respiratory physiology, the changes in transpulmonary pressure (force) multiplied by the change in lung volume (distance) may be used to quantitate the amount of work required to breathe (work = pressure × volume). Normally, about 5 percent of an individual's total energy output goes to the work of breathing.

Thus, because the patient may adopt a ventilatory pattern based on the **expenditure of energy** rather than the **efficiency of ventilation**, it cannot be assumed that the ventilatory pattern acquired by the patient in response to a certain respiratory disorder is the most efficient in terms of physiologic gas exchange. Such ventilatory patterns are usually seen in the more severe pulmonary disorders that cause lung compliance to decrease or airway resistance to increase.

The patient's adopted ventilatory pattern is frequently not seen in the clinical setting because of secondary heart or lung problems. For example, a patient with chronic emphysema, who has adopted a decreased ventilatory rate and an increased tidal volume because of increased R_{aw}, may demonstrate an increased ventilatory rate and a decreased tidal volume in response to a lung infection or pneumonia that causes lung compliance to decrease.

OVERVIEW OF SPECIFIC VENTILATORY PATTERNS

The following are ventilatory patterns frequently seen by the respiratory care practitioner in the clinical setting.

Apnea

Complete absence of spontaneous ventilation. This causes the $P_{A_{O_2}}$* and Pa_{O_2}† to rapidly decrease and the $P_{A_{CO_2}}$‡ and Pa_{CO_2}§ to increase. Death will ensue in minutes.

---

*$P_{A_{O_2}}$ = alveolar oxygen tension
†Pa_{O_2} = arterial oxygen tension
‡$P_{A_{CO_2}}$ = alveolar carbon dioxide tension
§Pa_{CO_2} = arterial carbon dioxide tension

Figure 2–32. *Biot's breathing: Short episodes of rapid, uniformly deep inspirations, followed by 10 to 30 seconds of apnea.*

Eupnea

Normal, spontaneous breathing (see Figure 2–27).

Biot's Breathing

Short episodes of rapid, uniformly deep inspirations, followed by 10 to 30 seconds of apnea (Figure 2–32). This pattern was first described in patients suffering from meningitis.

Hyperpnea

Increased depth (volume) of breathing with or without an increased frequency (Figure 2–33).

Figure 2–33. *Hyperpnea: Increased depth of breathing.*

Hyperventilation

Increased alveolar ventilation (produced by any ventilatory pattern that causes an increase in either the ventilatory rate or the depth of breathing) that causes the $P_{A_{CO_2}}$ and, therefore, the Pa_{CO_2} to decrease (Figure 2–34).

Hypoventilation

Decreased alveolar ventilation (produced by any ventilatory pattern that causes a decrease in either the ventilatory rate or the depth of breathing) that causes the $P_{A_{CO_2}}$ and, therefore, the Pa_{CO_2} to increase (Figure 2–35).

Tachypnea

A rapid rate of breathing.

Figure 2–34. *Hyperventilation: Increased rate (A) or depth (B), or some combination of both, of breathing that causes the $P_{A_{CO_2}}$ and, therefore, the Pa_{CO_2} to decrease.*

Figure 2–35.   *Hypoventilation: Decreased rate (A) or depth (B), or some combination of both, of breathing that causes the* PA_{CO_2}*, therefore, the* Pa_{CO_2} *to increase.*

Cheyne-Stokes Breathing

10 to 30 seconds of apnea, followed by a gradual increase in the volume and frequency of breathing, followed by a gradual decrease in the volume of breathing until another period of apnea occurs (Figure 2–36, page 98). As the depth of breathing increases, the PA_{O_2} and Pa_{O_2} rise and the PA_{CO_2} and Pa_{CO_2} fall. As the depth of breathing decreases, the PA_{O_2} and Pa_{O_2} fall and the PA_{CO_2} and Pa_{CO_2} rise. Cheyne-Stokes breathing is associated with cerebral disorders.

Kussmaul Breathing

Both an increased depth (hyperpnea) and rate of breathing (Figure 2–37, page 99). This ventilatory pattern causes the PA_{CO_2} and Pa_{CO_2} to decline and the PA_{O_2} and Pa_{O_2} to increase. Kussmaul breathing is commonly associated with diabetic acidosis (ketoacidosis).

Figure 2–36.   *Cheyne-Stokes breathing: A gradual increase and decrease in the volume and rate of breathing, followed by 10 to 30 seconds of apnea.*

Orthopnea

A condition in which an individual is able to breathe most comfortably only in the upright position.

Dyspnea

Difficulty in breathing, of which the individual is aware.

Time (seconds)

Figure 2–37. *Kussmaul breathing: Increased rate and depth of breathing. This breathing pattern causes the* $P_{A_{CO_2}}$ *and* Pa_{CO_2} *to decrease and* $P_{A_{O_2}}$ *and* Pa_{O_2} *to increase.*

CLINICAL APPLICATION 1

This 14-year-old female with a long history of asthma presented in the emergency room in moderate to severe respiratory distress. She appeared very frightened and tears were running down her face. She was sitting perched forward with her arms braced in a tripodlike position on the side of a gurney, hands clutching the edge of the gurney. She was using her accessory muscles of inspiration. When asked about her condition, she stated, "I can't get enough air." She could only speak two or three words at a time, between each breath.

The patient's skin appeared pale and bluish. She had a frequent and strong cough, productive of large amounts of thick, white secretions. Her vital signs were: blood pressure—

(continues)

151/93, heart rate—106 beats/min and strong, and respiratory rate—32 breaths/min. Wheezes were heard over both lung fields. The chest x-ray showed that her lungs were hyperinflated and that her diaphragm was depressed. Her peripheral oxygen saturation level (Sp_{O_2}), measured by pulse oximetry over the skin of her index finger, was 89 percent (normal is 97 percent).

The respiratory therapist working in the emergency room started the patient on oxygen via a 6-liter (6 L/min) nasal cannula, and on a bronchodilator continuously, via a hand-held aerosol. The therapist also remained at the patient's bedside to monitor the patient's response to treatment, and to encourage the patient to take slow, deep inspirations.

Forty-five minutes later, the patient had substantially improved. She was sitting up in bed and no longer appeared to be in respiratory distress. She could speak in longer sentences without getting short of breath. Her skin color was normal. Her vital signs were: blood pressure—126/83, heart rate—87 beats/min, and respiratory rate—14 breaths/min.

When instructed to cough, she generated a strong, nonproductive cough. Although wheezes could still be heard over the patient's lungs, they were not as severe as they were on admission. A second chest x-ray showed that her lungs were normal and her diaphragm was no longer depressed. Her Sp_{O_2} was 94 percent.

DISCUSSION

This case illustrates (1) an acute decreased lung compliance condition, (2) how *Poiseuille's law* can be used to demonstrate the effects of bronchial constriction and excessive airway secretions on bronchial gas flow and the work of breathing, (3) the effects of an increased *airway resistance* (R_{aw}) on *time constants,* and (4) the *frequency-dependent* effects of a decreased ventilatory rate on the ventilation of alveoli.

As the severity of the tracheobronchial tree constriction progressively increased, the patient's ability to exhale fully declined. This pathophysiologic process caused the patient's lungs to hyperinflate (but not with fresh air). As a result of the hyperinflation, the patient's work of breathing increased, because her lungs were functioning at the very top of their volume-pressure curve—the flat portion of the curve (see Figure 2–6). As the volume-pressure curve shows, lung compliance is very low on the upper, flat portion of the volume-pressure curve. Because of this, the patient was working extremely hard to breathe (i.e., generating large intrapleural pressure changes), with little or no change in her alveolar ventilation (volume), as shown in Figure 2–6.

In addition, as Poiseuille's law demonstrates, the tracheobronchial tree constriction and excessive airway secretions, both caused by the asthma attack, can have a tremendous impact on gas flow and on the patient's work of breathing. Poiseuille's law shows that gas flow is *directly* related to the fourth power of the radius (r^4) of the tracheobronchial tree, and pressure (e.g., intrapleural pressure changes) is *indirectly* related to the fourth power of the radius of the airways. Thus, if the patient's bronchial constriction and bronchial secretions decreased the radius of the airways by one-half, the flow of gas would decrease to 1/16 of the original flow (see Figure 2–20). Similarly, in order for the patient to maintain the same flow rate, she would have to increase her work of breathing to 16 times her original level (see Figure 2–22).

Airway resistance (R_{aw}) can be defined as the intrapleural pressure difference (ΔP) generated by the patient to move a volume of gas divided by the flow rate ($\dot{V}$). Again, according to Poiseuille's law, it can be seen that as the airways narrow, intrapleural pressure will increase significantly while, at the same time, gas flow through the airways will decrease. Since $R_{aw} = \Delta P \div \dot{V}$, it is easy to see mathematically how quickly airway resistance can increase during an asthmatic episode.

Finally, as the airway resistance (R_{aw}) increased, the alveoli distal to the bronchial constriction required a longer time to inflate. These alveoli are said to have a long *time constant* (see Figure 2–25). A product of the time constants is the measurement called *dynamic compliance,* which is the change in volume of the lungs divided by the change in the transpulmonary pressure during the time required for one breath (i.e., during a period of gas flow).

In the healthy lung, the dynamic compliance is approximately equal to static compliance at all breathing frequencies. In the patient with partially obstructed airways, however, the ratio of dynamic compliance to static compliance decreases as the respiratory rate increases. The alveoli distal to the airway obstruction do not have enough time to fully inflate as the breathing frequency rises. The compliance of these alveoli is said to be *frequency dependent.*

This is why it was important for the respiratory therapist to remain at the bedside and encourage the patient to take slow, deep breaths.

Because the patient was having trouble inhaling a normal volume of gas and because her oxygen saturation level (Sp_{O_2}) was below normal, oxygen therapy was clearly indicated. The continuous bronchodilator therapy was also indicated and worked to offset the effects of airway constriction (as described by Poiseuille's law), increased airway resistance, air trapping, and hyperinflation. As the lung hyperinflation progressively declined, lung compliance steadily increased, or returned to normal (i.e., returned back to the steep portion of the volume-pressure curve). The patient continued to improve and was discharged from the hospital the next afternoon.

CLINICAL APPLICATION

This 22-year-old white male motorcycle accident victim was brought to the emergency room with several facial, neck, and shoulder abrasions and lacerations, and multiple broken ribs. During each breath, the patient's right anterior chest moved inward during inspiration and outward during exhalation (clinically this is called a *flail chest*). The patient was alert, in pain, and stated, "I can't breathe. Am I going to die?"

The patient's skin was pale and blue. His vital signs were: blood pressure—166/93, heart rate—135 beats/min, and respiratory rate—26 breaths/min. and shallow. While on a simple oxygen mask, the patient's peripheral oxygen saturation level (Sp_{O_2}), measured over the skin of his index finger, was 79 percent (normal is 97

percent). His chest x-ray showed that the third, fourth, fifth, sixth, and seventh ribs were each broken in two or three places on the right anterior chest. The chest x-ray also revealed that his right lung was partially collapsed.

The patient was immediately transferred to the intensive care unit (ICU), sedated, intubated, and placed on a mechanical ventilator. The mechanical ventilator was set at a ventilatory rate of 12 breaths per minute, an oxygen concentration of 0.5, and a positive end-expiratory pressure (PEEP) of +5 cm H_2O.* No spontaneous breaths were present between the mandatory mechanical breaths.

Four hours later, the patient appeared comfortable and his skin color was normal. The ven-
(continues)

*At the end of a normal spontaneous expiration, the pressure in the alveoli is equal to the barometric pressure. A +5 cm H_2O of PEEP means that at the end of each exhalation, the patient's alveoli still had a positive pressure of 5 cm H_2O above atmospheric pressure. Therapeutically, this helps to re-expand collapsed alveoli or to prevent the collapse of alveoli.

tilator was set at a rate of 12 breaths per minute, an inspired oxygen concentration ($F_{I_{O_2}}$) of 0.3, and a PEEP of +5 cm H_2O. No spontaneous breaths were generated between each mechanical ventilation. During each mechanical breath, both the right and left side of the patient's chest expanded symmetrically. His blood pressure was 127/83 and his heart rate was 76 beats per minute. A second chest x-ray revealed that his right lung had re-expanded. His peripheral oxygen saturation level (Sp_{O_2}) was 97 percent.

DISCUSSION

This case illustrates (1) the effects on *transthoracic pressure* when the thorax is unstable, (2) how the excursions of the diaphragm affect the intrapleural pressure, (3) acute decreased lung compliance, and (4) the therapeutic effects of positive pressure ventilation in flail chest cases.

Under normal conditions, each time an individual inhales, the diaphragm moves downward and causes the intrapleural pressure and alveolar pressure to decrease (see Figure 2–5). In this case, however, the patient's ribs were broken on the right side and caved in during each inspiration when the intrapleural and alveolar pressure decreased. This caused the right lung to partially collapse—an acute decreased lung compliance condition (see Figure 2–6).

This pathophysiologic process was corrected when the patient was ventilated with positive pressure. The patient no longer had to generate negative pressure to inhale. During each positive pressure breath, the chest wall expanded evenly and returned to normal resting level at the end of each expiration. This process allowed the ribs to heal. After ten days, the patient was weaned from the ventilator; he was discharged three days later.

REVIEW QUESTIONS

1. The average compliance of the lungs and chest wall combined is
   a. 0.1 L/cm H_2O
   b. 0.2 L/cm H_2O
   c. 0.3 L/cm H_2O
   d. 0.4 L/cm H_2O
   e. 0.5 L/cm H_2O
2. Normally, the airway resistance in the tracheobronchial tree is about
   a. 0.5–1.0 cm H_2O/L/sec
   b. 1.0–2.0 cm H_2O/L/sec
   c. 2.0–3.0 cm H_2O/L/sec
   d. 3.0–4.0 cm H_2O/L/sec
   e. 4.0–5.0 cm H_2O/L/sec
3. In the normal individual in the upright position
   I. the negative intrapleural pressure is greater (i.e., more negative) in the upper lung regions
   II. the alveoli in the lower lung regions are larger than the alveoli in the upper lung regions
   III. ventilation is more effective in the lower lung regions

IV. the intrapleural pressure is always below atmospheric pressure during a normal ventilatory cycle
   a. I and II only
   b. II and III only
   c. II, III, and IV only
   d. I, III, and IV only
   e. I, II, III and IV

4. When lung compliance decreases, the patient commonly has
   I. an increased ventilatory rate
   II. a decreased tidal volume
   III. an increased tidal volume
   IV. a decreased ventilatory rate
     a. I only
     b. II only
     c. III only
     d. I and II only
     e. II and IV only

5. When arranged for flow ($\dot{V}$), Poiseuille's law states that $\dot{V}$ is
   I. inversely proportional to r^4
   II. directly proportional to P
   III. inversely proportional to η
   IV. directly proportional to l
     a. I only
     b. II only
     c. II and III only
     d. III and IV only
     e. II, III, and IV only

6. During a normal exhalation, the
   I. intra-alveolar pressure is greater than the atmospheric pressure
   II. intrapleural pressure is less than the atmospheric pressure
   III. intra-alveolar pressure is in equilibrium with the atmospheric pressure
   IV. intrapleural pressure progressively decreases
     a. I only
     b. IV only
     c. I and II only
     d. II and IV only
     e. II and III only

7. At rest, the normal intrapleural pressure change during quiet breathing is about
   a. 0–2 mm Hg
   b. 2–4 mm Hg
   c. 4–6 mm Hg
   d. 6–8 mm Hg
   e. 8–10 mm Hg

8. Normally, an individual's tidal volume is about
   a. 1–2 ml/lb
   b. 3–4 ml/lb

    c. 5–6 ml/lb

    d. 7–8 ml/lb

    e. 9–10 ml/lb

9. A rapid and shallow ventilatory pattern is called
   a. Hyperpnea
   b. Apnea
   c. Alveolar hyperventilation
   d. Tachypnea
   e. Kussmaul breathing

10. Assuming that pressure remains constant, if the radius of a bronchial airway through which gas flows at a rate of 400 L/min is reduced to one-half of its original size, the flow through the bronchial airway would change to
    a. 10 L/min
    b. 25 L/min
    c. 100 L/min
    d. 200 L/min
    e. 300 L/min

11. The difference between the alveolar pressure and the pleural pressure is called the
    a. transpulmonary pressure
    b. transthoracic pressure
    c. driving pressure
    d. transairway pressure
    e. transmural pressure

12. According to Laplace's law, if a bubble with a radius of 4 cm and a distending pressure of 10 cm H_2O is reduced to a radius of 2 cm, the new distending pressure of the bubble will be
    a. 5 cm H_2O
    b. 10 cm H_2O
    c. 15 cm H_2O
    d. 20 cm H_2O
    e. 25 cm H_2O

13. If alveolar Unit A has one-half the compliance of alveolar Unit B, the
    I. time constant of Unit A is essentially the same as Unit B
    II. volume in Unit B is two times greater than Unit A
    III. time constant of Unit B is twice as long as Unit A
    IV. volume in Unit B is essentially the same as the volume of Unit A
        a. I only
        b. III only
        c. IV only
        d. II and III only
        e. III and IV only

14. If a patient weighs 175 pounds and has a tidal volume of 550 ml and a respiratory rate of 17 breaths per minute, what is the patient's minute alveolar ventilation?

    Answer: _____

15. Lung compliance study

    Part I: If a patient generates a negative intrapleural pressure change of -8 cm H_2O during inspiration, and the lungs accept a new volume of 630 ml, what is the compliance of the lungs?

    Answer: _____

    Part II: If the same patient, 6 hours later, generates an intrapleural pressure of -12 cm H_2O during inspiration, and the lungs accept a new volume of 850 ml, what is the compliance of the lungs?

    Answer: _____

    Part III: In comparing Part II to Part I, the patient's lung compliance is
    a. increasing
    b. decreasing

16. If a patient produces a flow rate of 5 L/second during inspiration by generating a transairway pressure of 20 cm H_2O, what is the patient's R_{aw}?
    a. 1 cm H_2O/L/sec
    b. 2 cm H_2O/L/sec
    c. 3 cm H_2O/L/sec
    d. 4 cm H_2O/L/sec
    e. 5 cm H_2O/L/sec

17. As R_{aw} increases, the patient commonly manifests:
    I. a decreased ventilatory rate
    II. an increased tidal volume
    III. a decreased tidal volume
    IV. an increased ventilatory rate
       a. I only
       b. II only
       c. IV only
       d. III and IV only
       e. I and II only

18. If the radius of a bronchial airway, which has a driving pressure of 2 mm Hg, is reduced by 16% of its original size, what will be the new driving pressure required to maintain the same gas flow through the bronchial airway?
    a. 4 mm Hg
    b. 8 mm Hg
    c. 12 mm Hg
    d. 16 mm Hg
    e. 20 mm Hg

19. In the healthy lung, when the alveolus decreases in size during a normal exhalation, the:
    I. Surface tension decreases
    II. Surfactant to alveolar surface area increases
    III. Surface tension increases

IV. Surfactant to alveolar surface area decreases
    a. I only
    b. III only
    c. IV only
    d. I and II only
    e. III and IV only

20. At end-expiration, P_{ta} is:
    a. 0 mm Hg
    b. 2 mm Hg
    c. 4 mm Hg
    d. 6 mm Hg
    e. 8 mm Hg

CHAPTER THREE

THE DIFFUSION OF PULMONARY GASES

OBJECTIVES

By the end of this chapter, the student should be able to:

1. Define *diffusion*.
2. State the following gas laws:
   —Boyle's law
   —Charles' law
   —Gay-Lussac's law
   —Dalton's law
3. Identify the percentage and partial pressure of the gases that compose the *barometric pressure:*
   —Nitrogen
   —Oxygen
   —Argon
   —Carbon dioxide
4. Identify the partial pressure of the gases in the *air, alveoli,* and *blood:*
   —Oxygen (P_{O_2})
   —Carbon dioxide (P_{CO_2})
   —Nitrogen (P_{N_2})
   —Water (P_{H_2O})
5. Calculate the *ideal alveolar gas equation.*
6. Name the nine major structures of the *alveolar-capillary membrane* that a gas molecule must diffuse through.
7. Describe how oxygen and carbon dioxide normally diffuse across the alveolar-capillary membrane.
8. Explain how *Fick's law* relates to gas diffusion.
9. Describe how the following relate to the *diffusion constants* in Fick's law:
   —Henry's law
   —Graham's law
10. Describe how Fick's law can be applied to certain clinical conditions.
11. Define the meaning of *perfusion limited*, and explain how it relates to a gas like nitrous oxide.
12. Define the meaning of *diffusion limited*, and explain how it relates to a gas like carbon monoxide.
13. Describe how oxygen can be classified as perfusion or diffusion limited.
14. Complete the review questions at the end of this chapter.

As discussed in Chapter Two, the mass movement of air in and out of the lungs occurs by virtue of transpulmonary and transairway pressure changes that are generated by the action of the diaphragm. This mechanism carries oxygen from the atmosphere to the alveoli and carbon dioxide from the alveoli to the external environment. The process of ventilation, however, merely moves gases from one point to another (e.g., from the atmosphere to the alveoli); it does not move gas molecules across the alveolar-capillary membrane. This process occurs by means of **passive diffusion**.

Diffusion is defined as the movement of gas molecules from an area of relatively high concentration of gas to one of low concentration. Different gases each move according to their own individual partial pressure gradients. Diffusion continues until all the gases in the two areas are in equilibrium.

To aid in the understanding of how gases transfer (diffuse) across the alveolar-capillary membrane, a brief review of the physical principles governing the behavior of gases (gas laws) and the partial pressures of the atmospheric gases is appropriate.

GAS LAWS

IDEAL GAS LAW

The behavior of gases surrounding the earth is described in a mathematical relationship known as the *ideal gas law:*

$$PV = nRT$$

where P is pressure, V is volume, T is temperature on the Kelvin (K) scale,* n is the number of moles of gas molecules present, and R is the gas constant, which has a fixed value of 0.0821.

Assuming that the amount of gas remains constant (i.e., n remains unchanged), the ideal gas law can be used to predict specific changes of temperature, pressure, and volume under different conditions. In other words, if nR remains constant, then:

$$\frac{P_1 \times V_1}{T_1} = \frac{P_2 \times V_2}{T_2}$$

Thus, when any one of the above variables (P, V, T) is held constant while one of the others changes in value, the new value of the third variable can be calculated. The following laws illustrate the interrelationship of P, V, and T.

---

*Whenever the temperature of gases is involved in calculations, all temperatures must be converted to the Kelvin scale. Fahrenheit (°F) is converted first to Celsius (°C) as follows: 5 ÷ 9 (F − 32). Celsius is converted to Kelvin (K) by adding 273 to the Celsius temperature (e.g., 37°C + 273 = 310 K).

BOYLE'S LAW

Boyle's law ($P_1 \times V_1 = P_2 \times V_2$) states that if temperature remains constant, pressure will vary inversely to volume. For example, if an air-tight container, which has a volume of 200 ml and a pressure of 10 cm H_2O, has its volume reduced 50 percent (100 ml), the new pressure in the container can be computed as follows:

$$P_2 = \frac{P_1 \times V_1}{V_2}$$

$$= \frac{10 \text{ cm } H_2O \times 200 \text{ ml}}{100 \text{ ml}}$$

$$= 20 \text{ cm } H_2O$$

CHARLES' LAW

Charles' law ($V_1 \div T_1 = V_2 \div T_2$) states that if pressure remains constant, volume and temperature will vary directly. That is, if the temperature of the gas in a 3-liter balloon is increased from 250 K (Kelvin) to 300 K, the resulting volume of the balloon can be calculated as follows:

$$V_2 = \frac{V_1 \times T_2}{T_1}$$

$$= \frac{3 \text{ L} \times 300 \text{ K}}{250 \text{ K}}$$

$$= 3.6 \text{ L}$$

GAY-LUSSAC'S LAW

Gay-Lussac's law ($P_1 \div T_1 = P_2 \div T_2$) states that if the volume remains constant, pressure and temperature will vary directly. For instance, if the temperature of the gas in a closed container, having a pressure of 50 cm H_2O, is increased from 275 K to 375 K, the resulting pressure in the container can be calculated as follows:

$$P_2 = \frac{P_1 \times T_2}{T_1}$$

$$= \frac{50 \text{ cm } H_2O \times 375 \text{ K}}{275 \text{ K}}$$

$$= \frac{18750}{275}$$

$$= 68 \text{ cm } H_2O$$

DALTON'S LAW

Since the earth's atmosphere consists of several kinds of gases, it is essential to understand how these gases behave when they are mixed together. This is described by Dalton's law, which states that in a mixture of gases, the total pressure

Gas A
Pressure = 10

Gas B
Pressure = 5

Gas A+B
Pressure = 15

Figure 3–1. *Dalton's law.*

is equal to the sum of the partial pressures of each separate gas. In other words, if 10 molecules of gas are enclosed in a container, the total pressure may be expressed as 10; if 5 molecules of a different gas are enclosed in another container of equal volume, the total pressure may be expressed as 5; if both these gases are enclosed in a container of equal volume, the total pressure may be expressed as 15 (Figure 3–1).

It should be stressed that the pressure produced by a particular gas is completely unaffected by the presence of another gas. In short, each gas in a mixture will individually contribute to the total pressure created by the mixture of gas.

THE PARTIAL PRESSURES OF ATMOSPHERIC GASES

The atmospheric gases that surround the earth exert a force on the earth's surface called the *barometric pressure*. At sea level the barometric pressure is about 760 mm Hg and is a function of Dalton's law. The barometric pressure is primarily derived from the gases listed in Table 3–1.

The pressure between the external atmosphere and the alveoli is in equilibrium, except for slight changes (3–6 cm H_2O) that take place during inspiration or expiration. Within the circulatory system, however, the sum of the partial pressures is reduced, since the venous blood, which has a reduced P_{O_2} because of cellular metabolism, is not in equilibrium with the atmosphere.

It should also be noted that the barometric pressure decreases with an increase in altitude. For example, as one ascends a mountain, the barometric pressure steadily decreases. This is because the density of the different gas molecules surrounding the earth decreases with increased altitude. As the density of the various gases decreases, the partial pressure exerted by each gas also decreases. It should also be pointed out that, even though the barometric pressure varies with the altitude, the percent concentration of the atmospheric gases (see Table 3–1) is the same at both high and low elevations.

TABLE 3–1.   **Gases that Compose the Barometric Pressure**

GAS	% OF ATMOSPHERE	PARTIAL PRESSURE (mm Hg)
Nitrogen (N_2)	78.08	593
Oxygen (O_2)	20.95	159
Argon (Ar)	0.93	7
Carbon Dioxide (CO_2)	0.03	0.2

PARTIAL PRESSURES OF OXYGEN AND CARBON DIOXIDE

Table 3–2 shows the partial pressure of gases in dry air, alveolar air, arterial blood, and venous blood. Note that even though the total barometric pressure is the same in the atmosphere and in the alveoli, the partial pressure of oxygen in the atmosphere (159 mm Hg) is significantly higher than the partial pressure of oxygen in the alveoli (100 mm Hg). This is because alveolar oxygen must mix—or compete, in terms of partial pressures—with alveolar CO_2 pressure ($P_{A_{CO_2}} = 40$ mm Hg) and alveolar water vapor pressure ($P_{H_2O} = 47$ mm Hg), which are not nearly as high in the atmosphere. In short, by the time the oxygen molecules reach the alveoli, they are diluted by the addition of CO_2 and H_2O molecules. This must lead to a decrease in the partial pressure of oxygen in the alveoli ($P_{A_{O_2}}$).

WATER VAPOR PRESSURE

Depending on the surrounding temperature and pressure, water can exist as a liquid, gas, or solid. Water in the gaseous form is called *water vapor*, or *molecular water*. When water vapor is present in a volume of gas, it behaves according to the gas laws and exerts a partial pressure. Since alveolar gas is 100 percent humidified (saturated) at body temperature, the alveolar gas is assumed to have an *absolute*

TABLE 3–2.   **Partial Pressure (in mm Hg) of Gases in the Air, Alveoli, and Blood***

GASES	DRY AIR	ALVEOLAR GAS	ARTERIAL BLOOD	VENOUS BLOOD
P_{O_2}	159.0	100.0	95.0	40.0
P_{CO_2}	0.2	40.0	40.0	46.0
P_{H_2O} (water vapor)	0.0	47.0	47.0	47.0
P_{N_2} (and other gases in minute quantities)	600.8	573.0	573.0	573.0
Total	760.0	760.0	755.0	706.0

*The values shown are based upon standard pressure and temperature.

TABLE 3–3. **Relationship Between Temperature, Absolute Humidity, and Water Vapor Pressure***

TEMPERATURE	ABSOLUTE (MAXIMUM) HUMIDITY	WATER VAPOR PRESSURE
37°C	44.0 mg/L	47.0 mm Hg
35°C	39.6 mg/L	42.2 mm Hg
30°C	30.4 mg/L	31.8 mm Hg
27°C	25.8 mg/L	26.7 mm Hg
25°C	23.0 mg/L	23.8 mm Hg
20°C	17.3 mg/L	17.5 mm Hg

*At sea level (760 mm Hg).

humidity of 44 mg/L, and a *water vapor pressure* (P_{H_2O}) of 47 mm Hg—regardless of the humidity of the inspired air (Table 3–3).

THE IDEAL ALVEOLAR GAS EQUATION

Clinically, the alveolar oxygen tension $P_{A_{O_2}}$ can be computed from the **ideal alveolar gas equation**. A useful clinical approximation of the ideal alveolar gas equation is as follows:

$$P_{A_{O_2}} = [P_B - P_{H_2O}]F_{I_{O_2}} - P_{a_{CO_2}}(1.25)$$

where $P_{A_{O_2}}$ is the partial pressure of oxygen in the alveoli, P_B is the barometric pressure, P_{H_2O} is the partial pressure of water vapor in the alveoli ($P_{H_2O} = 47$ mm Hg), $F_{I_{O_2}}$ is the fractional concentration of inspired oxygen, and $P_{a_{CO_2}}$ is the partial pressure of arterial carbon dioxide. The number 1.25 is a factor that adjusts for alterations in oxygen tension due to variations in the *respiratory exchange ratio* (RR), which is the ratio of the amount of oxygen that moves into the pulmonary capillary blood to the amount of carbon dioxide that moves out of the pulmonary blood and into the alveoli. Normally, about 200 ml/minute of carbon dioxide move into the alveoli while about 250 ml/minute of oxygen move into the pulmonary capillary blood, making the respiratory exchange ratio about 0.8.

Thus, if a patient is receiving an $F_{I_{O_2}}$ of .40 on a day when the barometric pressure is 755 mm Hg, and if the $P_{a_{CO_2}}$ is 55 mm Hg, the patient's alveolar oxygen tension ($P_{A_{O_2}}$) can be calculated as follows:

$$P_{A_{O_2}} = [P_B - P_{H_2O}]F_{I_{O_2}} - P_{a_{CO_2}}(1.25)$$

$$= [755 - 47].40 - 55(1.25)$$

$$= [708].40 - 68.75$$

$$= [283.2] - 68.75$$

$$= 214.45$$

Clinically, when the Pa_{CO_2} is less than 60 mm Hg, and when the patient is receiving oxygen therapy, the following simplified version of the alveolar gas equation may be used:

$$PA_{O_2} = [PB - P_{H_2O}]FI_{O_2} - Pa_{CO_2}$$

THE DIFFUSION OF PULMONARY GASES

The process of diffusion is the passive movement of gas molecules from an area of high partial pressure to an area of low partial pressure until both areas are equal in pressure. Once gas equilibrium occurs, gas diffusion ceases.

In the lungs, a gas molecule must diffuse through the alveolar-capillary membrane (Figure 3–2), which is composed of (1) the liquid lining the intra-alveolar membrane, (2) the alveolar epithelial cell, (3) the basement membrane of the alveolar epithelial cell, (4) loose connective tissue (the interstitial space), (5) the basement membrane of the capillary endothelium, (6) the capillary endothelium, (7) the plasma in the capillary blood, (8) the erythrocyte membrane, and (9) the intracellular fluid in the erythrocyte until a hemoglobin molecule is encountered. Added together, the

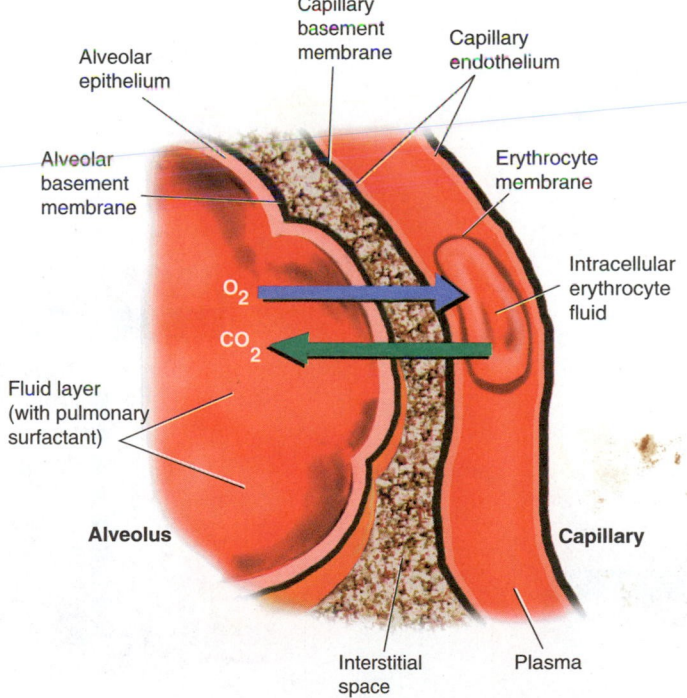

ALVEOLAR-CAPILLARY MEMBRANE

Figure 3–2. *The major barriers of the alveolar-capillary membrane through which a gas molecule must diffuse.*

thickness of these physical barriers is between 0.36 and 2.5 μ. Under normal circumstances, this is a negligible barrier to the diffusion of oxygen and carbon dioxide.

OXYGEN AND CARBON DIOXIDE DIFFUSION ACROSS THE ALVEOLAR-CAPILLARY MEMBRANE

In the healthy resting individual, venous blood entering the alveolar-capillary system has an average oxygen tension ($P\bar{v}_{O_2}$) of 40 mm Hg, and an average carbon dioxide tension ($P\bar{v}_{CO_2}$) of 46 mm Hg. As blood passes through the capillary, the average alveolar oxygen tension (PA_{O_2}) is about 100 mm Hg, and the average alveolar carbon dioxide tension (PA_{CO_2}) is about 40 mm Hg (see Table 3–2).

Thus, when venous blood enters the alveolar-capillary system, there is an oxygen pressure gradient of about 60 mm Hg and a carbon dioxide pressure gradient of about 6 mm Hg. As a result, oxygen molecules diffuse across the alveolar-capillary membrane into the blood while, at the same time, carbon dioxide molecules diffuse out of the capillary blood and into the alveoli (Figure 3–3).

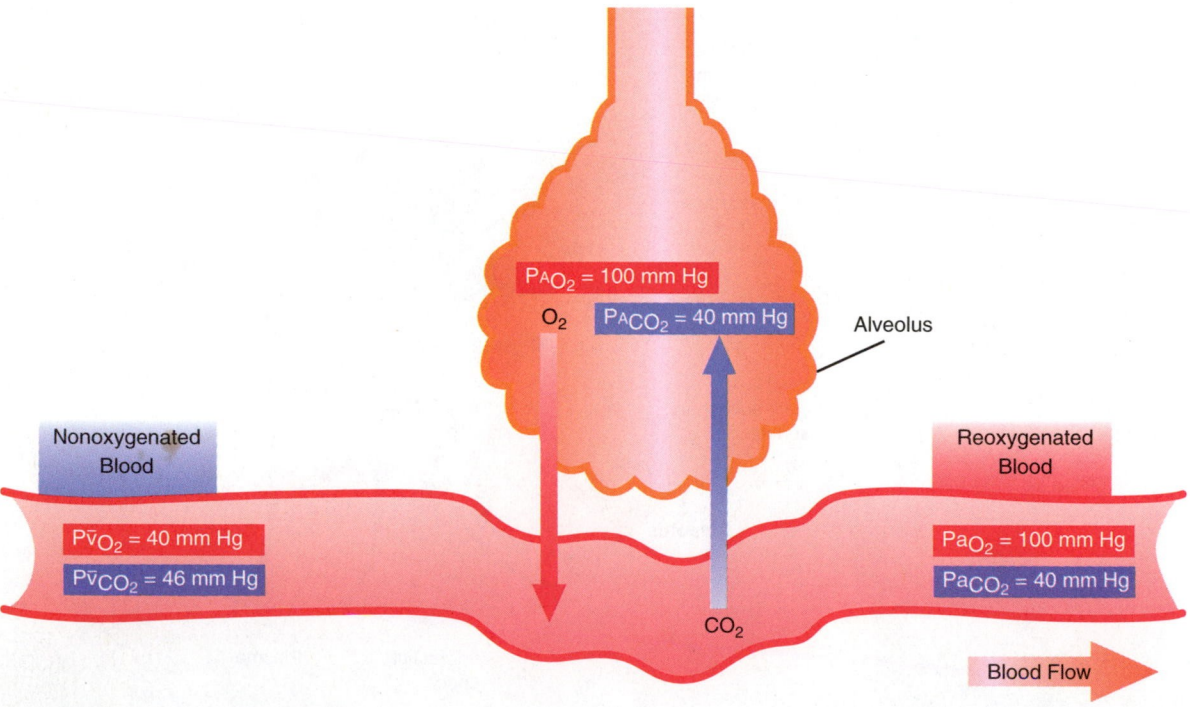

Figure 3–3. *Normal gas pressures for oxygen and carbon dioxide as blood moves through the alveolar-capillary membrane. $P\bar{v}_{O_2}$ = partial pressure of oxygen in mixed venous blood; $P\bar{v}_{CO_2}$ = partial pressure of carbon dioxide in mixed venous blood; PA_{O_2} = partial pressure of oxygen in alveolar gas; PA_{CO_2} = partial pressure of carbon dioxide in alveolar gas; Pa_{O_2} = partial pressure of oxygen in arterial blood; Pa_{CO_2} = partial pressure of carbon dioxide in arterial blood.*

Figure 3–4. *Under normal resting conditions, blood moves through the alveolar-capillary membrane in about 0.75 second. The oxygen pressure (P_{O_2}) and carbon dioxide pressure (P_{CO_2}) reach equilibrium in about 0.25 second—one-third of the time available. $P\bar{v}_{O_2}$ = partial pressure of oxygen in mixed venous blood; $P\bar{v}_{CO_2}$ = partial pressure of carbon dioxide in mixed venous blood; $P_{A_{O_2}}$ = partial pressure of oxygen in alveolar gas; $P_{A_{CO_2}}$ = partial pressure of carbon dioxide in alveolar gas; Pa_{O_2} = partial pressure of oxygen in arterial blood; Pa_{CO_2} = partial pressure of carbon dioxide in arterial blood.*

The diffusion of oxygen and carbon dioxide will continue until equilibrium is reached between the two gases; this is usually accomplished in about 0.25 second. Under normal resting conditions, the total transit time for blood to move through the alveolar-capillary system is about 0.75 second. Thus, the diffusion of oxygen and carbon dioxide is completed in about one-third of the time available (Figure 3–4, page 115).

In exercise, however, blood passes through the alveolar-capillary system at a much faster rate and, therefore, the time for gas diffusion decreases (i.e.,

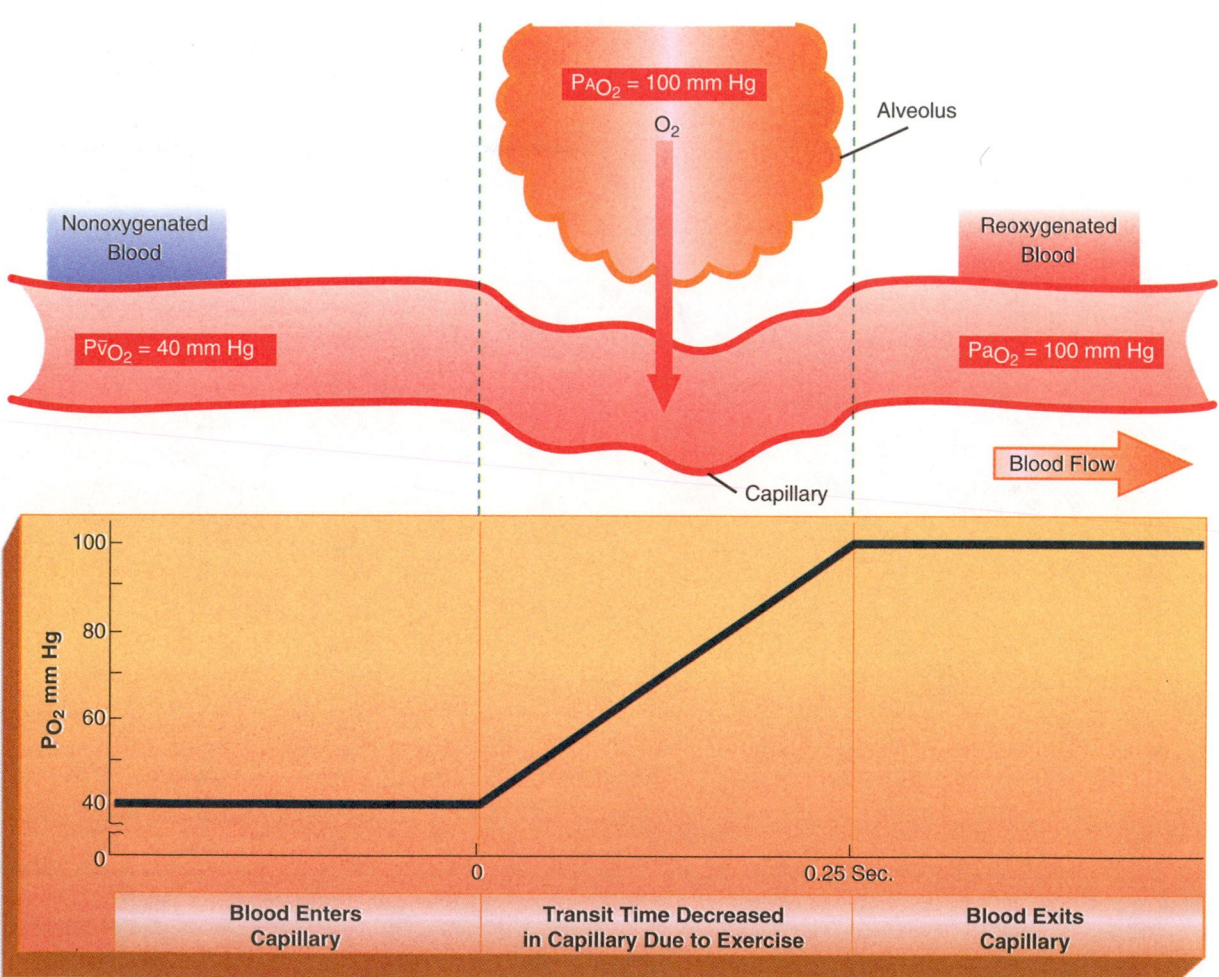

Figure 3–5. *During exercise or stress, the total transit time for blood through the alveolar-capillary membrane is less than normal (normal = 0.75 sec). In the healthy individual, however, oxygen equilibrium usually occurs. Pv_{O_2} = partial pressure of oxygen in mixed venous blood; PA_{O_2} = partial pressure of oxygen in alveolar gas; Pa_{O_2} = partial pressure of oxygen in arterial blood.*

the time available for gas diffusion is less than 0.75 second). In the healthy lung, oxygen equilibrium usually occurs in the alveolar-capillary system during exercise—in spite of the shortened transit time (Figure 3–5). In the presence of certain pulmonary diseases, however, the time required to achieve oxygen equilibrium in the alveolar-capillary system may not be adequate. Such diseases include alveolar fibrosis, alveolar consolidation, and pulmonary edema (Figure 3–6).

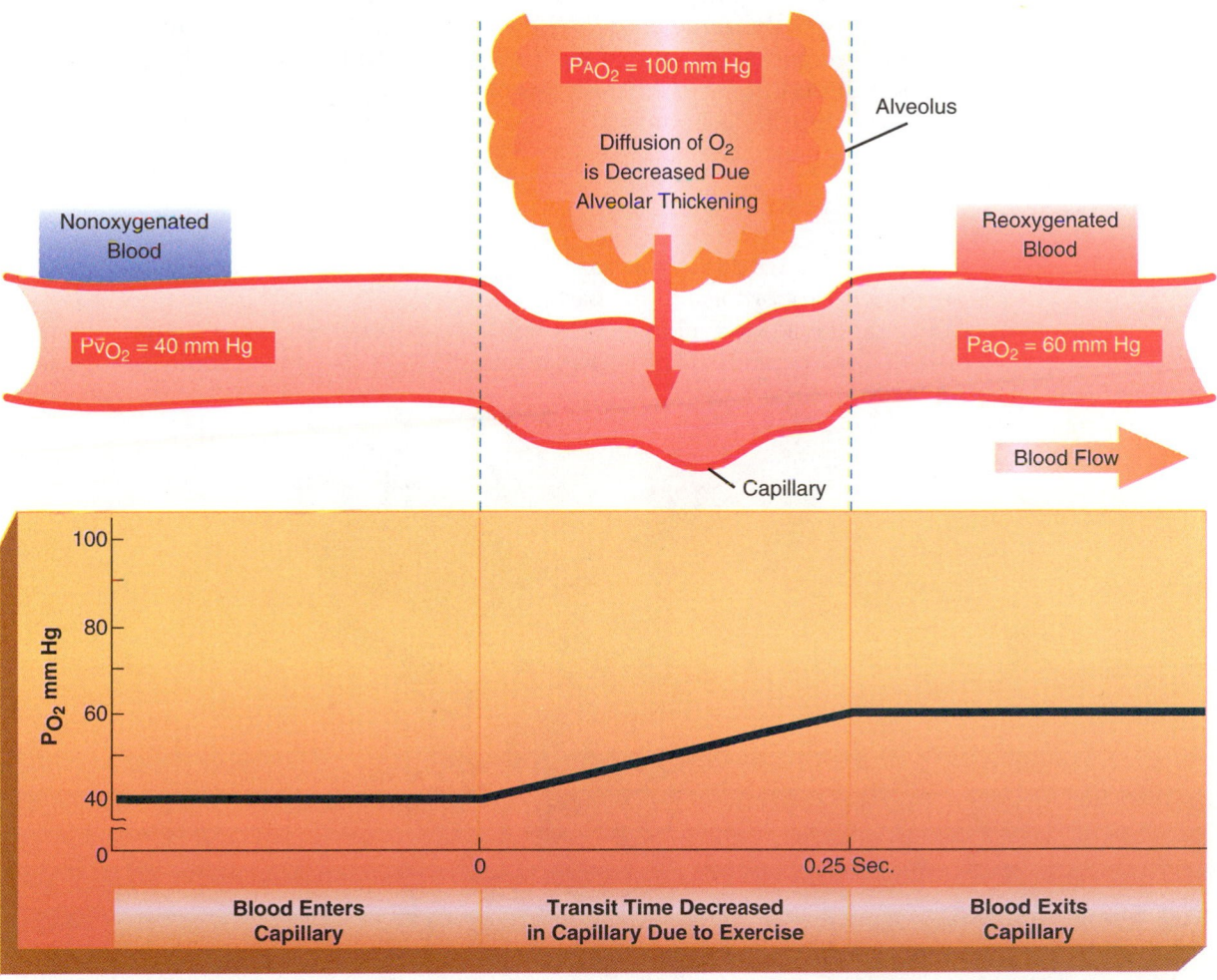

Figure 3–6. *When the rate of diffusion is decreased because of alveolar thickening, oxygen equilibrium will likely not occur when the total transit time is decreased as a result of exercise or stress.* Pv_{O_2} = *partial pressure of oxygen in mixed venous blood;* PA_{O_2} = *partial pressure of oxygen in alveolar gas;* Pa_{O_2} = *partial pressure of oxygen in arterial blood.*

GAS DIFFUSION

FICK'S LAW

The diffusion of gas takes place according to Fick's law, which is written as follows:

$$\dot{V} \text{ gas } \alpha \frac{A.D. (P_1 - P_2)}{T}$$

where $\dot{V}$ gas is the amount of gas that diffuses from one point to another, A is surface area, D is diffusion constants, $P_1 - P_2$ is the difference in partial pressure between two points, and T is thickness.

The law states that the rate of gas transfer across a sheet of tissue is directly proportional to the surface area of the tissue, to the diffusion constants, and to the difference in partial pressure of the gas between the two sides of the tissue and is inversely proportional to the thickness of the tissue (Figure 3–7).

The diffusion constants (D) noted in Fick's law are determined by Henry's law and Graham's law.

HENRY'S LAW

Henry's law states that the amount of a gas that dissolves in a liquid at a given temperature is proportional to the partial pressure of the gas. The amount of gas that can be dissolved by 1 ml of a given liquid at standard pressure (760 mm Hg) and specified temperature is known as the *solubility coefficient* of the liquid. At 37°C and

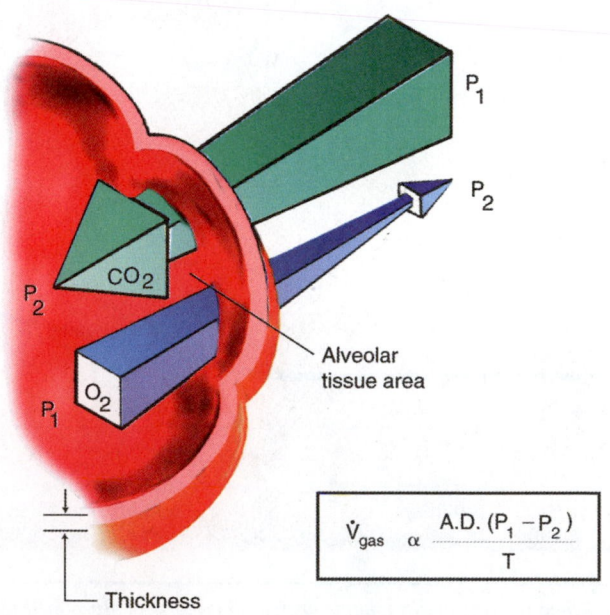

Figure 3–7. *Fick's law. See text for explanation.*

760 mm Hg pressure, the solubility coefficient of oxygen is 0.0244 ml/mm Hg/ml H_2O. The solubility coefficient of carbon dioxide is 0.592 ml/mm Hg/ml H_2O. The solubility coefficient varies inversely with temperature (i.e., if the temperature rises the solubility coefficient decreases in value).

On the basis of the solubility coefficients of oxygen and carbon dioxide, it can be seen that in a liquid medium (e.g., alveolar-capillary membrane) carbon dioxide is more soluble than oxygen:

$$\frac{\text{Solubility } CO_2}{\text{Solubility } O_2} = \frac{0.592}{0.0244} = \frac{24}{1}$$

GRAHAM'S LAW

Graham's law states that the rate of diffusion of a gas through a liquid is (1) directly proportional to the solubility coefficient of the gas and (2) inversely proportional to the square root of the gram-molecular weight (GMW) of the gas. In comparing the relative rates of diffusion to oxygen (GMW = 32) and carbon dioxide (GMW = 44), it can be seen that, since oxygen is the lighter gas, it moves faster than carbon dioxide:

$$\frac{\text{Diffusion rate for } CO_2}{\text{Diffusion rate for } O_2} = \frac{\sqrt{\text{GMW } O_2}}{\sqrt{\text{GMW } CO_2}} = \frac{\sqrt{32}}{\sqrt{44}}$$

$$= \frac{5.6}{6.6}$$

By combining Graham's and Henry's laws, it can be said that the rates of diffusion of two gases are directly proportional to the ratio of their solubility coefficients, and inversely proportional to the ratio of their gram-molecular weights. For example, when the two laws are used to determine the relative rates of diffusion of carbon dioxide and oxygen, it can be seen that carbon dioxide diffuses about 20 times faster than oxygen.

$$\frac{\text{Diffusion rate for } CO_2}{\text{Diffusion rate for } O_2} = \frac{5.6 \times 0.592}{6.6 \times 0.0244} = \frac{20}{1}$$

To summarize, the diffusion constant (D) for a particular gas is directly proportional to the solubility coefficients (S) of the gas, and inversely proportional to the square root of the gram-molecular weight (GMW) of the gas:

$$D = \frac{S}{\sqrt{GMW}}$$

Mathematically, by substituting the diffusion constants,

$$D = \frac{S}{\sqrt{GMW}}$$

into Fick's law:

$$\dot{V} \text{ gas } \alpha \frac{\text{A.D. } (P_1 - P_2)}{T}$$

then Fick's law can be rewritten as:

$$\dot{V} \text{ gas } \alpha \frac{\text{A.S. } (P_1 - P_2)}{\sqrt{\text{GMW}} \times \text{T}}$$

CLINICAL APPLICATION OF FICK'S LAW

Clinically, Fick's law is confirmed by the following general statements:

- The area (A) component of the law is verified in that a decreased alveolar surface area (e.g., caused by alveolar collapse or alveolar fluid) decreases the ability of oxygen to enter the pulmonary capillary blood.
- The $P_1 - P_2$ portion of the law is confirmed in that a decreased alveolar oxygen pressure ($P_{A_{O_2}}$ or P_1) (e.g., caused by high altitudes or alveolar hypoventilation) reduces the diffusion of oxygen into the pulmonary capillary blood.
- The thickness (T) factor is confirmed in that an increased alveolar tissue thickness (e.g., caused by alveolar fibrosis or alveolar edema) reduces the movement of oxygen across the alveolar-capillary membrane.

Fick's law also demonstrates how certain adverse pulmonary conditions may be improved. For example, when a patient's oxygen diffusion rate is decreased because of alveolar thickening, the administration of oxygen therapy to the patient will be beneficial. As the patient's fractional concentration of inspired oxygen ($F_{I_{O_2}}$) increases, the patient's alveolar oxygen pressure (i.e., $P_{A_{O_2}}$ or the P_1) also increases. This causes the movement of oxygen across the alveolar-capillary membrane to increase.

PERFUSION-LIMITED GAS FLOW

Perfusion limited means that the transfer of gas across the alveolar wall is a function of the amount of blood that flows past the alveoli. Nitrous oxide (N_2O) is an excellent gas to illustrate this concept: When N_2O moves across the alveolar wall and into the blood, it does not chemically combine with hemoglobin. Because of this, the partial pressure of N_2O in the blood plasma rises very quickly. It is estimated that the partial pressure of N_2O will equal that of the alveolar gas when the blood is only about one-tenth of the way through the alveolar-capillary system (Figure 3–8). Once the partial pressures of the N_2O in the blood and in the alveolar gas are equal, the diffusion of N_2O stops. In order for the diffusion of N_2O to resume, additional blood must enter the alveolar-capillary system. The rate of perfusion, therefore, limits the amount of diffusion of N_2O.

DIFFUSION-LIMITED GAS FLOW

Diffusion limited means that the movement of gas across the alveolar wall is a function of the integrity of the alveolar-capillary membrane itself. Carbon monoxide (CO) is an excellent gas to illustrate this concept: When CO moves across the

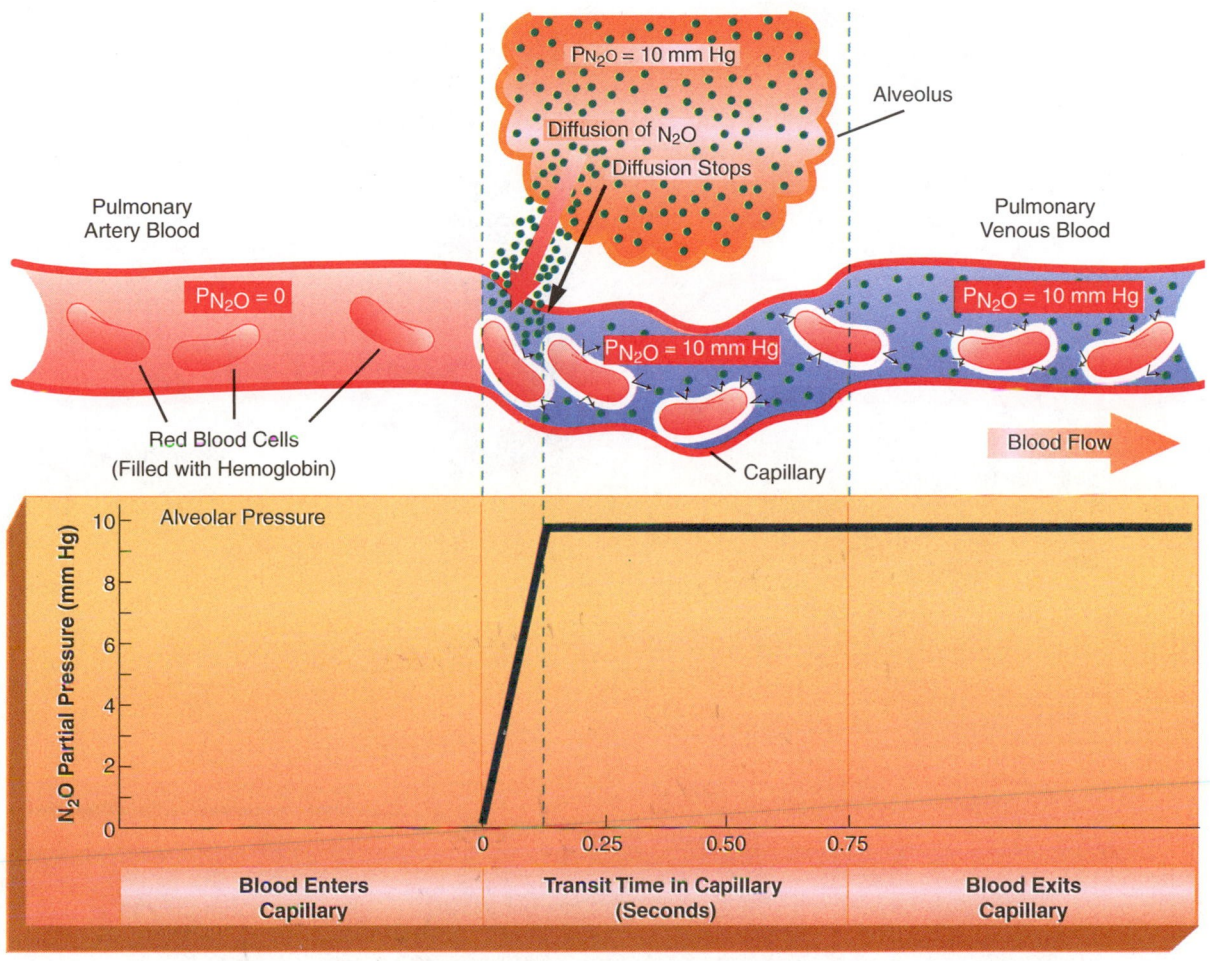

Figure 3–8. *Nitrous oxide (N$_2$O) quickly equilibrates with pulmonary blood. When equilibrium occurs, the diffusion of N$_2$O stops. In order for the diffusion of N$_2$O to resume, fresh blood (pulmonary artery blood) must enter the alveolar-capillary system. This phenomenon is called* perfusion limited. *P$_{N_2O}$ = partial pressure of nitrous oxide in the blood.*

alveolar wall and into the blood, it rapidly enters the red blood cell (RBC) and tightly bonds to hemoglobin (CO has an affinity for hemoglobin that is about 210 times greater than that of oxygen).

It should be noted that when gases are in chemical combination with hemoglobin, they no longer exert a partial pressure. Thus, since CO has a strong chemical attraction to hemoglobin, most of the CO enters the RBCs, combines with hemoglobin, and no longer exerts a partial pressure in the blood plasma. Because there is no appreciable partial pressure of CO in the blood plasma at any time (i.e., $P_2 - P_1$ stays constant), only the diffusion characteristics of the alveolar-capillary membrane, and not the amount of blood flowing through the capillary, limit the diffusion of CO (Figure 3–9, page 122).

Figure 3–9. *Carbon monoxide (CO) rapidly bonds to hemoglobin and, thus, does not generate an appreciable partial pressure (P_{CO}) in the blood plasma. As a result of this chemical relationship, blood flow (perfusion) does not limit the rate of CO diffusion. However, when the alveolar-capillary membrane is abnormal (e.g., in alveolar fibrosis), the rate of CO diffusion decreases. This phenomenon is called* diffusion limited. *In essence, diffusion limited means that the structure of the alveolar-capillary membrane alone limits the rate of gas diffusion.*

Clinically, this makes CO an excellent gas for evaluating the lung's ability to diffuse gases and is used in what is called the *diffusion capacity of carbon monoxide* (DL_{CO}) test. The DL_{CO} test measures the amount of CO that moves across the alveolar-capillary membrane into the blood in a given time. In essence, this test measures the physiologic effectiveness of the alveolar-capillary membrane. The normal diffusion capacity of CO is 25 ml/minute/mm Hg. Figure 3–10 shows clinical conditions that may cause problems in diffusion. See Figure 3–6 for an illustration of the diffusion of oxygen during a diffusion-limited state.

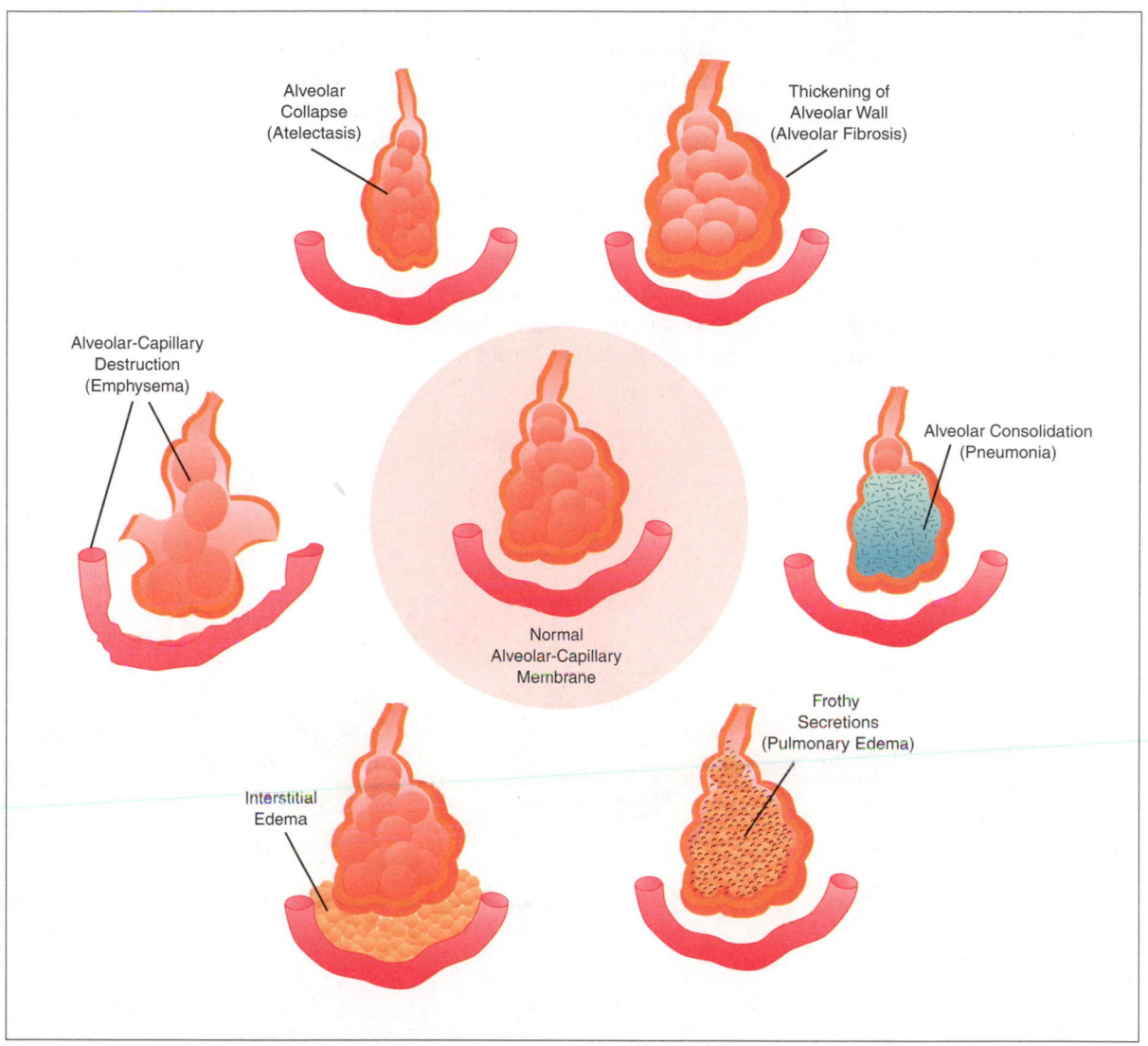

Figure 3–10. *Clinical conditions that decrease the rate of gas diffusion. These conditions are known as* diffusion-limited problems.

HOW OXYGEN CAN BE EITHER PERFUSION OR DIFFUSION LIMITED

When oxygen diffuses across the alveolar wall and into the blood, it enters the red blood cell and combines with hemoglobin—but not with the same avidity as carbon monoxide does. Hemoglobin quickly becomes saturated with oxygen and, once this happens, oxygen molecules in the plasma can no longer enter the red blood cell. This, in turn, causes the partial pressure of oxygen in the plasma to increase.

Under normal resting conditions, the partial pressure of oxygen in the capillary blood equals the partial pressure of oxygen in the alveolar gas when the blood is about one-third of the way through the capillary. Beyond this point, the transfer of oxygen is perfusion limited (Figure 3–11). When the patient has either a decreased cardiac output or a decreased hemoglobin level (anemia), the effects of perfusion limitation may become significant.

When the diffusion properties of the lungs are impaired (see Figure 3–10), however, the partial pressure of oxygen in the capillary blood may never equal the partial pressure of the oxygen in the alveolar gas during the normal alveolar-capillary transit time. Thus, under normal circumstances the diffusion of oxygen is perfusion limited, but under certain abnormal pulmonary conditions the transfer of oxygen may become diffusion limited.

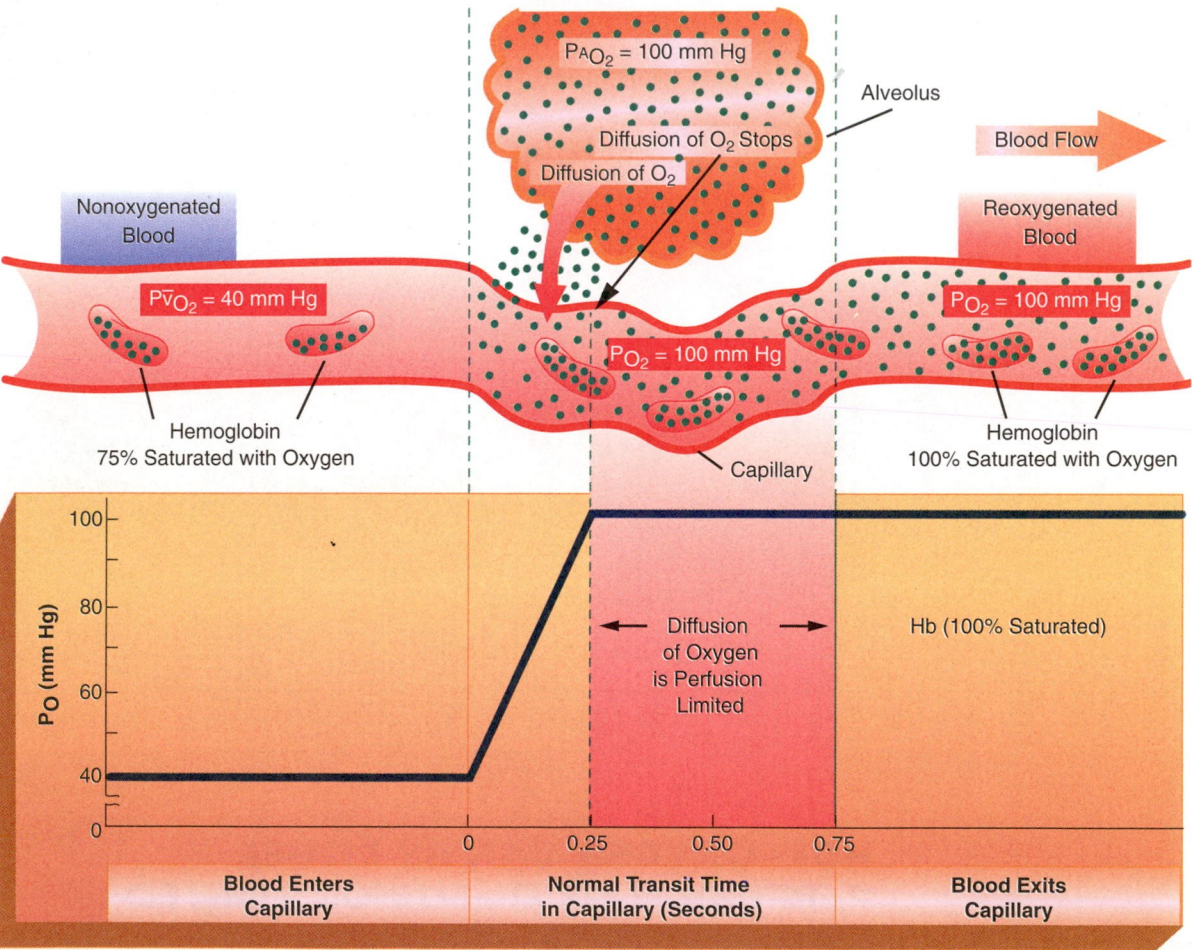

Figure 3–11. *Under normal resting conditions, the diffusion of oxygen across the alveolar-capillary membrane stops when blood is about one-third of the way through the capillary. This occurs because the partial pressure of oxygen in the capillary blood (P_{O_2}) equals the partial pressure of oxygen in the alveolus ($P_{A_{O_2}}$). Once oxygen equilibrium occurs between the alveolus and capillary blood, the diffusion of oxygen is* perfusion *limited.*

CLINICAL APPLICATION 1

This 68-year-old male entered the hospital in severe left ventricular heart failure and pulmonary edema.* He appeared very anxious and his lips and skin were blue. He had a frequent and strong cough, productive of moderate amounts of frothy, white and pink secretions. The patient's vital signs were: blood pressure—140/88, heart rate—93 beats/min and weak, and respiratory rate—28 breaths/min and shallow. On auscultation, crackles and rhonchi (fluid sounds) could be heard over both lung fields. His arterial oxygen pressure (Pa_{O_2}) was 53 mm Hg (normal range is 80–100 mm Hg).

The emergency room physician started the patient on several different heart medications and a diuretic. The respiratory therapist placed a continuous positive airway pressure (CPAP) mask over the patient's nose and mouth, and set the pressure at +10 cm H_2O and the fractional concentration of inspired oxygen (FI_{O_2}) at 0.4. One hour later the patient was breathing comfortably. His lips and skin no longer appeared blue, and his cough was not as frequent. No frothy or pink sputum was noted at this time. His vital signs were: blood pressure—126/78, heart rate—77 beats/min, and respiratory rate—16 breaths/min. On auscultation, his breath sounds were improved. His arterial oxygen pressure (Pa_{O_2}) was 86 mm Hg.

DISCUSSION

This case illustrates both the adverse and therapeutic effects of factors presented in Fick's law (see Figure 3–7). The patient presented in the emergency room in severe left ventricular heart failure and pulmonary edema. This means that the patient's left ventricle was failing to pump blood adequately and caused blood to back up into the patient's lungs. This pathologic process, in turn, caused the patient's pulmonary blood

pressure to increase. As the pulmonary blood pressure increased, fluid moved out of the pulmonary capillaries and into the extracapillary spaces, as well as into the alveoli and into the tracheobronchial tree. As a result of this process, the thickness of the alveolar-capillary membrane also increased (see Figure 3–2).

Because gas diffusion ($\dot{V}$) is *indirectly* related to thickness (T), the diffusion of oxygen across the alveolar-capillary membrane decreased (Fick's law). This fact was illustrated by the low Pa_{O_2} of 53 mm Hg when the patient first entered the hospital. The physician treated the original cause of this condition—the failing heart and fluid overload—with medications. As the cardiac function and fluid overload improved, the thickness of the alveolar-capillary membrane returned to normal. As the thickness of the alveolar-capillary membrane decreased, the diffusion of oxygen increased.

While the physician was treating the patient's failing heart, the respiratory therapist worked to offset the patient's poor oxygenation by increasing the patient's PA_{O_2} (P_1 of Fick's law). As Fick's law shows, the diffusion of gas is *directly* related to $P_1 - P_2$. The therapist increased the patient's PA_{O_2} by (1) increasing the patient's overall barometric pressure at the level of the alveoli with the CPAP mask, and (2) increasing the inspired FI_{O_2} to 0.4.

Thus, the reduction in alveolar-capillary membrane thickness (decreased via medications), the increased barometric pressure at the level of the alveoli (produced via CPAP), and the increased FI_{O_2} (increased P_1) all worked to enhance the diffusion of oxygen, as shown by the Pa_{O_2} of 86 mm Hg. The patient's cardiac condition progressively improved and he was discharged from the hospital two days later.

---

*Pulmonary edema refers to fluid accumulation in the alveoli and airways. Pulmonary edema is commonly associated with congestive heart failure.

CLINICAL APPLICATION

This 78-year-old female with a long history of chronic interstitial lung disease (alveolar thickening and fibrosis) was admitted to the hospital because of respiratory distress. She was well known to the hospital staff. She had been admitted to the hospital on several occasions, and for the past two years prior to this admission, she had been on continuous home oxygen (2L/min by nasal cannula). The home care respiratory therapist made regular visits to the patient's home to check on her equipment and to assess her respiratory status. In fact, it was the respiratory therapist who alerted the physician about the patient's poor respiratory status that prompted this hospitalization.

On admission, the patient appeared anxious and agitated. Her skin was pale and blue and felt cool and clammy. Her vital signs were: blood pressure—166/91, heart rate—105 beats/min, and respiratory rate—24 breaths/min. Her breath sounds were clear and loud. Although her chest x-ray regularly showed signs of increased alveolar density (white appearance) because of her lung fibrosis, this day's chest x-ray was markedly worse.

The physician on duty felt that the chest x-ray showed an acute inflammatory condition from an undetermined cause. The physician started the patient on steroids. The respiratory therapist noted that even though the patient's alveolar oxygen pressure ($P_{A_{O_2}}$) was calculated to be 165 mm Hg, the patient's arterial oxygen pressure (Pa_{O_2}) was only 57 mm Hg (normal is 80–100 mm Hg). In response to the low Pa_{O_2}, the therapist increased the patient's inspired oxygen concentration (FI_{O_2}) from 2 L/min via nasal cannula (an FI_{O_2} of about 0.28) to 0.5 via an oxygen Venturi mask.

Over the next 24 hours the patient progressively improved. She stated that she was breathing much better and her skin color returned to normal. Her skin no longer felt cold or wet. Her vital signs were: blood pressure—128/86, heart rate—76 beats/min, and respiratory rate—14 breaths/min. A second chest x-ray showed improvement when compared to the previous day's chest x-ray, and her Pa_{O_2} was 89 mm Hg, within normal limits.

DISCUSSION

This case illustrates both the acute and chronic effects of an increased alveolar-capillary membrane. As Fick's law states, the diffusion of gas is *indirectly* related to the thickness of the alveolar-capillary membrane, and *directly* related to $P_1 - P_2$ (see Figure 3–7). Because the patient had chronic alveolar fibrosis and thickening, her oxygen diffusion was low. This is why continuous oxygen (2 L/min) administered via nasal cannula at home was needed to offset this condition. Increasing the alveolar oxygen level (i.e., increasing the $P_{A_{O_2}}$ or P_1) enhanced oxygen diffusion. When the patient's usual chronic status was stable, the 2 L/min oxygen via cannula at home was usually adequate to oxygenate her alveolar-capillary blood.

However, because the patient had an acute alveolar inflammatory condition—on top of her chronic problem—her alveolar-capillary membrane became even thicker. As a result, her usual home oxygen administration was not enough to meet the new challenge. Over the course of her hospitalization, however, the steroid therapy reduced her alveolar inflammation. As the acute alveolar inflammation improved, the thickness of her alveolar-capillary membrane decreased. While this process was taking place, the increased oxygen concentration (P_1) worked to offset the patient's poor oxygenation status and thus worked to make the patient comfortable. The patient continued to improve and was discharged on day five of her hospital stay. She continued to use oxygen via nasal cannula at home.

REVIEW QUESTIONS

1. If a container having a volume of 375 ml and a pressure of 15 cm H_2O in it is suddenly reduced to a volume of 150 ml, what would be the pressure in the container?
   a. 17.5 cm H_2O
   b. 28 cm H_2O
   c. 37.5 cm H_2O
   d. 43 cm H_2O
   e. 56.5 cm H_2O

2. If the gas temperature in a closed container that has a pressure of 50 cm H_2O in it is increased from 125 absolute to 235 absolute, what would be the pressure in the container?
   a. 86 cm H_2O
   b. 94 cm H_2O
   c. 102 cm H_2O
   d. 117 cm H_2O
   e. 123 cm H_2O

3. Which of the following gas laws states that in a mixture of gases the total pressure is equal to the sum of the partial pressure of each gas?
   a. Dalton's law
   b. Gay-Lussac's law
   c. Charles' law
   d. Boyle's law
   e. Ideal gas law

4. At sea level, the normal percent of carbon dioxide in the atmosphere is
   a. 5%
   b. 40%
   c. 78%
   d. 0.40%
   e. 0.03%

5. At sea level, the alveolar water vapor pressure is normally about
   a. 0.2 mm Hg
   b. 47 mm Hg
   c. 0.0 mm Hg
   d. 40 mm Hg
   e. one-half the vapor pressure of the atmosphere

6. If a patient is receiving an F_{IO_2} of .60 on a day when the barometric pressure is 725 mm Hg, and if the Pa_{CO_2} is 50 mm Hg, what is the patient's alveolar oxygen tension (PA_{O_2})?
   a. 177 mm Hg
   b. 233 mm Hg
   c. 344 mm Hg
   d. 415 mm Hg
   e. 511 mm Hg

7. The normal transit time for blood through the alveolar-capillary system is about
   a. 0.25 sec
   b. 0.50 sec
   c. 0.75 sec
   d. 1.0 sec
   e. 1.5 sec

8. Under normal resting conditions, the diffusion of oxygen and carbon dioxide is usually completed in about
   I. 0.25 sec
   II. 0.50 sec
   III. 0.75 sec
   IV. 1.0 sec
   V. one-third of the time available
      a. I only
      b. II only
      c. III only
      d. IV and V only
      e. I and V only

9. Which of the following states that the rate of gas diffusion is inversely proportional to the weight of the gas?
   a. Graham's law
   b. Charles' law
   c. Henry's law
   d. Gay-Lussac's law
   e. Boyle's law

10. According to Fick's law, gas diffusion is
    I. directly proportional to the thickness of the tissue
    II. indirectly proportional to the diffusion constants
    III. directly proportional to the difference in partial pressure of the gas between the two sides
    IV. indirectly proportional to the tissue area
       a. I only
       b. III only
       c. IV only
       d. II and III only
       e. I, III, and IV only

CHAPTER FOUR

PULMONARY FUNCTION MEASUREMENTS

OBJECTIVES

By the end of this chapter, the student should be able to:

1. Define the following *lung volumes:*
   —Tidal volume
   —Inspiratory reserve volume
   —Expiratory reserve volume
   —Residual volume
2. Define the following *lung capacities:*
   —Vital capacity
   —Inspiratory capacity
   —Functional residual capacity
   —Total lung capacity
   —Residual volume/total lung capacity ratio
3. Identify the approximate lung volumes and capacities in milliliters in the average normal male and female between 20 and 30 years of age.
4. Define the following *expiratory flow rate measurements:*
   —Forced vital capacity
   —Forced expiratory volume timed
   —Forced expiratory flow$_{200-1200}$
   —Forced expiratory flow$_{25\%-75\%}$
   —Peak expiratory flow rate
   —Maximum voluntary ventilation
   —Forced expiratory volume$_{1\,sec}$/forced vital capacity ratio
   —Flow-volume curves

5. Identify the following average dynamic flow rate measurements for the healthy male and female between 20 and 30 years of age:
   —Forced expiratory volume timed for periods of 0.5, 1.0, 2.0, and 3.0 seconds
   —Forced expiratory flow$_{200-1200}$
   —Forced expiratory flow$_{25\%-75\%}$
   —Peak expiratory flow rate
   —Maximum voluntary ventilation
6. Describe the *effort-dependent portion* of a forced expiratory maneuver.
7. Describe the *effort-independent portion* of a forced expiratory maneuver.
8. Explain how the *dynamic compression mechanism* limits the flow rate during the last 70 percent of a forced vital capacity, and include the meaning of the *equal pressure point.*
9. Describe the diffusion capacity of carbon monoxide study.
10. Complete the review questions at the end of this chapter.

LUNG VOLUMES AND CAPACITIES

The total amount of air that the lungs can accommodate is divided into four separate volumes. Four specific combinations of these lung volumes are used to designate lung capacities (Figure 4–1). The volumes and capacities of the lungs are defined below.

LUNG VOLUMES

Tidal Volume (V_T)

The volume of air that normally moves into and out of the lungs in one quiet breath.

Inspiratory Reserve Volume (IRV)

The maximum volume of air that can be inhaled after a normal tidal volume inhalation.

Expiratory Reserve Volume (ERV)

The maximum volume of air that can be exhaled after a normal tidal volume exhalation.

Residual Volume (RV)

The amount of air remaining in the lungs after a maximal exhalation.

Figure 4–1. *Normal lung volumes and capacities. IRV = inspiratory reserve volume; V_T = tidal volume; RV = residual volume; ERV = expiratory reserve volume; TLC = total lung capacity; VC = vital capacity; IC = inspiratory capacity; FRC = functional residual capacity.*

LUNG CAPACITIES
Vital Capacity (VC)

The maximum volume of air that can be exhaled after a maximal inspiration ($IRV + V_T + ERV$). There are two major VC measurements: slow vital capacity (SVC), in which exhalation is performed slowly; and forced vital capacity (FVC), in which a maximal effort is made to exhale as rapidly as possible.

Inspiratory Capacity (IC)

The volume of air that can be inhaled after a normal exhalation ($V_T + IRV$).

Functional Residual Capacity (FRC)

The volume of air remaining in the lungs after a normal exhalation ($ERV + RV$).

Total Lung Capacity (TLC)

The maximum amount of air that the lungs can accommodate ($IC + FRC$).

Residual Volume/Total Lung Capacity Ratio (RV/TLC $\times$ 100)

The percentage of the TLC occupied by the RV.

The amount of air that the lungs can accommodate varies with the age, race, weight, height, and sex of the individual. Table 4–1 lists the normal lung volumes and capacities of the average man and woman between 20 and 30 years of age.

Changes in lung volumes and capacities are seen in trauma and disease. Such changes are commonly classified as either an obstructive lung disorder or a restrictive lung disorder.

TABLE 4–1. **Approximate Lung Volumes and Capacities in the Average Normal Subject Between 20 and 30 Years of Age**

MEASUREMENT	MALE Approx. ml	MALE % of TLC	FEMALE Approx. ml	FEMALE % of TLC
Tidal Volume (V_T)	500	8–10	400–500	8–10
Inspiratory Reserve Volume (IRV)	3100	50	1900	30
Expiratory Reserve Volume (ERV)	1200	20	800	20
Residual Volume (RV)	1200	20	1000	25
Vital Capacity (VC)	4800	80	3200	75
Inspiratory Capacity (IC)	3600	60	2400	60
Functional Residual Capacity (FRC)	2400	40	1800	40
Total Lung Capacity (TLC)	6000	—	4200	—
Residual Volume/Total Lung	1200	20	1000	25
Capacity Ratio (RV/TLC $\times$ 100)	6000		4200	

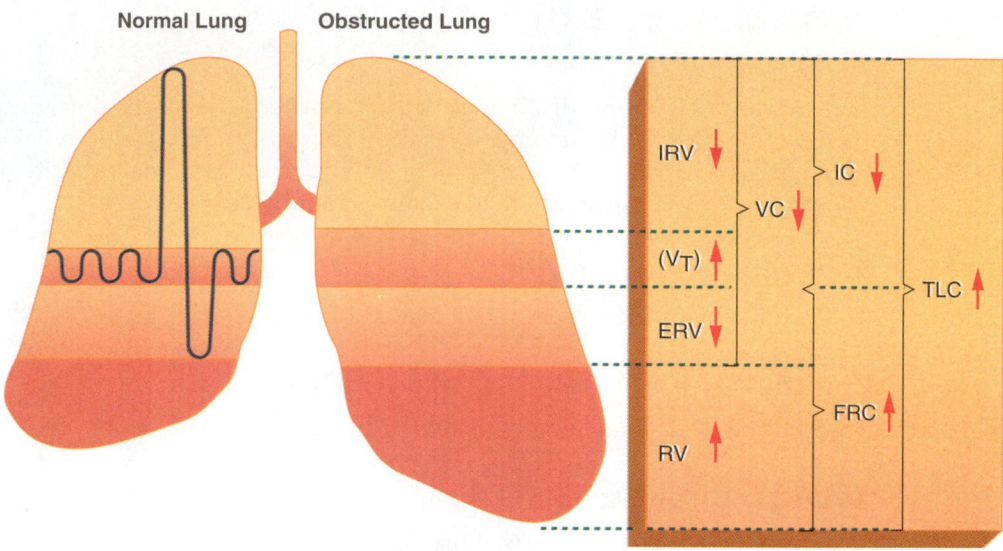

Figure 4–2.   *How obstructive lung disorders alter lung volumes and capacities. IRV = inspiratory reserve volume; V_T = tidal volume; RV = residual volume; ERV = expiratory reserve volume; TLC = total lung capacity; VC = tidal capacity; IC = inspiratory capacity; FRC = functional residual capacity.*

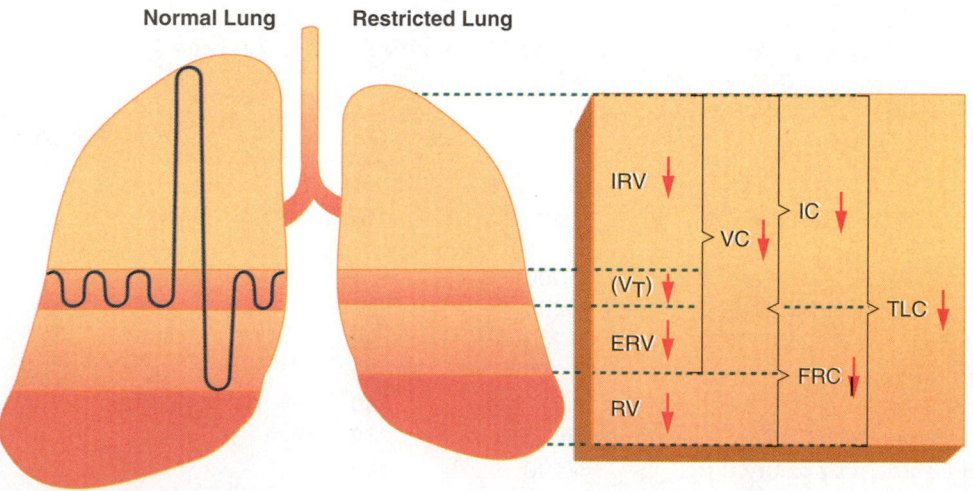

Figure 4–3.   *How restrictive lung disorders alter lung volumes and capacities. IRV = inspiratory reserve volume; V_T = tidal volume; RV = residual volume; ERV = expiratory reserve volume; TLC = total lung capacity; VC = vital capacity; FRC = functional residual capacity.*

In an obstructive lung disorder, the RV, V_T, FRC, and RV/TLC ratio are increased; and the VC, IC, IRV, and ERV are decreased (Figure 4–2). In a restrictive lung disorder, the VC, IC, RV, FRC, V_T, and TLC are all decreased (Figure 4–3).

PULMONARY MECHANICS

In addition to measuring volumes and capacities, one can also measure the rate at which gas flows into and out of the lungs. Expiratory flow rate measurements provide data on the integrity of the airways and the severity of airway impairment, as well as indicating whether the patient has a large airway or a small airway problem. Collectively, the tests for measuring expiratory flow rates are referred to as the pulmonary mechanic measurements and are described below.

PULMONARY MECHANIC MEASUREMENTS

Forced Vital Capacity (FVC)

The maximum volume of gas that can be exhaled as forcefully and rapidly as possible after a maximal inspiration. Normally FVC equals VC. In obstructive lung disease, however, the FVC is less than the VC (Figure 4–4). The FVC decreases with age.

Forced Expiratory Volume Timed (FEV_T)

The maximum volume of gas that can be exhaled over a specific time period. This measurement is obtained from an FVC. The most frequently used time period

Figure 4–4. *Forced vital capacity (FVC). A = point of maximal inspiration and the starting point of an FVC.*

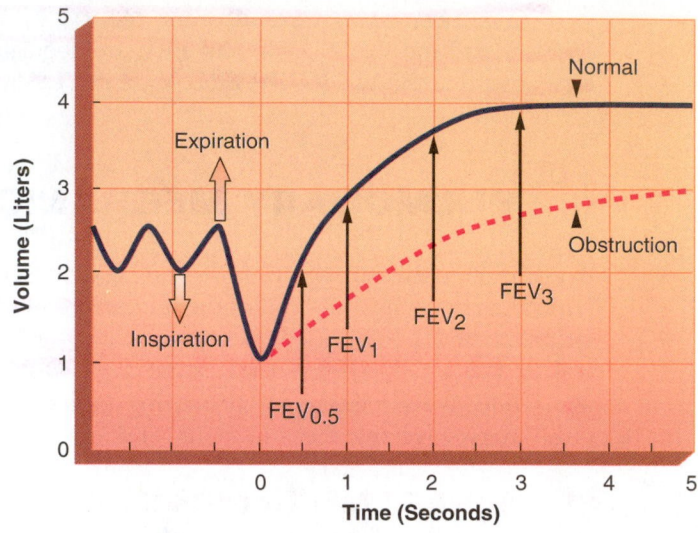

Figure 4–5. *Forced expiratory volume timed (FEV$_T$).*

is 1.0 second; other commonly used periods are 0.5, 2.0, and 3.0 seconds. Normally, the percentage of the total volume exhaled during these time periods is as follows: FEV$_{0.5}$, 60 percent; FEV$_{1.0}$, 83 percent; FEV$_{2.0}$, 94 percent; and FEV$_{3.0}$, 97 percent.

In obstructive disease, the FEV$_T$ decreases (Figure 4–5). The FEV$_T$ normally decreases with age.

Forced Expiratory Flow$_{200-1200}$ (FEF$_{200-1200}$)

The average rate of airflow between 200 and 1200 ml of the FVC (Figure 4–6); formerly known as the *maximum expiratory flow rate* (MEFR). The first 200 ml of the FVC is usually exhaled slower than the average flow rate because of (1) the inertia involved in the respiratory maneuver, and (2) the general unreliability of the equipment response time. Because the FEF$_{200-1200}$ measures expiratory flows at high lung volumes (i.e., the initial part, or the *effort-dependent portion*,* of the FVC), it is a good index of the integrity of large airway function. The average FEF$_{200-1200}$ for the healthy male between 20 and 30 years of age is about 8 L/sec (480 L/min), and for the female between 20 and 30 years of age is about 5.5 L/sec (330 L/min). In obstructive lung disease, however, flow rates as low as 1 L/sec (60 L/min) have been reported. The FEF$_{200-1200}$ decreases with age and in obstructive lung disease. Conceptually, the FEF$_{200-1200}$ is similar to measuring, and then averaging, the flow rate from a water faucet when 200 ml and 1200 ml have accumulated in a measuring container (Figure 4–7).

---

*See The Effort-Dependent Portion of a Forced Expiratory Maneuver, later in this chapter.

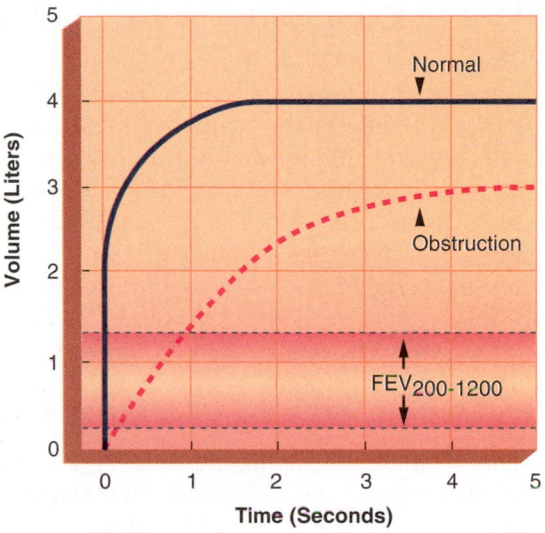

Figure 4–6. *Forced expiratory flow$_{200-1200}$ (FEF$_{200-1200}$).*

Figure 4–7. *The FEF$_{200-1200}$ is similar to measuring, and then averaging, the flow rate of water from a faucet at the precise moment when 200 ml and 1200 ml of water have accumulated in a container. Picture the flow rate from the faucet being measured when 200 ml of water have entered the container (A). Again, picture the flow rate from the faucet being measured when 1200 ml of water have entered the container (B). Taking the average of the two flow rates would be similar to the FEF$_{200-1200}$, which measures, and then averages, the flow rate at the precise point when 200 ml and 1200 ml of gas have been exhaled during an FVC maneuver.*

Forced Expiratory Flow$_{25\%-75\%}$ (FEF$_{25\%-75\%}$)

The average flow rate during the middle 50 percent of an FVC measurement (Figure 4–8); also known as the *maximum midexpiratory flow rate* (MMFR). This measurement reflects the status of medium- to small-sized airways. The average FEF$_{25\%-75\%}$ for the normal healthy male between 20 and 30 years old is about 4.5 L/sec (270 L/min), and for the female about 3.5 L/sec (210 L/min). In obstructive lung disease, flow rates as low as 0.3 L/sec (18 L/min) have been reported. The FEF$_{25\%-75\%}$ decreases progressively with age and in obstructive lung disease. Conceptually, the FEF$_{25\%-75\%}$ is similar to measuring, and then averaging, the flow rate from a water faucet when 25% and 75% of a specific volume of water has accumulated in a measuring container (Figure 4–9).

Peak Expiratory Flow Rate (PEFR)

The maximum flow rate that can be achieved; also known as *peak flow rate*. The PEFR can be obtained from the FVC (Figure 4–10). The average PEFR for the normal healthy male between 20 and 30 years is about 10 L/sec (600 L/min), and for the female about 7.5 L/sec (450 L/min). The PEFR decreases with age and in obstructive lung disease.

Maximum Voluntary Ventilation (MVV)

The largest volume of gas that can be breathed voluntarily in and out of the lungs in 1 minute (the patient actually performs the test for only 12 or 15 seconds); also known as *maximum breathing capacity* (MBC). The MVV is a general test that evaluates the performance of the respiratory muscles, the compliance of the lung and

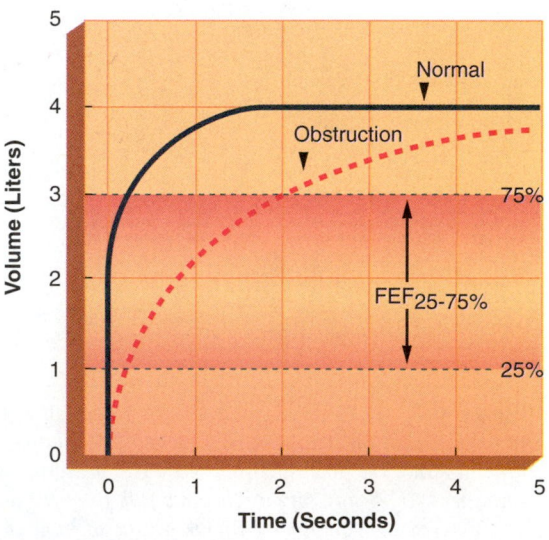

Figure 4–8.   *Forced expiratory flow$_{25\%-75\%}$ (FEF$_{25\%-75\%}$).*

Figure 4–9. *The FEF$_{25\%-75\%}$ is similar to measuring, and then averaging, the flow rate from a faucet when one liter and three liters of water have accumulated in a four-liter container. Picture the flow rate from the faucet being measured when one liter (25%) of water has entered a four-liter container (A). Again, picture the flow rate from the faucet being measured when three liters (75%) of water have entered the container (B). Taking the average of the two flow rates would be similar to the FEF$_{25\%-75\%}$, which measures, and then averages, the flow rate when an individual exhales 25% and 75% of their FVC.*

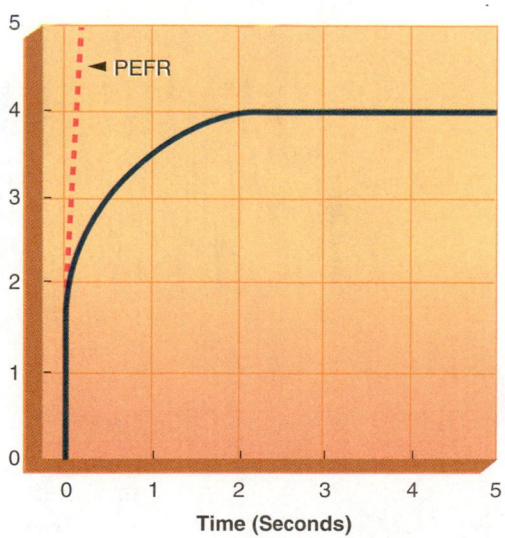

Figure 4–10. *Peak expiratory flow rate (PEFR).*

thorax, and the resistance generated by the airways and tissues. The average MVV for the healthy male between 20 and 30 years old is about 170 L/min, and for the female about 110 L/min. In patients with chronic obstructive disease, the MVV is decreased. The MVV decreases with age (Figure 4–11).

Forced Expiratory Volume$_{1\ Sec}$/Forced Vital Capacity Ratio (FEV$_1$/FVC ratio)

The ratio of the volume of gas that can be forcefully exhaled in 1 second to the total volume of gas that can be forcefully exhaled after a maximum inspiration. A decreased FEV$_1$/FVC ratio is a broad indicator of airway obstruction, but the absence of a decrease does not exclude the presence of airway obstruction.

Flow-volume Curve

The flow-volume curve is a graphic presentation of a forced vital capacity (FVC) maneuver followed by a forced inspiratory volume (FIV) maneuver. When the FVC and FIV are plotted together, the graphic illustration produced by the two curves is called a **flow-volume loop**. The flow-volume loop compares both the flow rates and volume changes produced at different points of an FVC and FIV maneuver. Depending on the sophistication of the equipment, the following measurements can be obtained from the flow-volume loop (Figure 4–12):

- Peak expiratory flow rate (PEFR)
- Peak inspiratory flow rate (PIFR)
- Forced vital capacity (FVC)

Figure 4–11. *Maximum voluntary ventilation (MVV).*

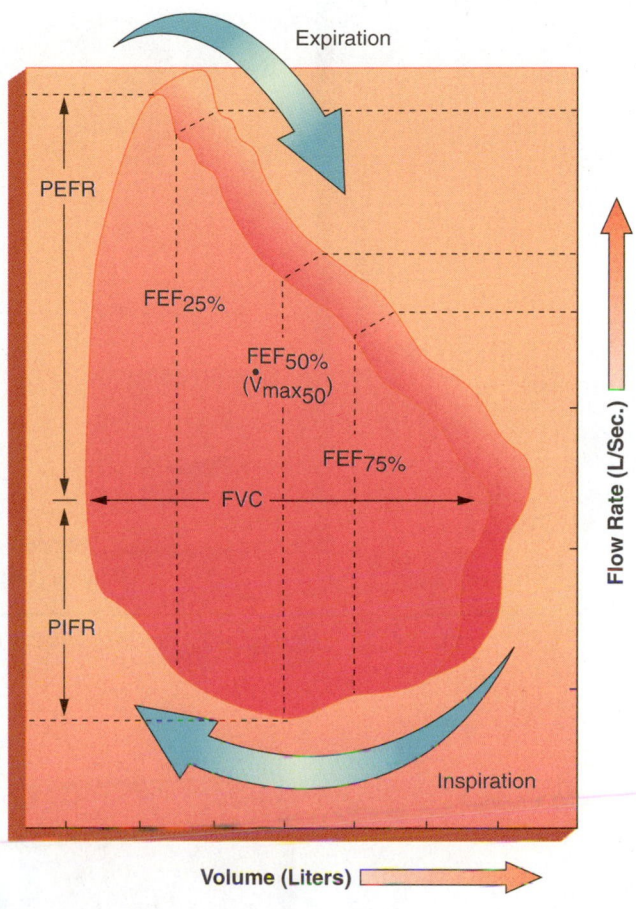

Figure 4–12. *Normal flow-volume loop. PEFR = peak expiration flow rate; PIFR = peak in-spiratory flow rate; FVC = forced vital capacity; $FEF_{25\%-75\%}$ = forced expiratory $flow_{25\%-75\%}$; $FEF_{50\%}$ = forced expiratory $flow_{50\%}$ (also called $\dot{V}max_{50}$).*

- Forced expiratory volume timed (FEV_T)
- Forced expiratory $flow_{25\%-75\%}$ ($FEF_{25\%-75\%}$)
- Forced expiratory $flow_{50\%}$ ($FEF_{50\%}$); also called the $\dot{V}max_{50}$. In the normal subject, the $FEF_{50\%}$ has a straight-line appearance, since the expiratory flow decreases linearly with volume throughout most of the VC range. In subjects with obstructive lung disease, however, flow frequently decreases at low lung volumes, causing the $FEF_{50\%}$ line to appear cuplike or scooped out.

Flow-volume loop measurements graphically illustrate both obstructive (Figure 4–13, page 140) and restrictive lung problems (Figure 4–14, page 140). Table 4–2 (see page 141) summarizes the average dynamic flow rate values found in the healthy male and female between 20 and 30 years of age.

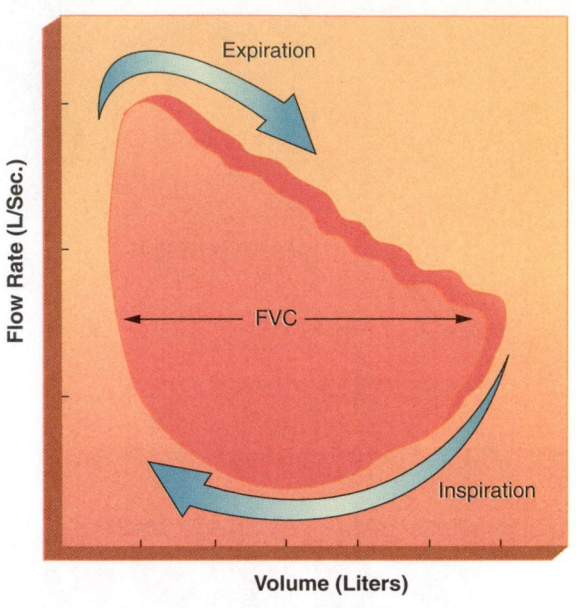

Figure 4–13. *Flow-volume loop, obstructive pattern. FVC = forced vital capacity.*

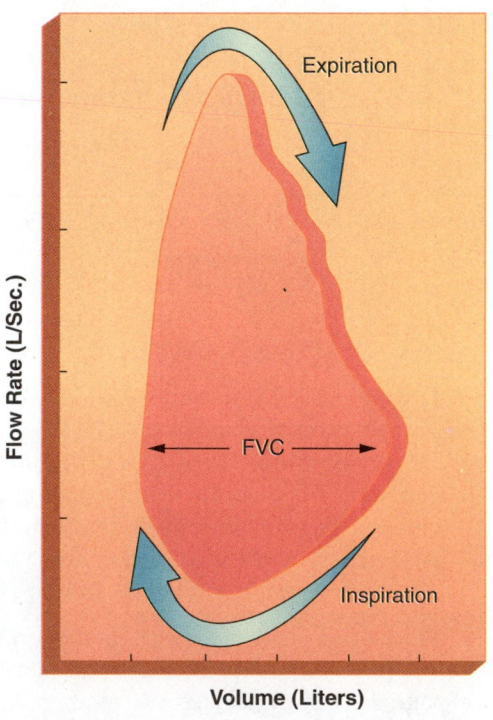

Figure 4–14. *Flow-volume loop, restrictive pattern. FVC = forced vital capacity.*

TABLE 4–2.	Average Dynamic Flow Rate Measurements of the Healthy Male and Female Between 20 and 30 Years of Age	
MEASUREMENT	**MALE**	**FEMALE**
FEV$_T$		
FEV$_{0.5}$	60%	60%
FEV$_{1.0}$	83%	83%
FEV$_{2.0}$	94%	94%
FEV$_{3.0}$	97%	97%
FEF$_{200-1200}$	8 L/sec (480 L/min)	5.5 L/sec (330 L/min)
FEF$_{25\%-75\%}$	4.5 L/sec (270 L/min)	3.5 L/sec (210 L/min)
PEFR	10 L/sec (600 L/min)	7.5 L/sec (450 L/min)
MVV	170 L/min	110 L/min

*See text for explanation of abbreviations.

HOW THE EFFECTS OF DYNAMIC COMPRESSION DECREASE EXPIRATORY FLOW RATES

THE EFFORT-DEPENDENT PORTION OF A FORCED EXPIRATORY MANEUVER

Normally, during approximately the first 30 percent of a forced vital capacity maneuver, the maximum peak flow rate is dependent on the amount of muscular effort exerted by the individual. Therefore, the first 30 percent of a forced expiratory maneuver is referred to as effort dependent.

THE EFFORT-INDEPENDENT PORTION OF A FORCED EXPIRATORY MANEUVER

The flow rate during approximately the last 70 percent of a forced vital capacity maneuver is effort independent. That is, once a maximum flow rate has been attained, the flow rate cannot be increased by further muscular effort.

The lung volume at which the patient initiates a forced expiratory maneuver also influences the maximum flow rate. As lung volumes decline, flow also declines. The reduced flow, however, is the maximum flow for that particular volume.

Figure 4–15 (see page 142) illustrates where the effort-dependent and effort-independent portions of a forced expiratory maneuver appear on a flow-volume loop.

DYNAMIC COMPRESSION OF THE BRONCHIAL AIRWAYS

The limitation of the flow rate that occurs during the last 70 percent of a forced vital capacity maneuver is due to the dynamic compression of the walls of the airways.

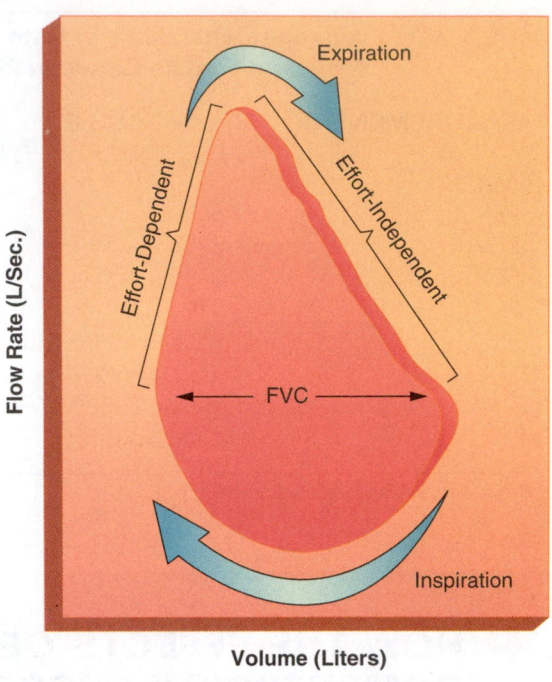

Figure 4–15. *The effort-dependent and effort-independent portions of a forced expiratory maneuver in a flow-volume loop measurement. FVC = forced vital capacity.*

As gas flows through the airways from the alveoli to the atmosphere during passive expiration, the pressure within the airways diminishes to zero (Figure 4–16A).

During a forced expiratory maneuver, however, as the airway pressure decreases from the alveoli to the atmosphere, there is a point at which the pressure within the lumen of the airways equals the pleural pressure surrounding the airways. This point is called the **equal pressure point**.

Downstream (i.e., toward the mouth) from the equal pressure point, the lateral pressure within the airway becomes less than the surrounding pleural pressure. Consequently, the airways are compressed. As muscular effort and pleural pressure increase during a forced expiratory maneuver, the equal pressure point moves upstream (i.e., toward the alveolus). Ultimately, the equal pressure point becomes fixed where the individual's flow rate has achieved maximum (Figure 4–16B). In essence, once dynamic compression occurs during a forced expiratory maneuver, increased muscular effort merely augments airway compression, which in turn increases airway resistance.

As the structural changes associated with certain respiratory diseases (e.g., chronic obstructive pulmonary diseases) intensify, the patient commonly responds by increasing intrapleural pressure during expiration to overcome the increased airway resistance produced by the disease. By increasing intrapleural pressure during expiration, however, the patient activates the dynamic compression mechanism, which in turn further reduces the diameter of the bronchial airways. This results in an even greater increase in airway resistance.

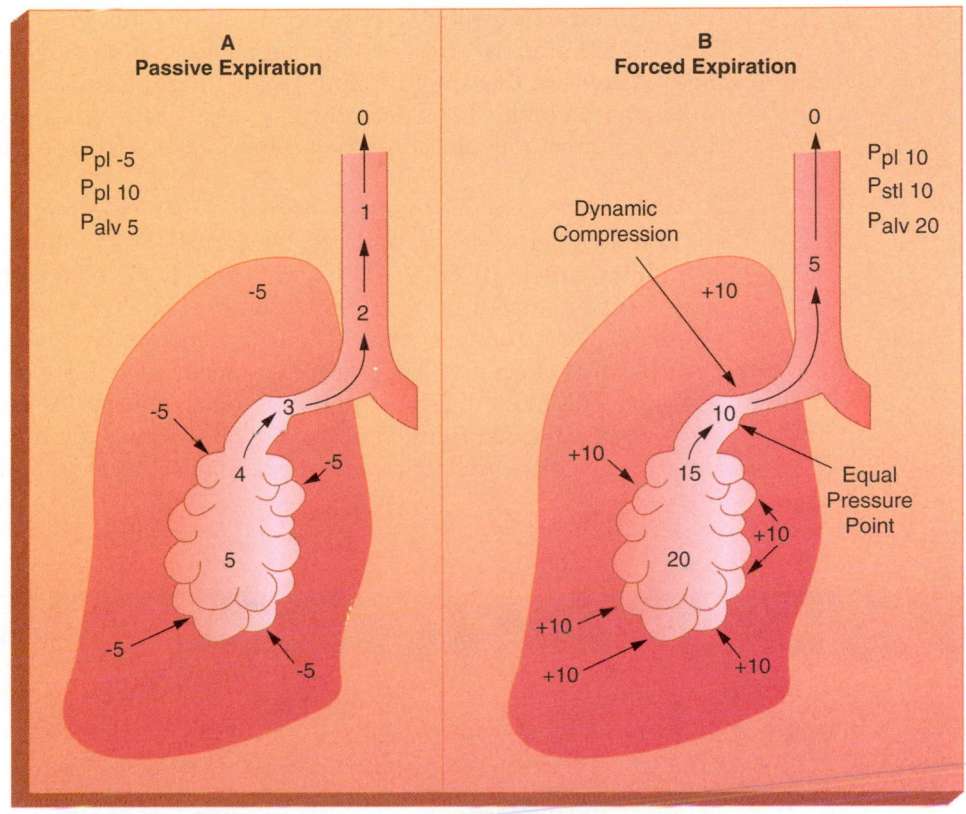

Figure 4–16. *The dynamic compression mechanism. (A) During passive expiration, static elastic recoil pressure of the lungs (P_{stL}) is 10, pleural pressure (P_{pl}) at the beginning of expiration is −5, and alveolar pressure (P_{alv}) is +5. In order for gas to move from the alveolus to the atmosphere during expiration, the pressure must decrease progressively in the airways from +5 to 0. As A shows, P_{pl} is always less than the airway pressure. (B) During forced expiration, P_{pl} becomes positive (+10 in this illustration). When this P_{pl} is added to the P_{stL} of +10, P_{alv} becomes +20. As the pressure progressively decreases during forced expiration, there must be a point at which the pressures inside and outside the airway wall are equal. This point is the* **equal pressure point.** *Airway compression occurs downstream (toward the mouth) from this point because the lateral pressure is less than the surrounding wall pressure.*

Flow is normally not limited to effort during inspiration. This is because the airways widen as greater inspiratory efforts are generated. This action enhances gas flow (see Figure 4–12).

DIFFUSION CAPACITY OF CARBON MONOXIDE (D$_{L_{CO}}$)

The D$_{L_{CO}}$ study measures the amount of carbon monoxide (a diffusion-limited gas*) that moves across the alveolar-capillary membrane. Carbon monoxide (CO)

---

*See diffusion limited, page 120.

has an affinity for hemoglobin that is about 210 times greater than that of oxygen. Thus, in individuals who have normal amounts of hemoglobin and normal ventilatory function, the only limiting factor to the diffusion of CO is the alveolar-capillary membrane. In essence, the $D_{L_{CO}}$ study measures the physiologic status of the various anatomic structures that compose the alveolar-capillary membrane (see Figure 4–2).

The carbon monoxide single-breath technique is commonly used for this measurement. Under normal conditions, the average $D_{L_{CO}}$ value for the resting male is 25 ml/min/mm Hg (STPD). This value is slightly lower in females, presumably because of their smaller normal lung volumes. The $D_{L_{CO}}$ may increase three-fold in healthy subjects during exercise. The $D_{L_{CO}}$ generally decreases in response to lung disorders that effect the alveolar-capillary membrane. For example, the $D_{L_{CO}}$ is decreased in emphysema because of the alveolar-capillary destruction associated with this lung disease. See Figure 3–10 (page 123) for other common lung disorders that affect the alveolar-capillary membrane and cause the $D_{L_{CO}}$ to decrease.

CLINICAL APPLICATION 1

This 16-year-old female with a long history of asthma became short of breath while playing volleyball during her high school gym class. The head coach took her out of the game and had an assistant coach watch her closely. Even though the patient inhaled a total of four puffs of the bronchodilator Ventolin® (albuterol) from her metered-dose inhaler over the next thirty minutes, her condition progressively worsened. Concerned, the coach called the patient's mother. Because the patient had to be given mechanical ventilation on two different occasions, the patient's mother asked the coach to take her daughter directly to the emergency department of the local hospital.

In the emergency room, the patient was observed to be in severe respiratory distress. Her skin was blue and she was using her accessory muscles of inspiration. The patient stated, "My asthma is really getting bad." Her vital signs were: blood pressure—180/110, heart rate—130 beats/min, respiratory rate—36 breaths/min, and oral temperature 37°C. While on 4 L/min oxygen via nasal cannula, her hemoglobin oxygen saturation (Sp_{O_2}), measured by pulse oximetry over the skin of her index finger, was 83 percent.

A portable chest x-ray showed that her lungs were hyperinflated and that her diaphragm was depressed. With a bedside spirometer, the respiratory therapist measured the patient's forced vital capacity (FVC), which in turn provided the following data:

BEDSIDE SPIROMETRY

Parameter*	Predicted	Actual
FVC	2800 ml	1220 ml
FEV$_1$	<83%	44%
PEFR	400 L/min	160 L/min

*FVC = forced vital capacity; FEV$_1$ = forced expiratory volume in 1 second (see text); PEFR = peak expiratory flow rate.

Because the respiratory therapist felt that the patient did not produce a good effort on her first FVC test, a second test was done. Even though the patient appeared to exhale much more forcefully during the second FVC, the spirometry results were identical to the previous findings. The patient's mother stated that her daughter's "personal best" peak expiration flow rate (PEFR) at home was 360 L/min. While the patient was in the emergency room, the nurse started an intravenous (IV) line. The respiratory therapist increased the patient's oxygen via nasal cannula to 6 L/min and then started the patient on a continuous bronchodilator therapy via a hand-held nebulizer per the respiratory care protocol. The medical director of the respiratory care department was notified and a mechanical ventilator was placed on standby.

One hour later, the patient stated that she was breathing easier. Her skin appeared normal and pink and she was no longer using her accessory muscles of inspiration. Her vital signs were: blood pressure—122/76, heart rate—82 beats/min, and respiratory rate—14 breaths/min. On 2 L/min oxygen via nasal cannula her Sp_{O_2} was 97 percent. Her bedside spirometry results at this time were as follows:

BEDSIDE SPIROMETRY

Parameter*	Predicted	Actual
FVC	2800 ml	2375 ml
FEV_1	<83%	84%
PEFR	400 L/min	345 L/min

*FVC = forced vital capacity; FEV_1 = forced expiratory volume in 1 second; PEFR = peak expiratory flow rate.

The patient continued to improve and her oxygen therapy, bronchodilator therapy, and IV were all discontinued the next morning. Her bedside spirometry results were FVC 2810 ml, FEV_1 87 percent, and a PEFR of 355 L/min. She was discharged on the afternoon of the second day. During her exit interview, she was instructed to use her metered-dose inhaler about fifteen minutes before her gym class in the future.

DISCUSSION

This case illustrates (1) how the measurement of a patient's pulmonary mechanics can serve as an important clinical monitor; and (2) the effects and interrelationships of the following on the bronchial airways during a forced expiratory maneuver: the *effort-independent* portion of a forced expiratory maneuver, *dynamic compression,* and the *equal pressure point.*

When the patient was in the emergency room, the fact that her mother knew her daughter's "personal best" PEFR served as an important clinical indicator of the severity of the patient's asthma attack. Today, asthma patients commonly monitor their own PEFR at home to evaluate the severity of an asthmatic episode. Some physicians instruct their patients to call them or to go directly to the hospital when their PEFR decreases to a specific level.

The fact that the respiratory therapist obtained the same bedside spirometry results on the second test demonstrated the effects of *effort-independent flow rate, dynamic compression,* and the *equal pressure point* on the bronchial airways during a forced vital capacity (FVC) maneuver. Remember, approximately the last 70 percent of an FVC maneuver is effort independent because of the dynamic compression of the bronchial airways. When the patient made a stronger muscular effort on the second FVC test, she only moved the equal pressure point (and dynamic compression) of her airways closer to the alveoli—which in turn further increased airway resistance and offset any increase in her FVC (see Figure 4–16).

CLINICAL APPLICATION

This 29-year-old male with no previous history of pulmonary disease went to his family doctor's office complaining of a frequent cough and shortness of breath. He stated that his cough had started about two weeks prior to this admission as a result of breathing paint fumes while working in a small and confined area. Even though the patient stated that he had stopped painting in the enclosed area immediately, his cough and his ability to breathe progressively worsened. At the time of this office visit, he had been too ill to work for two days. Concerned, the physician admitted the patient to the hospital and requested a pulmonary consultation.

In the hospital, the patient appeared as a well-nourished male in severe respiratory distress. His skin was blue and his hospital gown was damp from perspiration. He had a frequent and weak cough. During each coughing episode, he produced a moderate amount of thick, white and yellow sputum. His vital signs were: blood pressure—155/96, heart rate—90 beats/min, and respiratory rate—26 breaths/min. Dull percussion notes were elicited over the lower lobe of the patient's left lung. Rhonchi (wet, gurgle-like sounds) were heard over both lung fields during exhalation, and loud bronchial breath sounds were heard over the left lower lobe.

On 4 L/min oxygen by nasal cannula, the patient's arterial oxygen pressure (Pa_{O_2}) was 63 mm Hg (normal is 80–100 mm Hg). A chest x-ray showed several patches of alveolar collapse (*atelectasis*) throughout the left lower lobe. A pulmonary function study revealed the following results:

PULMONARY FUNCTION STUDY NO. 1

Parameter*	Predicted	Actual
FVC	4600 ml	2990 ml
FEV_1	<83%	67%
$FEF_{200-1200}$	470 L/min	306 L/min
PEFR	<400 L/min	345 L/min
VC	4600 ml	2900 ml
RV	1175 ml	764 ml
FRC	2350 ml	1528 ml

*FVC = forced vital capacity; FEV_1 = forced expiratory volume in first second of an FVC maneuver; $FEF_{200-1200}$ = forced expiratory flow$_{200-1200}$, see text; PEFR = peak expiratory flow rate; VC = vital capacity; RV = residual volume; FRC = functional residual capacity.

In the patient's chart, the physician documented that the excessive bronchial secretions were a result of an acute tracheobronchial tree inflammation (acute bronchitis) caused by the inhalation of noxious paint fumes. The physician also wrote that the patches of atelectasis (see Figure 3–10) identified in the patient's left lower lung lobe were most likely caused by excessive airway secretions and mucus plugging.

The respiratory therapist working with the patient obtained a sputum sample and sent it to the laboratory to determine the source of the possible infection. To help mobilize and clear the excessive bronchial secretions and to offset the mucus plugging, the patient was started on aggressive bronchial hygiene therapy, which consisted of coughing and deep breathing, chest physical therapy, and postural drainage. To treat the atelectasis in the left lower lobe, the patient received lung expansion therapy (also called hyperinflation therapy), which consisted of incentive spirometry, coughing and deep breathing, and continuous positive airway pressure (CPAP) via a face mask.

Three days later, the patient's general appearance had improved significantly and he no longer appeared to be in respiratory distress. His skin was pink and normal. He no longer had a cough. When the patient was asked to cough, the cough was strong and nonproductive. At this time, he was receiving antibiotic therapy for a streptococcal infection that had been identified from a sputum culture. His vital signs were: blood pressure—116/66, heart rate—64 beats/min, respiratory rate—12 breaths/min, and oral temperature of 37°C. Normal percussion notes were elicited over both lungs. Normal bronchial vesicular breath sounds were heard over both lung fields.

On room air, the patient's Pa_{O_2} was 96 mm Hg. A chest x-ray showed no remarkable problems. A second pulmonary function study revealed the results shown in the table at right.

The patient was discharged the following day.

DISCUSSION

This case illustrates both an obstructive and restrictive lung disorder. Because of the excessive bronchial secretions produced by the inhalation of paint fumes and the subsequent streptococcal infection, the patient's FVC, FEV_1, $FEF_{200-1200}$, and PEFR (dynamic flow rate measurements) were all decreased at the time of admission.

In addition, the excessive bronchial secretions (and the patient's weak cough effort)

PULMONARY FUNCTION STUDY NO. 2

Parameter*	Predicted	Actual
FVC	4600 ml	4585 ml
FEV_1	<83%	83%
$FEF_{200-1200}$	470 L/min	458 L/min
PEFR	<400 L/min	455 L/min
VC	4600 ml	4585 ml
RV	1175 ml	1165 ml
FRC	2350 ml	2329 ml

*FVC = forced vital capacity; FEV_1 = forced expiratory volume in first second of an FVC maneuver; $FEF_{200-1200}$ = forced expiratory flow$_{200-1200}$, see text; PEFR = peak expiratory flow rate; VC = vital capacity; RV = residual volume; FRC = functional residual capacity.

caused mucus pooling, and mucus plugging, of the bronchial airways in the left lower lobe. As a result of the mucus plugging, the alveoli distal to the bronchial obstructions could not be ventilated and eventually collapsed. This condition was verified by the chest x-ray and by the decreased VC, RV, and FRC.

Fortunately, his respiratory problems were reversible with aggressive bronchial hygiene therapy and lung expansion therapy. Once the bronchial secretions were cleared, the obstructive problem was no longer present. This was verified by the increased values shown of the FVC, FEV_1, $FEF_{200-1200}$, and PEFR. When the mucus plugs were cleared and the lungs were re-expanded, the restrictive problem was no longer present. This was verified by the increased values of the VC, FRC, and RV.

REVIEW QUESTIONS

1. The volume of air that can be exhaled after a normal tidal volume exhalation is the
   a. IRV
   b. FRC

    c. FVC

    d. ERV

    e. TLC

2. In an obstructive lung disorder, the

    I. FRC is decreased

    II. RV is increased

    III. VC is decreased

    IV. IRV is increased

        a. I and III only

        b. II and III only

        c. II and IV only

        d. II, III, and IV only

        e. I, II, and III only

3. The PEFR in the normal healthy male between 20 and 30 years of age may exceed

    a. 200 L/min

    b. 300 L/min

    c. 400 L/min

    d. 500 L/min

    e. 600 L/min

4. Which of the following can be obtained from a flow-volume loop study?

    I. FVC

    II. PEFR

    III. FEV_T

    IV. $FEF_{25\%-75\%}$

        a. IV only

        b. I and II only

        c. II and III only

        d. I, III, and IV only

        e. I, II, III and IV

5. The MVV in the normal healthy male between 20 and 30 years of age is

    a. 60 L/min

    b. 100 L/min

    c. 170 L/min

    d. 240 L/min

    e. 400 L/min

6. Approximately how much of a forced expiratory maneuver is effort dependent?

    a. 20%

    b. 30%

    c. 40%

    d. 50%

    e. 60%

7. Which of the following forced expiratory measurements reflects the status of medium to small-sized airways?

    a. $FEF_{200-1200}$

    b. PEFR

    c. MVV

    d. $FEF_{25\%-75\%}$

    e. FEV_1/FVC ratio

8. Normally, the percentage of the total volume exhaled during an FEV_1 by a 20-year-old individual is

    a. 60%

    b. 83%

    c. 94%

    d. 97%

    e. 100%

9. Which of the following forced expiratory measurements is a good index of the integrity of large airway function?

    a. FEV_T

    b. $FEF_{200-1200}$

    c. $FEF_{25\%-75\%}$

    d. MVV

    e. FEV_1/FVC

10. The residual volume/total lung capacity ratio in the healthy male between 20 and 30 years old is

    a. 15%

    b. 20%

    c. 25%

    d. 30%

    e. 35%

11. A 73-year-old male, with a long history of smoking, demonstrates the following clinical data on a pulmonary function test (PFT):

PULMONARY FUNCTION STUDY

PFT	BELOW NORMAL	NORMAL	ABOVE NORMAL
VC	X		
RV			X
FRC			X
ERV	X		
FEV_T	X		
$FEF_{25\%-75\%}$	X		
PEFR	X		
MVV	X		

Based upon the above information, the patient appears to have:

a. an obstructive lung disorder

b. a restrictive lung disorder

c. both an obstructive and restrictive lung disorder

d. neither an obstructive or restrictive lung disorder

5

THE CIRCULATORY SYSTEM

OBJECTIVES

By the end of this chapter, the student should be able to:

1. Describe the function of the following specialized cells of the plasma:
   —Erythrocytes
   —Leukocytes
   —Thrombocytes
2. List the chemical components of plasma.
3. Describe the structure and function of the following components of the heart:
   —Inferior and superior venae cavae
   —Right and left atria
   —Right and left ventricles
   —Pulmonary trunk
   —Pulmonary arteries
   —Pulmonary veins
   —Tricuspid valve
   —Bicuspid valve (mitral valve)
   —Pulmonary valve
   —Aortic valve
   —Chordae tendineae
   —Papillary muscles
4. Describe how blood flows through the heart.
5. Identify the major blood vessels that nourish the heart.
6. Describe the location and function of the following components of the *conduction system* of the heart:
   —Sinoatrial node

—Atrioventricular node
—Bundle of His
—Right and left bundle branches
—Purkinje fibers
7. Explain how the following components of the autonomic nervous system coordinate the moment-to-moment *rhythmicity* of the heart:
   —Cardioinhibitor center
   —Cardioaccelerator center
8. Describe the following components of an *electrocardiogram:*
   —P wave
   —QRS complex
   —T wave
9. Identify the *average heart rate* of the normal adult and infant.
10. Describe the following components of the *pulmonary* and *systemic vascular systems:*
    —Arteries
    —Arterioles
    —Capillaries
    —Venules
    —Veins
11. Explain the *neural control* of the vascular systems.
12. Describe the function of the *baroreceptors.*

(continues)

13. Define the following types of *pressures:*
    —Intravascular pressure
    —Transmural pressure
    —Driving pressure
14. Describe how the following relate to the *cardiac cycle* and *blood pressure:*
    —Ventricular systole
    —Ventricular diastole
15. List the *intraluminal blood pressures* throughout the pulmonary and systemic vascular systems.
16. Describe how blood volume affects blood pressure, and include the following:
    —Stroke volume
    —Heart rate
    —Cardiac output
17. Identify the percentage of blood found throughout the various parts of the pulmonary and systemic systems.
18. Describe the influence of *gravity* on blood flow, and include how it relates to
    —Zone 1
    —Zone 2
    —Zone 3
19. Define the following *determinants of cardiac output:*
    —Ventricular preload
    —Ventricular afterload
    —Myocardial contractility
20. Define *vascular resistance.*
21. Describe how the following affect the pulmonary vascular resistance:
    —Active mechanisms
      • Abnormal blood gas values
      • Pharmacologic stimulation
      • Pathologic conditions
    —Passive mechanisms
      • Increased pulmonary arterial pressure
      • Increased left atrial pressure
      • Lung volume and transpulmonary pressure changes
      • Blood volume changes
      • Blood viscosity changes
22. Complete the review questions at the end of this chapter.

The delivery of oxygen to the cells of the body is a function of blood flow. Thus, when the flow of blood is inadequate, good alveolar ventilation is of little value.

The circulatory system consists of the blood, the heart (pump), and the vascular system.

BLOOD

Blood consists of numerous specialized cells that are suspended in a liquid substance called plasma. The cells in the plasma include the erythrocytes (red blood cells), leukocytes (white blood cells), and thrombocytes (or platelets, which are actually cell fragments) (Figure 5–1).

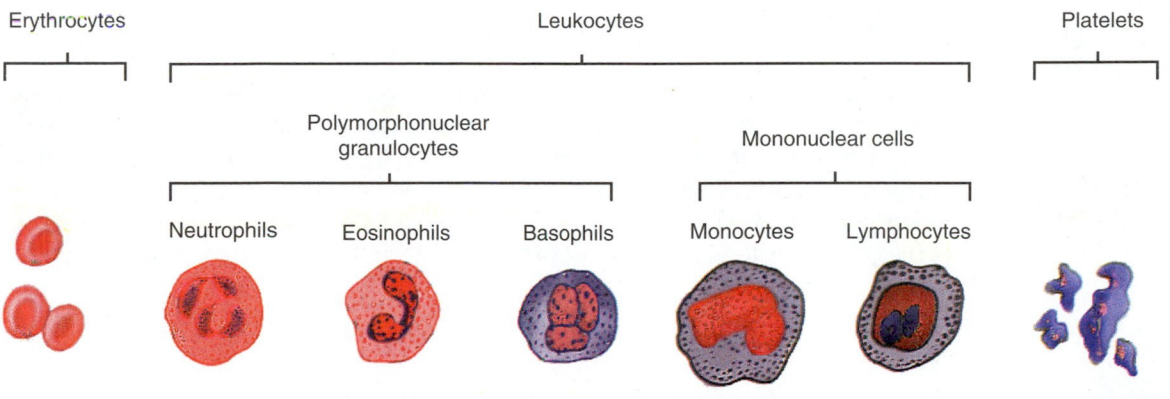

Figure 5–1. *The cells in the blood plasma.*

ERYTHROCYTES

The erythrocytes constitute the major portion of the blood cells. In the healthy adult male there are about 5 million red blood cells (RBCs) in each cubic millimeter of blood. The healthy adult female has about 4 million RBCs in each cubic millimeter of blood. The percentage of RBCs in relation to the total blood volume is known as the hematocrit. The normal hematocrit is approximately 45 percent in the adult male (Figure 5–2) and 42 percent in the adult female. In the normal newborn, the hematocrit ranges between 45 and 60 percent.

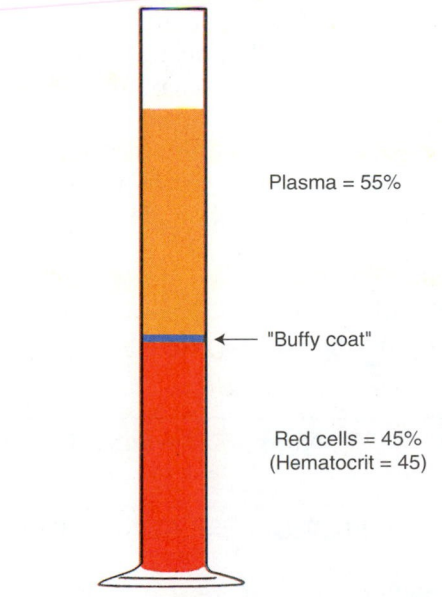

Plasma = 55%

← "Buffy coat"

Red cells = 45%
(Hematocrit = 45)

Figure 5–2. *When a blood-filled capillary tube is centrifuged, the red blood cells become packed at the bottom of the test tube, leaving the fluid plasma at the top of the tube. White cells and platelets form a thin, light-colored "buffy coat" at the interface between the packed red blood cells and the plasma.*

Microscopically, the RBCs appear as biconcave discs, averaging about 7.5 μ in diameter and 2.5 μ in thickness. They are produced in the red bone marrow in the spongy bone of the cranium, bodies of vertebrae, ribs, sternum, and proximal epiphyses of the humerus and femur. It is estimated that the RBCs are produced at the astonishing rate of 2 million cells per second. An equal number of worn-out RBCs are destroyed each second by the spleen and liver. The life span of a RBC is about 120 days. The major constituent of the RBCs is hemoglobin, which is the primary substance responsible for the transport of oxygen and carbon dioxide.

LEUKOCYTES

The primary function of the leukocytes is to protect the body against the invasion of bacteria and other foreign agents that can harm the body. Leukocytes fall into two major groups: (1) the polymorphonuclear granulocytes, which include the neutrophils, eosinophils, and basophils; and (2) the mononuclear or nongranulated cells, which include the monocytes and lymphocytes. The polymorphonuclear granulocytes are produced in the red bone marrow, and the mononuclear cells develop from lymphoid and myeloid tissue.

The leukocytes are far less numerous than the red blood cells, averaging between 5000 to 9000 cells per cubic millimeter of blood. Because the general function of the leukocytes is to combat inflammation and infection, the clinical diagnosis of an injury or infection often entails what is called a *differential count*, which is the determination of the number of each type of white cell in 100 white blood cells. Table 5–1 shows a normal differential count.

The neutrophils are the most active white cells in response to tissue destruction by bacteria. They are one of several types of cells called phagocytes that ingest and destroy particulate matter. They also release an enzyme called lysozyme, which destroys certain bacteria. Thus, a high neutrophil count suggests a bacterial infection.

An elevated eosinophil count indicates an allergic condition, such as an allergic asthmatic episode. Eosinophils are thought to combat the allergen responsible for the allergic reaction. Basophils are also believed to combat allergic reactions.

An elevated number of monocytes indicates a chronic infection (e.g., tuberculosis). Monocytes, which are also phagocytes, take a longer time to reach the site of infection than do neutrophils, but when they do arrive they do so in greater

---

TABLE 5–1. Normal Differential Count

POLYMORPHONUCLEAR GRANULOCYTES		MONONUCLEAR CELLS	
Neutrophils	60–70%	Lymphocytes	20–25%
Eosinophils	2–4%	Monocytes	3–8%
Basophils	0.5–1%		

numbers and destroy more bacteria. Lymphocytes are involved in the production of **antibodies**, which are special proteins that inactivate antigens.

THROMBOCYTES

Thrombocytes, or *blood platelets*, are the smallest of the formed elements in the plasma (see Figure 5–1). The normal platelet count in each cubic millimeter of blood ranges between 250,000 and 500,000. The function of the platelets is to prevent blood loss from a traumatized area of the body involving the smallest blood vessels. They do this by virtue of an activator substance called **platelet factor**, which is a sticky substance that causes blood clotting at the traumatized site. The platelets also contain *serotonin*, which, when released, causes smooth muscle constriction and reduced blood flow.

PLASMA

When all the cells are removed from the blood, a straw-colored liquid called plasma remains. Plasma constitutes about 55 percent of the total blood volume (see Figure 5–2). Approximately 90 percent of plasma consists of water. The remaining 10 percent is composed of proteins, electrolytes, food substances, respiratory gases, hormones, vitamins, and waste products. Table 5–2 outlines the chemical composition of plasma. Blood serum is plasma without its fibrinogen and several other proteins involved in clotting.

TABLE 5–2.   Chemical Composition of Plasma

Water		Food Substances	
	93% of plasma weight	Amino acids	40 mg/100 ml
		Glucose/carbohydrates	100 mg/100 ml
Proteins		Lipids	500 mg/100 ml
Albumins	4.5 g/100 ml	Individual vitamins	0.0001–2.5 mg/100 ml
Globulins	2.5 g/100 ml		
Fibrinogen	0.3 g/100 ml	**Respiratory Gases**	
		O_2	0.3 ml/100 ml
Electrolytes		CO_2	2 ml/100 ml
Cations		N_2	0.9 ml/100 ml
Na^+	143 mEq/L		
K^+	4 mEq/L	**Individual Hormones**	
Ca^{2+}	2.5 mEq/L		0.000001–0.05 mg/100 ml
Mg^{2+}	1.5 mEq/L		
Anions		**Waste Products**	
Cl^-	103 mEq/L	Urea	34 mg/100 ml
PO_4^{3-}	1 mEq/L	Creatinine	1 mg/100 ml
SO_4^{2-}	0.5 mEq/L	Uric Acid	5 mg/100 ml
HCO_3^-	27 mEq/L	Bilirubin	0.2–1.2 mg/100 ml

THE HEART

The **heart** is a hollow, four-chambered, muscular organ that consists of the upper right and left **atria** and the lower right and left **ventricles** (Figure 5–3). The atria are separated by a thin muscular wall called the **interatrial septum**; the ventricles are separated by a thick muscular wall called the **interventricular septum**. The heart actually functions as two separate pumps. The right atrium and ventricle act as one

Right common carotid artery

Left common carotid artery

Right subclavian artery

Left internal jugular vein

Right internal jugular vein

Left subclavian artery

Right subclavian vein

Left subclavian vein

Brachiocephalic artery

Aorta

Ligamentum arteriosum

Superior vena cava

Left pulmonary artery

Right pulmonary artery

Right pulmonary veins

Left pulmonary veins

Left atrium

Pulmonary trunk

Left coronary artery

Right atrium

Circumflex branch

Right coronary artery (posterior descending branch)

Left anterior descending branch

Left ventricle

Right ventricle

Apex

Figure 5–3. *Anterior view of the heart.*

pump to propel unoxygenated blood to the lungs. At the same time, the left atrium and ventricle act as another pump to propel oxygenated blood throughout the systemic circulation.

BLOOD FLOW THROUGH THE HEART

As shown in Figure 5–4, the right atrium receives venous blood from the inferior and superior venae cavae. This blood is low in oxygen and high in carbon dioxide. A one-way valve called the tricuspid valve lies between the right atrium and the right ventricle. The tricuspid valve gets its name from its three valve leaflets, or cusps. The tricuspid leaflets are held in place by tendinous cords called chordae tendineae. The chordae tendineae are secured to the ventricular wall by the papillary muscles. When the ventricles contract, the tricuspid valve closes and blood leaves the right ventricle through the pulmonary trunk and enters the lungs by way of the right and left pulmonary arteries. The pulmonary valve separates the right ventricle from the pulmonary trunk.

Figure 5–4. *Blood flow through the heart.*

After blood passes through the lungs, it returns to the left atrium by way of the pulmonary veins. The returning blood is high in oxygen and low in carbon dioxide. The bicuspid valve (also called the mitral valve) lies between the left atrium and the left ventricle. The bicuspid valve, which consists of two cusps, prevents blood from returning to the left atrium during ventricular contraction. Similarly to the tricuspid valve, the bicuspid valve is also held in position by chordae tendineae and papillary muscles. The left ventricle pumps blood through the ascending aorta. The aortic valve, which lies at the base of the ascending aorta, has semilunar cusps that close in response to the increased pressure in the aorta and thus prevents the backflow of blood into the left ventricle (see Figure 5–4).

BLOOD SUPPLY OF THE HEART

The blood supply that nourishes the heart originates directly from the aorta by means of two arteries—the left coronary artery and the right coronary artery (see Figure 5–3).

The left coronary artery divides into the circumflex and anterior descending branches. The circumflex branch, which runs posteriorly, supplies the lateral wall of the left ventricle and the diaphragmatic surface of the left ventricle. The anterior descending branch supplies the anterior wall of the left ventricle and portions of the right ventricle and interventricular septum.

The right coronary artery supplies the right ventricle and the posterior portion of the septum. The posterior descending branch of the right coronary artery supplies portions of the diaphragmatic surface of the left ventricle.

At rest, the heart receives about 5 percent of the total cardiac output. Most of the blood delivered to the heart returns to the right atrium via the coronary sinus. Some of the venous blood returns to the ventricular chambers via the Thebesian veins. The function of the Thebesian veins, however, is controversial: some investigators feel that, in the left ventricle at least, the Thebesian vein carries oxygenated blood from the ventricular chamber backward into the muscular walls to supply the inner musculature with nutrients.

THE CONDUCTIVE SYSTEM OF THE HEART

The cardiac muscle possesses an intrinsic rhythmicity that enables the heart to initiate the heartbeat without extrinsic stimulation. This unique autorhythmicity is a function of the conductive system of the heart. The components of the conductive system are the sinoatrial node (SA node), atrioventricular node (AV node of AV junction), bundle of His, the right and left bundle branches, and the Purkinje fibers (Figure 5–5).

The SA node, or *pacemaker*, is located in the upper portion of the right atrium. The SA node initiates the cardiac contraction by producing an electrical impulse that travels through the muscle strands of the atria, causing them to contract simultaneously. This action forces the atrial blood into the ventricles. The AV node, located in the lower portion of the right interatrial septum, receives the electrical impulse and relays it to the ventricles via the bundle of His, the right and left bundle branches, and the Purkinje fibers. Stimulation of the Purkinje fibers causes the ventricles to contract simultaneously.

Figure 5–5. *Conductive system of the heart.*

Although the cardiac muscle has an intrinsic rhythmicity, it is also controlled by the *autonomic nervous system,* which enables the heart to respond to the ever-changing needs of the body. Two areas in the medulla oblongata that are responsible for coordinating the moment-to-moment activity of the heart are called the **cardioinhibitor center** and the **cardioaccelerator center;** collectively, they are known as the **cardiac centers**. When activated, the cardioaccelerator center increases the heart rate and increases the strength of contraction by sending sympathetic impulses to the heart. In contrast, the cardioinhibitor center slows the heart and decreases the strength of contraction by sending parasympathetic (vagal) impulses to the heart.

THE ELECTROCARDIOGRAM

The electrical impulses that travel through the conductive system of the heart can be recorded as an **electrocardiogram** (ECG) by means of electrodes placed on the surface of the body. The ECG represents the electrical changes of the heart that result from the depolarization and repolarization of the cardiac muscle (Figure 5–6, page 160).

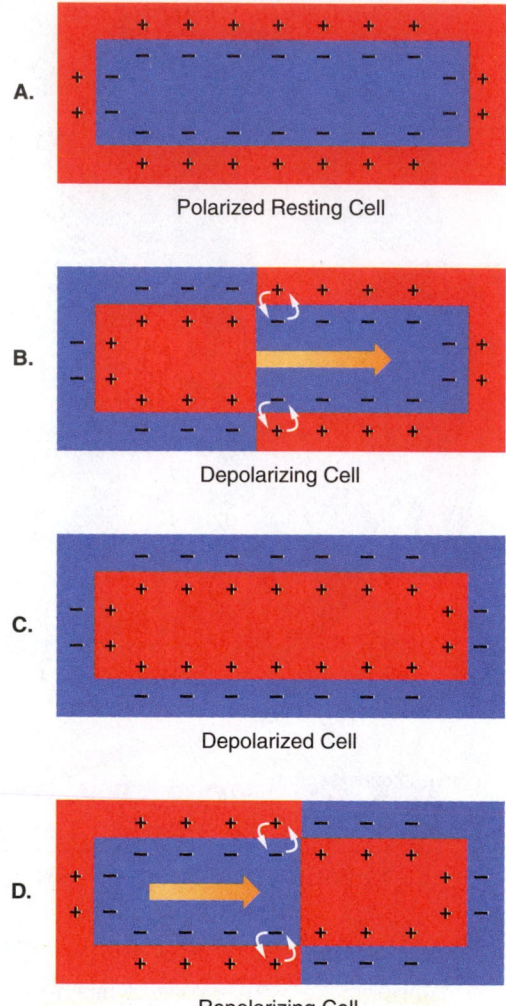

Figure 5–6. *Depolarization and repolarization. A) Polarized resting cell. The heart muscle is in the resting, or polarized, state: that is, the cell carries an electrical charge, with the inside negatively charged with potassium and the outside positively charged with sodium. B) Depolarizing cell. When the muscle cell is stimulated, the cell begins to depolarize: that is, the positively charged ions flow into the cell, and the negatively charged ions flow out of the cell. C) Depolarized cell. During the period that the cell is depolarized, all the positively charged ions are on the inside of the cell, and all the negatively charged ions are on the outside of the cell. D) Repolarizing cell. After the muscle cell has depolarized, it begins to return to the resting state: that is, the negatively charged ions flow into the cell, and the positively charged ions flow out of the cell.*

Figure 5–7 illustrates the ECG of a normal cardiac cycle. The P wave represents the depolarization of the atria, the QRS complex represents ventricular depolarization (the P wave repolarizes during the QRS complex and is not seen on the ECG tracing), and the T wave represents ventricular repolarization. The normal

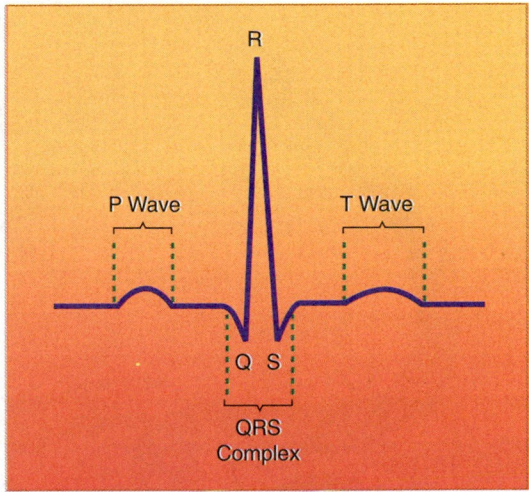

Figure 5–7. *Normal electrocardiogram (ECG) tracing.*

adult heart rate is 60 to 100 beats per minute; it is reduced in well-trained athletes (see Chapter Fourteen). The normal infant heart rate is 130 to 150 beats per minute.

THE PULMONARY AND SYSTEMIC VASCULAR SYSTEMS

The vascular network of the circulatory system is composed of two major subdivisions: the **systemic system** and the **pulmonary system** (Figure 5–8, page 162). The pulmonary system begins with the pulmonary trunk and ends in the left atrium. The systemic system begins with the aorta and ends in the right atrium. Both systems are composed of arteries, arterioles, capillaries, venules, and veins (see Figure 1–24, page 33).

Arteries are vessels that carry blood away from the heart. The arteries are strong, elastic vessels that are well suited for carrying blood under high pressures in the systemic system. The arteries subdivide as they move away from the heart into smaller vessels and, eventually, into vessels called **arterioles**. Arterioles play a major role in the distribution and regulation of blood pressure and are referred to as the **resistance vessels**.

Gas exchange occurs in the **capillaries**. In the capillaries of the pulmonary system, gas exchange is called **external respiration** (gas exchange between blood and air). In the capillaries of the systemic system, gas exchange is called **internal respiration** (gas exchange between blood and tissues).

The **venules** are tiny veins continuous with the capillaries. The venules empty into the veins, which carry blood back to the heart. The veins differ from the arteries in that they are capable of holding a large amount of blood with very little

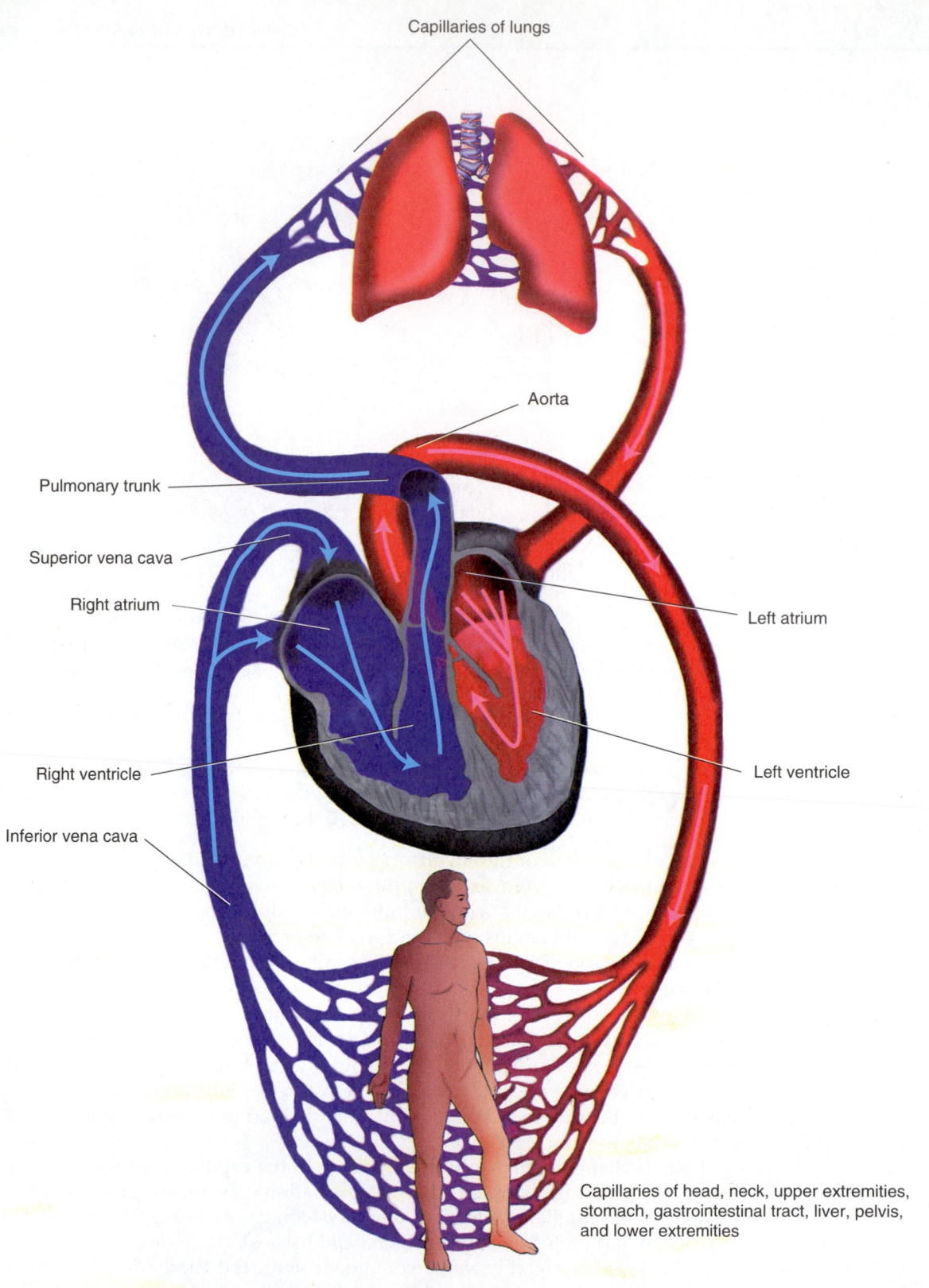

Capillaries of lungs

Aorta

Pulmonary trunk

Superior vena cava

Right atrium

Left atrium

Right ventricle

Left ventricle

Inferior vena cava

Capillaries of head, neck, upper extremities, stomach, gastrointestinal tract, liver, pelvis, and lower extremities

Figure 5–8. *Pulmonary and systemic circulation. The pulmonary circulation is indicated by pink arrows; the systemic circulation is indicated by blue arrows.*

pressure change. Because of this unique feature, the veins are called **capacitance vessels**. Approximately 60 percent of the body's total blood volume is contained within the venous system.

NEURAL CONTROL OF THE VASCULAR SYSTEM

The pulmonary arterioles and most of the arterioles in the systemic circulation are controlled by sympathetic impulses. Sympathetic fibers are found in the arteries, arterioles, and, to a lesser degree, in the veins (Figure 5–9). The **vasomotor center**, which is located in the medulla oblongata, governs the number of sympathetic impulses sent to the vascular systems. Under normal circumstances, the vasomotor center transmits a continual stream of sympathetic impulses to the blood vessels, maintaining the vessels in a moderate state of constriction all the time. This state of vascular contraction is called the **vasomotor tone**.

The vasomotor center coordinates both vasoconstriction and vasodilation by controlling the number of sympathetic impulses that leave the medulla. For example, when the vasomotor center is activated to constrict a particular vascular region (i.e., more than the normal state of constriction), it does so by increasing the number of sympathetic impulses to that vascular area. In contrast, the vasomotor center initiates vasodilation by reducing the number of sympathetic impulses sent to a certain vascular region. (The major vascular beds in the systemic system that are *not* controlled by this mechanism are the arterioles of the heart, brain, and skeletal muscles. Sympathetic impulses to these vessels cause vasodilation.) In addition to the sympathetic control, blood flow through the large veins can be affected by abdominal and intrathoracic pressure changes.

Working together, the vasomotor center and the cardiac centers in the medulla oblongata regulate the arterial blood pressure in response to signals received from special pressure receptors located throughout the body. These pressure receptors are called **arterial baroreceptors**.

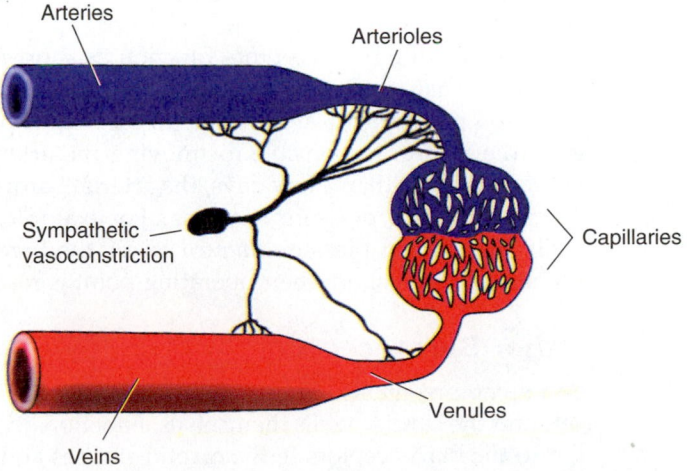

Figure 5–9.   *Neural control of the vascular system. Sympathetic neural fibers to the arterioles are especially abundant.*

THE BARORECEPTOR REFLEX

Specialized stretch receptors called baroreceptors (also called *pressoreceptors*) are located in the walls of the carotid arteries and the aorta. In the carotid arteries, the baroreceptors are found in the carotid sinuses high in the neck where the common carotid arteries divide into the external and internal carotid arteries (Figure 5–10). The walls of the carotid sinuses are thin and contain a large number of branching, vinelike nerve endings that are sensitive to stretch or distortion. The afferent fibers from the carotid sinuses travel with the glossopharyngeal nerve (ninth cranial) to the medulla. In the aorta, the baroreceptors are located in the aortic arch (see Figure 5–10). The afferent fibers from the aortic arch baroreceptors travel with the vagus nerve (tenth cranial).

The baroreceptors regulate the arterial blood pressure by initiating reflex adjustments to deviations in blood pressure. For example, when the arterial pressure decreases, the neural impulses transmitted from the baroreceptors to the vasomotor and cardiac centers in the medulla also decrease. This causes the medulla to increase its sympathetic activity, which, in turn, causes an increase in the following:

- Heart rate
- Myocardial force of contraction
- Arterial constriction
- Venous constriction

The net result is (1) an increased cardiac output (because of an increased heart rate and stroke volume), (2) an increase in the total peripheral resistance (primarily induced by arterial constriction), and (3) the return of blood pressure toward normal. The vascular constriction occurs primarily in the abdominal region (including the liver, spleen, pancreas, stomach, intestine, kidneys, skin, and skeletal muscles).

In contrast, when the blood pressure increases, the neural impulses from the arterial baroreceptors increase. This causes the medulla to decrease its sympathetic activity, which in turn reduces both the cardiac output and the total peripheral resistance.

Finally, the baroreceptors function as short-term regulators of arterial blood pressure. That is, they respond instantly to any blood pressure change to restore the blood pressure toward normal (to the degree possible in the situation). If, however, the factors responsible for moving the arterial pressure away from normal persist for more than a few days, the arterial baroreceptors will eventually come to "accept" the new pressure as normal. For example, in individuals who have chronically high blood pressure (*hypertension*), the baroreceptors still operate, but at a higher level—in short, their operating point is reset at a higher level.

Other Baroreceptors

Baroreceptors are also found in the large arteries, large veins, and pulmonary vessels and the cardiac walls themselves. Functionally, most of these receptors are similar to the baroreceptors in the carotid sinuses and aortic arch in that they send an increased rate of neural transmissions to the medulla in response to increased pressure. By means of these additional receptors, the medulla gains a further degree of

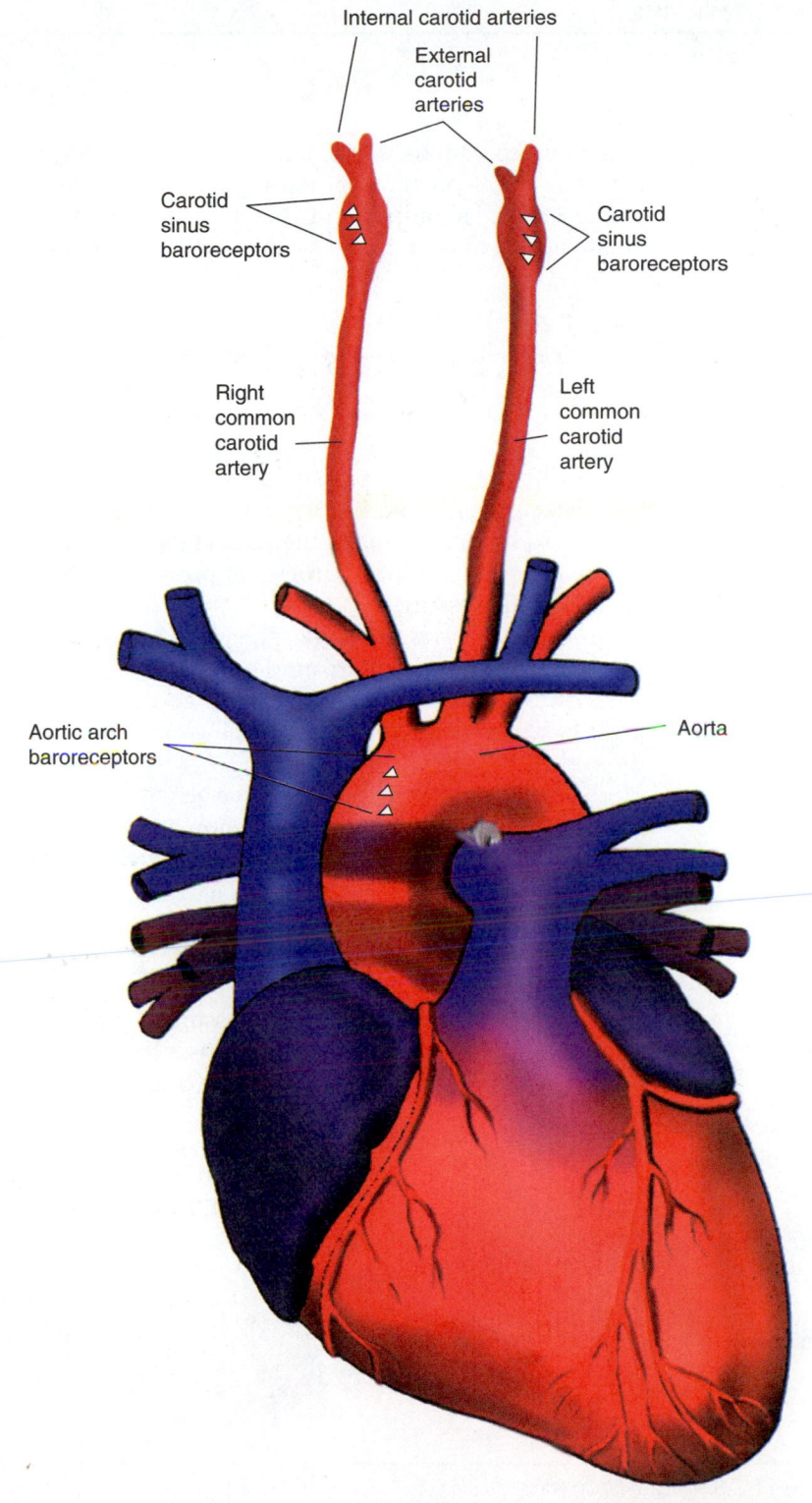

Figure 5–10. *Location of the arterial baroreceptors.*

sensitivity to venous, atrial, and ventricular pressures. For example, a slight decrease in atrial pressure initiates sympathetic activity even before there is a decrease in cardiac output and therefore, a decrease in the arterial blood pressure great enough to be detected by the aortic and carotid baroreceptors.

PRESSURES IN THE PULMONARY AND SYSTEMIC VASCULAR SYSTEMS

Three different types of pressures are used to study the blood flow: (1) intravascular, (2) transmural, and (3) driving pressures.

Intravascular pressure is the actual blood pressure in the lumen of any vessel at any point, relative to the barometric pressure. This pressure is also known as the intraluminal pressure.

Transmural pressure is the difference between the intravascular pressure of a vessel and the pressure surrounding the vessel. The transmural pressure is *positive* when the pressure inside the vessel exceeds the pressure outside the vessel, and *negative* when the pressure inside the vessel is less than the pressure surrounding the vessel.

Driving pressure is the difference between the pressure at one point in a vessel and the pressure at any other point downstream in the vessel.

Figure 5–11 illustrates the different types of pressures used to study the flow of blood.

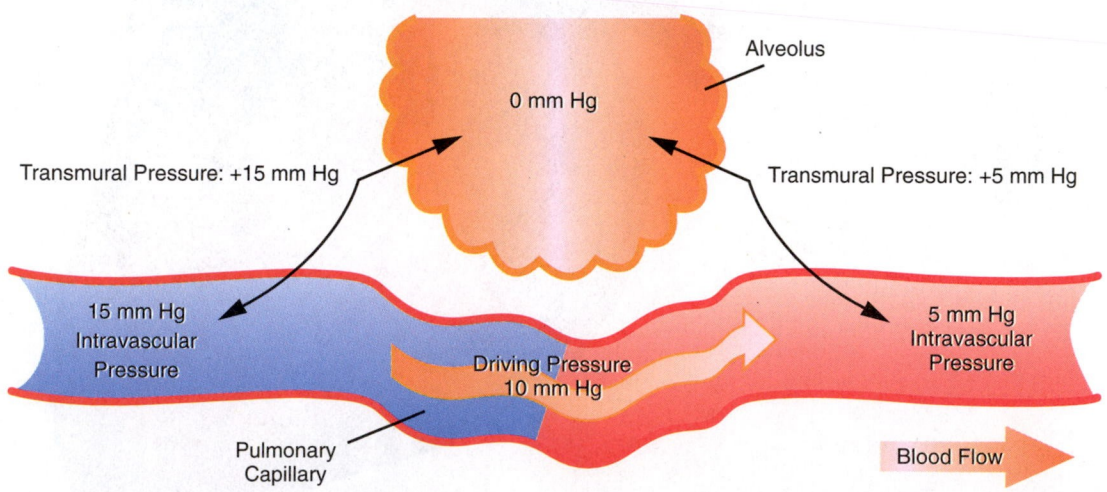

Figure 5–11. *Schematic illustration of a blood vessel and an alveolus showing the types of blood pressures used to study flood flow. Within the blood vessel, the* intravascular pressure *at point A is 15 mm Hg, and the intravascular pressure at point B is 5 mm Hg. The pressure within the alveolus (which represents the pressure surrounding the blood vessel) is zero. In view of these numbers, the following can be stated: (1) the* transmural pressure *at point A is a positive 15 mm Hg, (2) the* transmural pressure *at point B is a positive 5 mm Hg, and (3) the* driving pressure *between point A and point B is 10 mm Hg.*

THE CARDIAC CYCLE AND ITS EFFECT ON BLOOD PRESSURE

The arterial blood pressure rises and falls in a pattern that corresponds to the phases of the cardiac cycle. When the ventricles contract (ventricular systole), blood is forced into the pulmonary artery and the aorta, and the pressure in these arteries rises sharply. The maximum pressure generated during ventricular contraction is the systolic pressure. When the ventricles relax (ventricular diastole), the arterial pressure drops. The lowest pressure that remains in the arteries prior to the next ventricular contraction is the diastolic pressure (Figure 5–12). In the systemic system, normal systolic pressure is about 120 mm Hg and normal diastolic pressure is about 80 mm Hg. In the pulmonary system, the normal systolic pressure is about 25 mm Hg and the normal diastolic pressure is about 8 mm Hg (Figure 5–13, page 168).

The pulmonary circulation is a low-pressure system. The mean pressure in the pulmonary artery is about 15 mm Hg, and the mean pressure in the left atrium is about 5 mm Hg. Thus, the driving pressure needed to move blood through the lungs is 10 mm Hg. In contrast, the mean intraluminal pressure in the aorta is about 100 mm Hg and the mean right atrial pressure is about 2 mm Hg, making the driving pressure through the systemic system about 98 mm Hg. Compared to the pulmonary circulation, the pressure in the systemic system is about 10 times greater. Figure 5–14 (page 169) shows the mean intraluminal blood pressures throughout both the pulmonary and systemic vascular systems.

The surge of blood rushing into the arterial system during each ventricular contraction causes the elastic walls of the arteries to expand. When the ventricular contraction stops, the pressure drops almost immediately and the arterial walls

Figure 5–12.   *Sequence of cardiac contraction. A) Ventricular diastole and atrial systole; B) Ventricular systole and atrial diastole.*

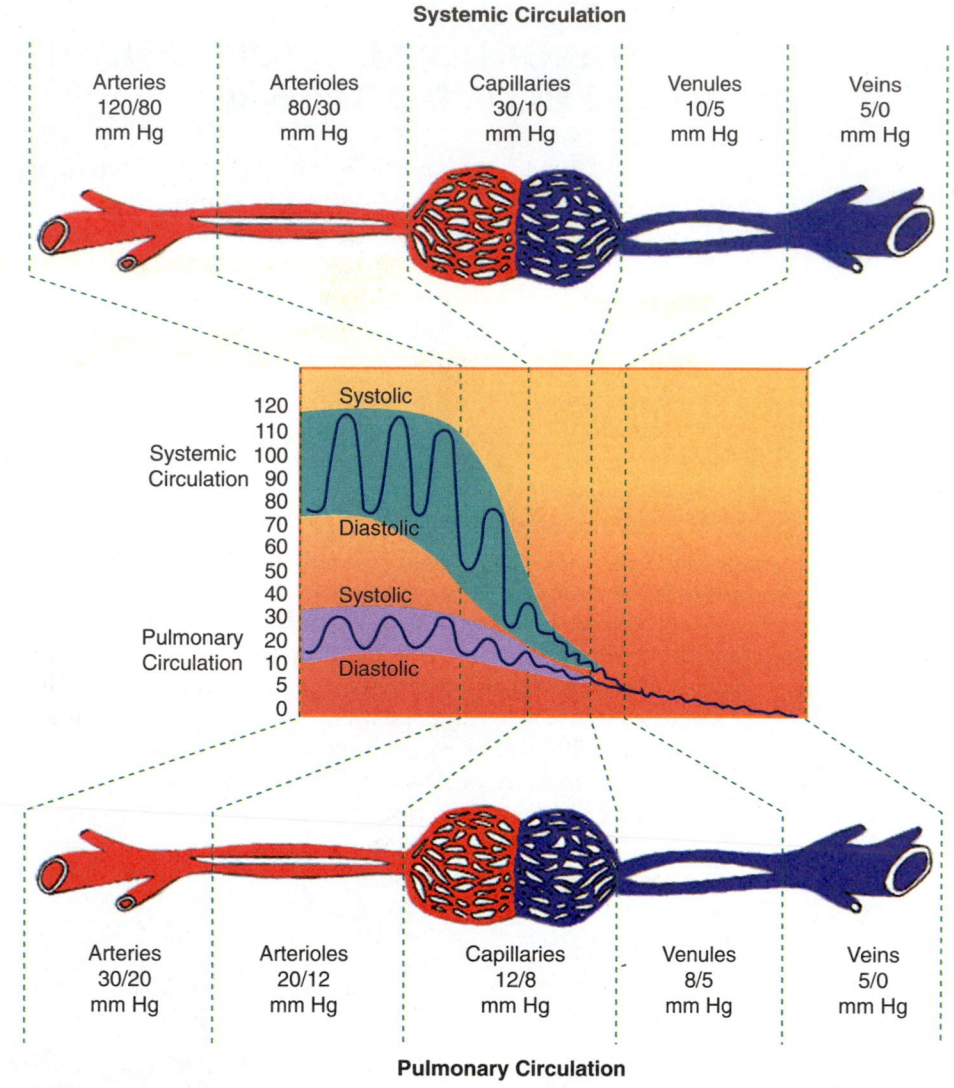

Figure 5–13. *Summary of diastolic and systolic pressures in various segments of the circulatory system.*

recoil. This alternating expansion and recoil of the arterial wall can be felt as a pulse in several systemic arteries that run close to the skin's surface. Figure 5–15 (page 170) shows the major sites where a pulse can be detected by palpation.

THE BLOOD VOLUME AND ITS EFFECT ON BLOOD PRESSURE

The volume of blood ejected from the ventricle during each contraction is called the stroke volume. Normally, the stroke volume ranges between 40 ml and 80 ml. The total volume of blood discharged from the ventricles per minute is called cardiac

Figure 5–14. *Mean intraluminal blood pressure at various points in the pulmonary and systemic circulation.*

output. The cardiac output (CO) is calculated by multiplying the stroke volume (SV) by the heart rate (HR) per minute (CO = SV × HR). Thus, if the stroke volume is 70 ml, and the heart rate is 72 beats per minute, the cardiac output is 5040 ml per minute.

Under normal circumstances, the cardiac output directly influences blood pressure. In other words, *when either the stroke volume or heart rate increases, the blood pressure increases.* Or conversely, when the stroke volume or heart rate decreases, the blood pressure decreases.

Although the total blood volume varies with age, body size, and sex, the normal adult volume is about 5 liters. Of this volume, about 75 percent is in the systemic circulation, 15 percent in the heart, and 10 percent in the pulmonary circulation. Overall, about 60 percent of the total blood volume is in the veins, and about

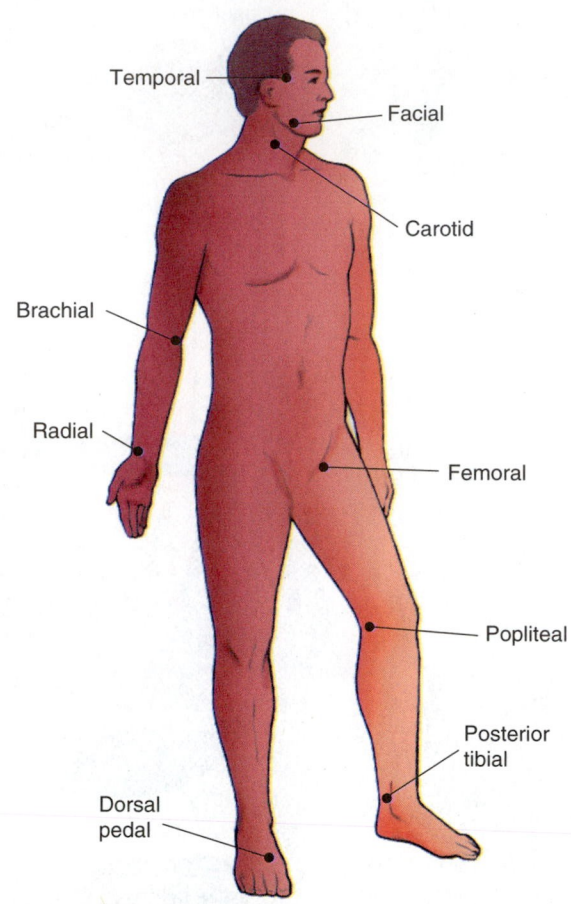

Temporal

Facial

Carotid

Brachial

Radial

Femoral

Popliteal

Posterior tibial

Dorsal pedal

Figure 5–15.   *Major sites where an arterial pulse can be detected.*

10 percent is in the arteries. Normally, the pulmonary capillary bed contains about 75 ml of blood, although it has the capacity for about 200 ml.

THE DISTRIBUTION OF PULMONARY BLOOD FLOW

In the upright lung, blood flow progressively decreases from the base to the apex (Figure 5–16). This linear distribution of blood is a function of (1) gravity, (2) cardiac output, and (3) pulmonary vascular resistance.

GRAVITY

Because blood is a relatively heavy substance, it is gravity dependent; i.e., it naturally moves to the portion of the body, or portion of the organ, that is closest to the

Figure 5–16. *Distribution of pulmonary blood flow. In the upright lung, blood flow steadily increases from the apex to the base.*

ground. In the average lung, there is a distance of about 30 centimeters (cm) between the base and the apex. The blood that fills the lung from the bottom to the top is analogous to a column of water 30 cm long and, therefore, exerts a pressure of about 30 cm H_2O (22 mm Hg) between the base and apex. Because the pulmonary artery enters each lung about midway between the top and bottom of the lung, the pulmonary artery pressure has to be greater than 15 cm H_2O (11 mm Hg) to overcome the gravitational force and, thereby, supply blood to the lung apex. For this reason, most of the blood flows through (or falls into) the lower half of the lung—the gravity-dependent portion of the lung.

As a result of the gravitational effect on blood flow, the intraluminal pressures of the vessels in the gravity-dependent area (lower lung region) are greater than the intraluminal pressures in the least gravity-dependent area (upper lung region). The high intraluminal pressure of the vessels in the gravity-dependent area causes the vessels to distend. As the vessels widen, the vascular resistance decreases and, thus, permits blood flow to increase. The fact that blood flow is enhanced as the vascular system widens is according to Poiseuille's law for flow ($\dot{V} \simeq Pr^4$).

The position of the body can significantly change the gravity-dependent portion of the lungs. For example, when an individual is in the supine position (lying on the back), the gravity-dependent area is the posterior portion of the lungs; when an individual is in the prone position (lying on the stomach), the gravity-dependent region is the anterior portion of the lungs; when the person is lying on the side, the lower, lateral half of the lung nearest the ground is gravity dependent; when an individual is suspended upside down, the apices of the lungs become gravity dependent (Figure 5–17, page 172).

Figure 5–18 (page 173) uses a three-zone model to illustrate the effects of gravity and alveolar pressure on the distribution of pulmonary blood flow:

In **Zone 1** (the least gravity-dependent area), the alveolar pressure is sometimes greater than both the arterial and the venous intraluminal pressures. As a

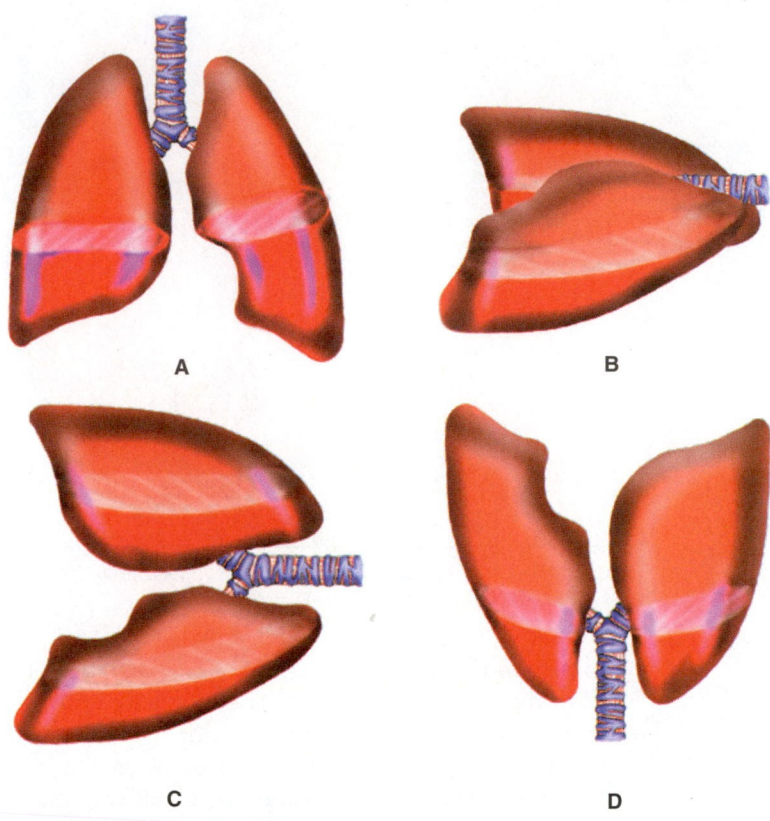

Figure 5–17. *Blood flow normally moves into the gravity-dependent areas of the lungs. Thus, body position affects the distribution of the pulmonary blood flow as illustrated in the erect (A), supine (B), lateral (C), and upside-down (D) positions.*

result, the pulmonary capillaries can be compressed and blood is prevented from flowing through this region. Under normal circumstances, this situation does not occur, since the pulmonary arterial pressure (generated by the cardiac output) is usually sufficient to raise the blood to the top of the lungs and to overcome the alveolar pressure. There are, however, a variety of conditions—such as severe hemorrhage, dehydration, and positive pressure ventilation—that can result in the alveolar pressure being higher than the arterial and venous pressures. When the alveoli are ventilated but not perfused, no gas exchange can occur and **alveolar dead space** is said to exist (see Figure 2–28, page 88).

In **Zone 2**, the arterial pressure is greater than the alveolar pressure and, therefore, the pulmonary capillaries are perfused. Because the alveolar pressure is greater than the venous pressure, the effective driving pressure for blood flow is determined by the pulmonary arterial pressure minus the alveolar pressure—not the normal arterial-venous pressure difference. Thus, because the alveolar pressure is essentially the same throughout all the lung regions, and because the arterial pressure progressively increases toward the gravity-dependent areas of the lung, the effective driving pressure (arterial pressure minus alveolar pressure) steadily

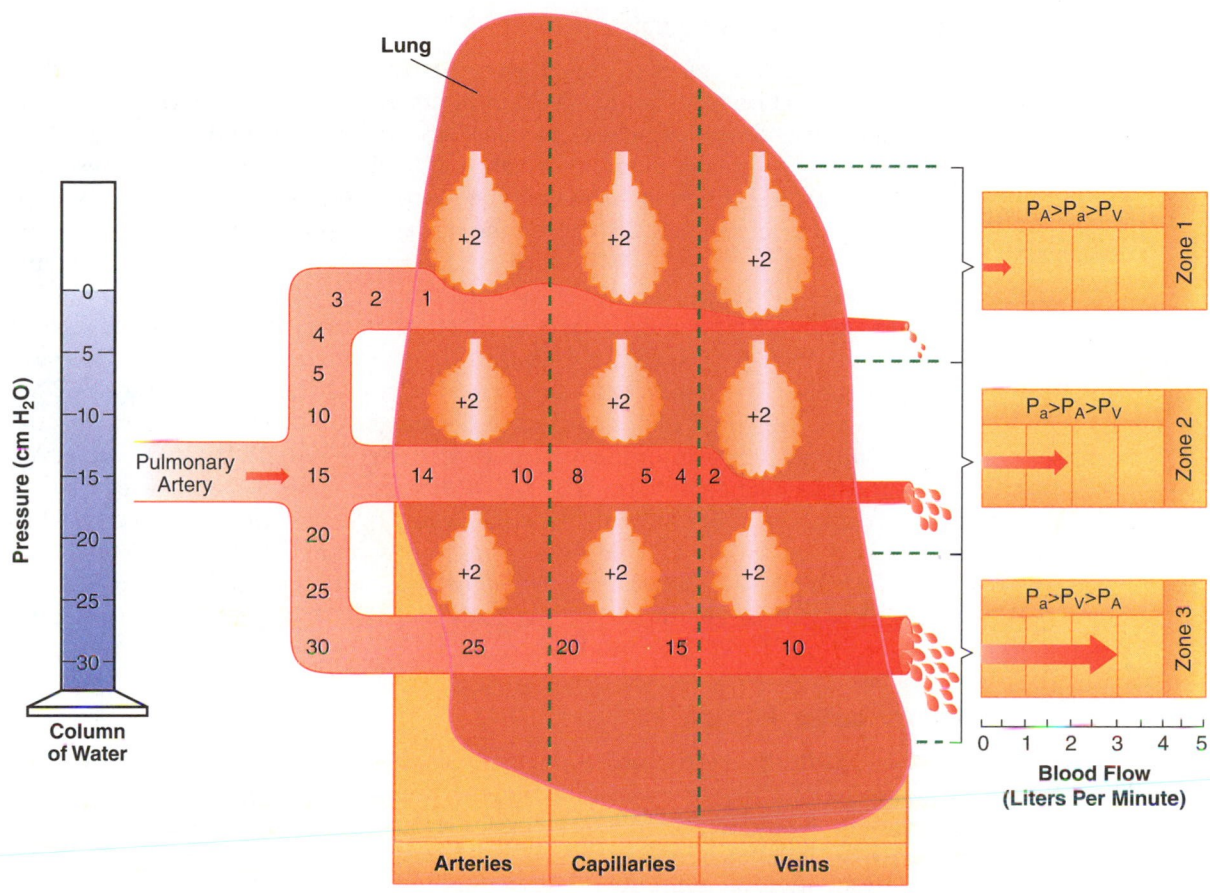

Figure 5–18. *Relationship between gravity, alveolar pressure (PA), pulmonary arterial pressure (Pa), and pulmonary venous pressure (Pv̄) in different lung zones. Note: The +2 cm H₂O pressure in the alveoli (e.g., during expiration) was arbitrarily selected for this illustration.*

increases down the vertical axis of Zone 2. As a result, from the beginning of the upper portion of Zone 2 (the point at which the arterial pressure equals the alveolar pressure) to the lower portion of Zone 2 (the point at which the venous pressure equals the alveolar pressure) the flow of blood progressively increases.

In **Zone 3** (gravity-dependent area), both the arterial and the venous pressures are greater than the alveolar pressure, and therefore blood flow through this region is constant. Because the arterial pressure and venous pressure both increase equally downward in Zone 3, the arterial-venous pressure difference and, therefore, blood flow is essentially the same throughout all of Zone 3.

DETERMINANTS OF CARDIAC OUTPUT

As described earlier, the cardiac output is equal to the stroke volume times the heart rate. The stroke volume is determined by (1) ventricular preload, (2) ventricular afterload, and (3) myocardial contractility.

Ventricular Preload

Ventricular preload refers to the degree that the myocardial fiber is stretched prior to contraction (*end-diastole*). Within limits, the more the myocardial fiber is stretched during diastole (*preload*), the more strongly it will contract during systole, and therefore the greater the myocardial contractility will be. This mechanism enables the heart to convert an increased venous return into an increased stroke volume. Beyond a certain point, however, the cardiac output does not improve as the preload increases.

Because the degree of myocardial fiber stretch (*preload*) is a function of the pressure generated by the volume of blood returning to the ventricle during diastole, ventricular preload is reflected in the **ventricular end-diastolic pressure (VEDP)**—which, in essence, reflects the **ventricular end-diastolic volume (VEDV)**. In other words, as the VEDV increases or decreases, the VEDP (and, therefore, the cardiac output) increases or decreases, respectively. It should be noted, however, that, similar to lung compliance (C_L), VEDP and VEDV are also influenced by ventricular compliance. For example, when the ventricular compliance is decreased as a result of disease, the VEDP increases significantly more than the VEDV.

The relationship between the VEDP (degree of myocardial stretch) and cardiac output (stroke volume) is known as the **Frank-Starling relationship** (Figure 5–19).

Ventricular Afterload

Ventricular afterload is defined as the force against which the ventricles must work to pump blood. It is determined by several factors, including (1) the volume and viscosity of the blood ejected, (2) the peripheral vascular resistance, and (3) the total cross-sectional area of the vascular space into which blood is ejected. The arterial systolic blood pressure best reflects the ventricular afterload. For example, as the arterial systolic pressure increases, the resistance (against which the heart must work to eject blood) also increases. Clinically, this condition is particularly serious in the patient with a failing heart and low stroke volume. By reducing the peripheral resistance (*afterload reduction*) in such patients, the stroke volume increases with little or no change in the blood pressure. This is because blood pressure (BP) is a function of the cardiac output (CO) times the systemic vascular resistance (SVR) (BP = CO × SVR).

Myocardial Contractility

Myocardial contractility may be regarded as the force generated by the myocardium when the ventricular muscle fibers shorten. In general, when the contractility of the heart increases or decreases, the cardiac output increases or decreases, respectively.

There is no single measurement that defines contractility in the clinical setting. Changes in contractility, however, can be inferred through clinical assessment (e.g., pulse, blood pressure, skin temperature) and serial hemodynamic measurements (discussed in Chapter Six). An increase in myocardial contractility is referred to as **positive inotropism**. A decrease in myocardial contractility is referred to as **negative inotropism**.

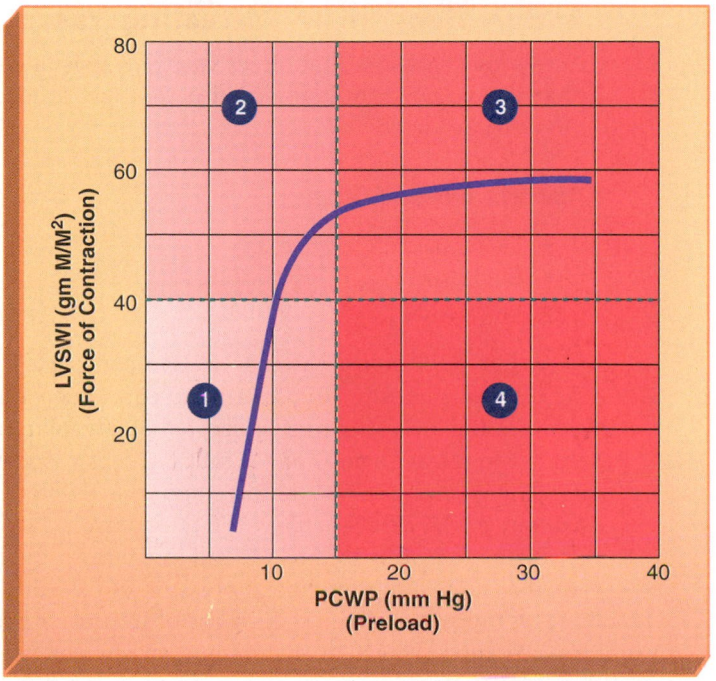

Figure 5–19.   *Frank-Starling curve. The Frank-Starling curve shows that the more the myocardial fiber is stretched as a result of the blood pressure that develops as blood returns to the chambers of the heart during diastole, the more the heart muscle will contract during systole. In addition, it will contract with greater force. The stretch produced within the myocardium at end-diastole is called preload.* Clinically, it would be best to determine the preload of the left ventricle by measuring the end-diastolic pressure of the left ventricle or left atrium. However, since it is impractical to measure this at the patient's bedside, the best preload approximation of the left heart is the pulmonary capillary wedge pressure (PCWP). As shown in this illustration, the relationship of the PCWP (preload) to the left ventricular stroke work index (LVSWI) (force of contraction) may appear in four quadrants: (1) hypovolemia, (2) optimal function, (3) hypervolemia, and (4) cardiac failure.*

VASCULAR RESISTANCE

Circulatory resistance is derived by dividing the mean blood pressure (BP) by the cardiac output (CO):

$$\text{Resistance} = \frac{\text{BP}}{\text{CO}}$$

In general, when the vascular resistance increases, the blood pressure increases (which, in turn, increases the ventricular afterload). Because of this relationship, blood pressure monitoring can be used to reflect pulmonary or systemic resistance. That is, when resistance increases or decreases, the blood pressure will likely increase or decrease.

In the pulmonary system, there are several known mechanisms that change the vascular resistance. Such mechanisms are classified as either *active* or *passive mechanisms.*

Active Mechanisms Affecting Vascular Resistance

Active mechanisms that affect vascular resistance include abnormal blood gases, pharmacologic stimulation, and pathologic conditions that have a direct effect on the vascular system.

Abnormal Blood Gases

- Decreased P_{O_2} (Hypoxia)
- Increased P_{CO_2} (Hypercapnia)
- Decreased pH (Acidemia)

The pulmonary vascular system constricts in response to a decreased alveolar oxygen pressure (hypoxia). The exact mechanism of this phenomenon is unclear. Some investigators suggest that alveolar hypoxia causes the lung parenchyma to release a substance that produces vasoconstriction. It is known, however, that the partial pressure of oxygen in the *alveoli* ($P_{A_{O_2}}$)—not the partial pressure of oxygen of the *capillary blood* ($P_{C_{O_2}}$)—controls this response. The effect of hypoxic vasoconstriction is to direct blood away from the hypoxic lung regions to lung areas that have a higher partial pressure of oxygen.

Clinically, when the number of hypoxic regions becomes significant (e.g., in the advanced stages of emphysema or chronic bronchitis), generalized pulmonary vasoconstriction can develop. This can cause a substantial increase in the pulmonary vascular resistance and in the work of the right heart. This in turn leads to right ventricular hypertrophy, or *cor pulmonale*.

Pulmonary vascular resistance increases in response to an acute increase in the P_{CO_2} level (hypercapnia). It is believed, however, that the vasoconstriction that occurs is most likely due to the increased hydrogen ion (H^+) concentration (*respiratory acidosis*) that develops from a sudden increase in the P_{CO_2} level, rather than to the P_{CO_2} itself. This is supported by the fact that pulmonary vasoconstriction does not occur when hypercapnia is accompanied by a normal pH (*compensated respiratory acidosis*).

Pulmonary vasoconstriction develops in response to decreased pH (increased H^+ concentration), or acidemia, of either metabolic or respiratory origin.

Pharmacologic Stimulation. The pulmonary vessels constrict in response to various pharmacologic agents, including:

- Epinephrine (Adrenalin®)
- Norepinephrine (Levophed®, Levarterenol®)
- Dobutamine (Dobutrex®)
- Dopamine (Intropin®)
- Phenylephrine (Neo-Synephrine®)

Constricted pulmonary vessels relax in response to the following agents:

- Oxygen
- Isoproterenol (Isuprel®)
- Aminophylline
- Calcium-blocking agents

Pathologic Conditions.   Pulmonary vascular resistance increases in response to a number of pathologic conditions. Some of the more common ones are:

- Vessel blockage or obstruction—e.g., caused by a thrombus or an embolus (blood clot, fat cell, air bubble, or tumor mass)
- Vessel wall diseases—e.g., sclerosis, polyarteritis, or scleroderma
- Vessel destruction or obliteration—e.g., emphysema or pulmonary interstitial fibrosis
- Vessel compression—e.g., pneumothorax, hemothorax, or tumor mass

Pathologic disturbances in the pulmonary vasculary system can develop in the arteries, arterioles, capillaries, venules, or veins. When increased vascular resistance originates in the venules or veins, the transmural pressure increases and, in severe cases, causes the capillary fluid to spill into the alveoli. This is called pulmonary edema. Left ventricular failure will cause the same pathologic disturbances. When the resistance originates in the arteries or arterioles, the pulmonary artery pressure will increase but the pulmonary capillary pressure will be normal or low. Regardless of the origin of the pathologic disturbance, a severe and persistent pulmonary vascular resistance is ultimately followed by an elevated right ventricular pressure, right ventricular strain, right ventricular hypertrophy, and right heart failure.

Passive Mechanisms Affecting Vascular Resistance

The term *passive mechanism* refers to a secondary change in pulmonary vascular resistance that occurs in response to another mechanical change. In other words, when a mechanical factor in the respiratory system changes, a passive increase or decrease in the caliber of the pulmonary blood vessels also occurs. Some of the more common passive mechanisms are:

Pulmonary Arterial Pressure Changes.   As pulmonary arterial pressure increases (either by increasing the height of the perfusion reservoir or by increasing blood flow), the pulmonary vascular resistance decreases (Figure 5–20, page 178). This is assuming that lung volume and left atrial pressure remain constant. The pulmonary vascular resistance decreases because of the increase in intraluminal distending pressure, which increases the total cross-sectional areas of the pulmonary vascular system through the mechanisms of recruitment and distension.

As shown in Figure 5–21 (page 178), *recruitment* entails the opening of vessels that were closed or not being utilized for blood flow before the vascular pressure increased. *Distension*, on the other hand, entails the stretching or widening of vessels that were open, but not to their full capacity. Both of these mechanisms increase the total cross-sectional area of the vascular system, which, in turn, reduces the vascular resistance. These mechanisms, however, have their limits.

Left Atrial Pressure Changes.   As the left atrial pressure increases, while the lung volume and pulmonary arterial pressure are held constant, pulmonary vascular resistance decreases.

Figure 5–20. *Increased mean pulmonary arterial pressure decreases pulmonary vascular resistance.*

Figure 5–21. *Schematic drawing of the mechanisms that may be activated to decrease pulmonary vascular resistance when the mean pulmonary artery pressure increases. (A) A group of pulmonary capillaries, one-half of which are not perfused. (B) The previously unperfused capillaries shown in A are recruited (i.e., opened) in response to the increased pulmonary artery pressure. (C) The increased blood pressure has distended the capillaries that are already open.*

Lung Volume Changes.   The effect of changes in lung volume on pulmonary vascular resistance varies according to the location of the vessel. Two major groups of vessels must be considered: (1) alveolar vessels—those vessels that surround the alveoli (*pulmonary capillaries*)— and (2) extra-alveolar vessels—the larger arteries and veins.

Alveolar Vessels.   Because the pulmonary capillary vessels are so thin, intrapleural pressure changes directly affect the anatomy of the capillaries. During normal inspiration, the alveolar vessels progressively stretch and flatten. During expiration, the alveolar vessels shorten and widen. Thus, as the lungs are inflated, the resistance offered by the alveolar vessels progressively increases (Figure 5–22). During the inspiratory phase of mechanical ventilation (*positive pressure phase*), moreover, the resistance generated by the alveolar vessels may become excessively high and, as a result, restrict the flow of pulmonary blood. The pressure difference between the alveoli and the inside of the pulmonary capillaries is called the *transmural pressure* (see Figure 5–11).

Extra-alveolar Vessels.   The extra-alveolar vessels (the large arterioles and veins) are also exposed to the intrapleural pressure. However, they behave differently from the pulmonary capillaries (alveolar vessels) when subjected to volume and pressure changes. That is, as the lung volume increases in response to a more negative intrapleural pressure during inspiration, the transmural pressure increases (i.e., the pressure within the vessels becomes more positive) and the extra-alveolar vessels distend (Figure 5–22). A second factor that dilates the extra-alveolar vessels at higher lung volumes is the radial traction generated by the connective tissue and by the alveolar septa that hold the larger vessels in place throughout the lung.

Another type of extra-alveolar vessel is the so-called "corner vessel," located at the junction of the alveolar septa. As the lung volume increases, the corner

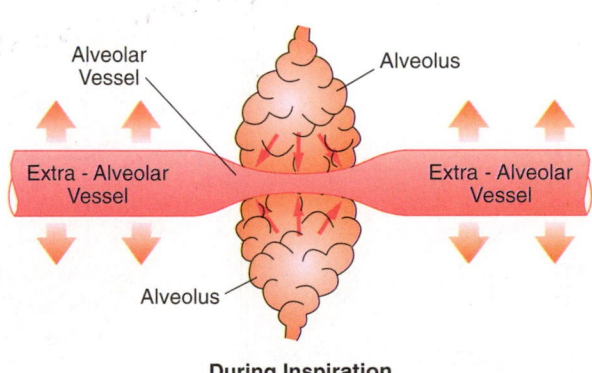

During Inspiration

Figure 5–22.   *Schematic illustration of pulmonary vessels during inspiration. The alveolar vessels (pulmonary capillaries) are exposed to the intrapleural pressure change and are stretched and flattened. The extra-alveolar vessels expand as the intrapleural pressure becomes more negative during inspiration.*

vessels are also pulled open (dilated to a greater radius) by the radial traction force created by the expansion of the alveoli (Figure 5–23).

To summarize, at low lung volumes (low distending pressures), the extra-alveolar vessels narrow and cause the vascular resistance to increase. The alveolar vessels, however, widen and cause the vascular resistance to decrease. In contrast, at high lung volumes (high distending pressures), the extra-alveolar vessels dilate and cause the vascular resistance to decrease. The alveolar vessels, however, flatten and cause the vascular resistance to increase.

PULMONARY VASCULAR RESISTANCE

Low Lung Volume

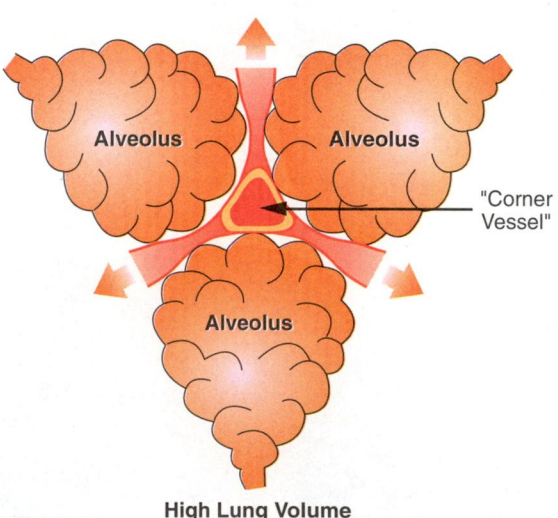

High Lung Volume

Figure 5–23. *Schematic drawing of the extra-alveolar "corner vessels" found at the junction of the alveolar septa. Expansion of the alveoli generates radial traction on the corner vessels, causing them to dilate. The alveolar vessels are compressed and flattened at high lung volumes.*

Finally, because the alveolar and extra-alveolar vessels are all part of the same vascular system, the resistance generated by the two groups of vessels is additive at any lung volume. The effect of changes in lung volume on the total pulmonary vascular resistance demonstrates a U-shaped curve (Figure 5–24). Thus, the pulmonary vascular resistance (PVR) is lowest near the functional residual capacity (FRC) and increases in response to both high and low lung volumes.

Blood Volume Changes. As blood volume increases, the recruitment and distension of pulmonary vessels will ensue, and pulmonary vascular resistance will tend to decrease (see Figure 5–21).

Blood Viscosity Changes. The viscosity of blood is derived from the hematocrit, the integrity of red blood cells, and the composition of plasma. As blood viscosity increases, the pulmonary vascular resistance increases. Table 5–3 (page 182) summarizes the active and passive mechanisms of vascular resistance.

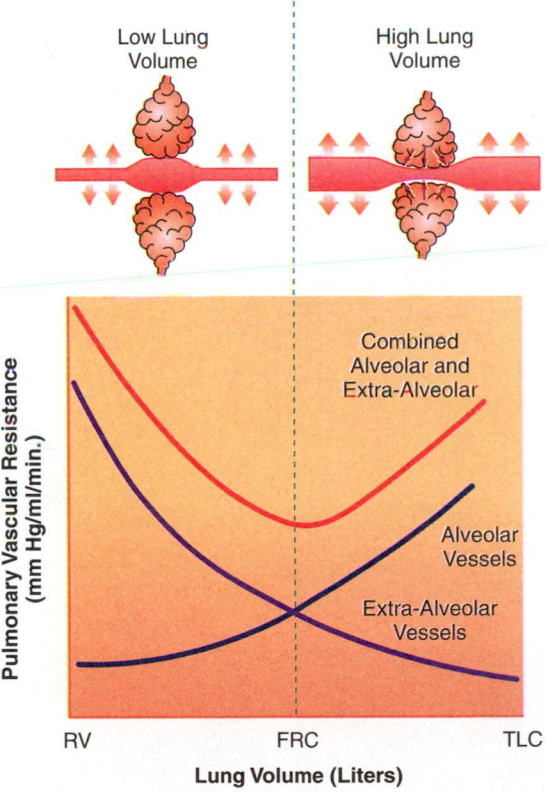

Figure 5–24. *At low lung volumes, the extra-alveolar vessels generate a greater resistance to pulmonary blood flow; at high lung volumes, the alveolar vessels generate a greater resistance to pulmonary blood flow. When added together, the resistances of the extra-alveolar and alveolar vessels demonstrate a U-shaped curve. Pulmonary vascular resistance (PVR) is lowest near the functional residual capacity (FRC) and increases at both high and low lung volumes. RV = residual volume; TLC = total lung capacity.*

TABLE 5–3. Summary of Active and Passive Mechanisms on Vascular Resistance

	↑ RESISTANCE (VASCULAR CONSTRICTION)	↓ RESISTANCE (VASCULAR DILATION)
ACTIVE MECHANISMS		
Abnormal Blood Gases		
↓PO_2	X	
↑P_{CO_2}	X	
↓pH	X	
Pharmacologic Stimulation		
Epinephrine (Adrenalin®)	X	
Norepinephrine (Levophed®)	X	
Dobutamine (Dobutrex®)	X	
Dopamine (Intropin®)	X	
Phenylephrine (Neo-Synephrine®)	X	
Oxygen		X
Isoproterenol (Isuprel®)		X
Aminophylline		X
Calcium-blocking Agents		X
Pathologic Conditions		
Vessel Blockage/Obstruction	X	
Vessel Wall Disease	X	
Vessel Destruction	X	
Vessel Compression	X	
PASSIVE MECHANISMS		
↑Pulmonary Arterial Pressure		X
↑Left Atrial Pressure		X
↑Lung Volume (Extreme)	X	
↓Lung Volume (Extreme)	X	
↑Blood Volume		X
↑Blood Viscosity	X	

↑ = increased; ↓ = decreased.

CLINICAL APPLICATION *1*

This 16-year-old female was involved in an automobile accident on the way home from school during a freezing rain. As she drove over a bridge, her car hit a patch of ice, spun out of control, and hit a cement embankment. It took the 911 team almost an hour to cut her out of her car with the "Jaws of Life." She was stabilized at the accident scene and then transported to the trauma center.

In the emergency room, the patient was unconscious and hypotensive. It was obvious that she had lost a lot of blood; her shirt and pants were soaked with blood. She had several large lacerations on her forehead, face, neck, left arm, and left leg. Immediately, the patient's head was lowered and her legs were elevated. The emergency room nurse inserted an intravenous (IV) line and started infusing Ringer's lactate solution. The respiratory therapist placed a nonrebreathing oxygen mask on the patient's face and drew an arterial blood gas sample. The radiologic technician took several portable x-rays.

The patient had several large bruises and abrasions over her left anterior chest that were most likely caused by the steering wheel when her car hit the cement embankment. Her four upper front teeth were broken off at the gum line. Her skin was pale and blue. Her vital signs were: blood pressure—78/42, heart rate—145 beats/min and weak, and respiratory rate—22 breaths/min and shallow. Her breath sounds were diminished bilaterally. Her arterial oxygen pressure (Pa_{O_2}) was 72 mm Hg.

Although her chest x-ray showed no broken ribs, patches of pulmonary infiltrates (increased alveolar density) could be seen over the left anterior lung. Additional x-rays showed she had a broken left humerus and left tibia. She was taken to surgery to have her lacerations and broken bones repaired. Five hours later, she was transferred to the surgical intensive care unit (ICU) with her left arm and left leg in a cast.

To offset the increased alveolar density noted on the chest x-ray, the respiratory therapist administered continuous positive airway pressure (CPAP) via a face mask for 20 minutes every hour. Between the CPAP treatments, the patient continued to receive oxygen via a nonrebreathing mask. Two hours later, the patient was conscious and talking to her parents. Her skin appeared normal and her vital signs were: blood pressure—115/82, heart rate—75 beats/min and strong, and respiratory rate—14 breaths/min. Normal vesicular breath sounds were heard throughout both lungs. Her fractional concentration of inspired oxygen (Fi_{O_2}) was decreased to 0.4, and her Pa_{O_2} on this setting was 94 mm Hg.

The patient's cardiopulmonary status progressively improved and she was discharged on her sixth day of hospitalization. Although her broken bones healed adequately, she had trouble walking normally for some time after the accident. Because of this problem, she continued to receive physical therapy twice a week for six months on an outpatient basis. At the time of her high school graduation, she had completely recovered.

DISCUSSION

This case study illustrates (1) the activation of the baroreceptor reflex, (2) hypovolemia and how it relates to preload, (3) negative transmural pressure, and (4) the effects of gravity on blood flow.

As shown in this chapter, the specialized stretch receptors called *baroreceptors* (see Figure 5–10) regulate the arterial blood pressure by initiating reflex adjustments to changes in blood pressure. In this case scenario, as the patient's blood pressure decreased from the loss of blood, neural impulses transmitted from the baroreceptors to the vasomotor and cardiac centers in the medulla decreased. This action, in turn, likely caused the patient's medulla to

(continues)

increase its sympathetic activity, which increased the heart rate (her pulse was 145 beats per minute in the emergency room).

Because *ventricular preload* is a function of the blood pressure generated by the volume of blood returning to the left or right ventricle during diastole, it can easily be seen why the patient's ventricular preload decreased as she became hypovolemic from the loss of blood. In the emergency room, the fact that the patient's ventricular preload was low was reflected by her low blood pressure (78/42). It should be noted that as preload decreases, cardiac output decreases.

Finally, as the patient's preload decreased (from blood loss), the *transmural pressure* in her least gravity-dependent lung areas became more and more negative. *Transmural pressure* is the difference between the intraluminal pressure of a vessel and the pressure surrounding the vessel (see Figure 5–11). The transmural pressure is negative when the pressure surrounding the vessel is greater than the pressure inside the vessel. In this case, this pathophysiologic process was offset by (1) lowering the patient's head and elevating her legs, which used the effects of gravity to move blood to the patient's lungs, and (2) replacing the volume of blood lost by administering Ringer's lactate solution through the patient's IV. These two procedures worked to change the negative transmural pressures to positive transmural pressures in the lung regions.

CLINICAL APPLICATION

This 72-year-old female presented in the intensive care unit (ICU) with left ventricular heart failure and pulmonary edema (also called congestive heart failure). She had no history of respiratory disease. The patient's husband stated that she had gone to bed with no remarkable problems, but awoke with severe dyspnea after several hours of sleep. Concerned, her husband called 911.

On observation, the patient's skin appeared cyanotic and she was in obvious respiratory distress. Her neck veins were distended and her ankles were swollen. Her vital signs were: blood pressure—214/106, heart rate—90 beats/min, and respiratory rate—28 breaths/min. On auscultation, rales and rhonchi (wet sounds) were heard over both lung fields. She had a frequent cough, productive of frothy white secretions. Her arterial oxygen pressure (Pa_{O_2}) on 3 L/min oxygen via nasal cannula was 48 mm Hg. A portable chest x-ray showed dense, fluffy opacities (white areas) that spread outward from the hilar areas to the peripheral borders of the lungs. The chest x-ray also showed that her left ventricle was enlarged (ventricular hypertrophy).

The physician prescribed (1) *positive inotropic agents* (see Table 6–3, page 193) to improve the strength of the left ventricular contraction and cardiac output, and (2) a systemic *vasodilator* (see Table 6–6, page 197) to decrease the patient's elevated blood pressure. Diuretic agents were also administered to promote fluid excretion. The respiratory therapist increased the patient's oxygen levels with a partial rebreathing mask.

Two hours later, the patient's cardiopulmonary status had significantly improved. Her skin appeared normal and her neck veins were no longer distended. Her peripheral edema was no longer present. Her vital signs were: blood pressure—130/87, heart rate—81 beats/min, and respiratory rate—14 breaths/min. Her

Pa_{O_2} on 2 L/min oxygen via nasal cannula was 103 mm Hg. A second chest x-ray showed that her lungs were clear and that the left ventricle had returned to normal size.

DISCUSSION

This case illustrates the effects of high blood pressure on (1) ventricular afterload, (2) ventricular contractility, (3) ventricular preload, and (4) transmural pressure.

Ventricular afterload is defined as the force against which the ventricles must work to pump blood. In this case, the patient's left ventricular afterload was very high because of increased peripheral vascular resistance. Clinically, this was reflected by the patient's high blood pressure of 214/106. Because of the high blood pressure and high left ventricular afterload, the patient's left ventricle eventually weakened and began to fail. As the ability of the left ventricle to pump blood decreased, the blood volume (and pressure) in the left ventricle increased. Even though the preload was increased, the left ventricle was unable to meet the increased demands created by the increased blood volume.

As this condition worsened, blood backed up into the patient's lungs. This pathophysiologic process caused the *transmural pressure* in the pulmonary capillary to increase significantly. As a result of the excessively high transmural pressure, fluid leaked out of the pulmonary capillaries and into the alveoli and airways. Clinically, this was verified by the rales and rhonchi (wet sounds) heard during auscultation, and by the white, frothy secretions produced when the patient coughed. As fluid accumulated in the patient's alveoli, the diffusion of oxygen into the pulmonary capillaries decreased. This was verified by the decreased Pa_{O_2} of 48 mm Hg.

Finally, as the blood volume and the transmural pressure in the pulmonary capillaries increased, the right ventricular afterload increased. This pathologic process, in turn, decreased the ability of the right ventricle to pump blood, in spite of the fact that the preload increased. This condition was reflected by the patient's distended neck veins and peripheral edema.

Fortunately, in this case the patient responded well to the positive inotropic agents, vasodilator, and diuretics. The vasodilator and diuretics worked to reduce the right and left ventricular afterloads, and the inotropic agents increased the ability of the ventricles to pump blood. The patient rapidly improved and was discharged on the fourth day of her hospital stay. Presently, she is seen by her family physician every two months.

REVIEW QUESTIONS

1. Which of the following are polymorphonuclear granulocytes?
   I. Neutrophils
   II. Monocytes
   III. Eosinophils
   IV. Lymphocytes
   V. Basophils
      a. I only
      b. II only
      c. V only

    d. II and IV only

    e. I, III, and V only

2. In the normal male, the hematocrit is about
   a. 25%
   b. 35%
   c. 45%
   d. 65%
   e. 75%

3. Which of the following agents cause pulmonary vascular constriction?
   I. Isoproterenol
   II. Epinephrine
   III. Oxygen
   IV. Dopamine
       a. I only
       b. III only
       c. II and IV only
       d. I, II, and IV only
       e. I, II, III, and IV

4. If the pressure in the pulmonary artery is 34 mm Hg, and the pressure in the left atrium is 9 mm Hg, what is the driving pressure?
   a. 9 mm Hg
   b. 17 mm Hg
   c. 25 mm Hg
   d. 34 mm Hg
   e. 43 mm Hg

5. The tricuspid valve lies between the
   a. right atrium and the right ventricle
   b. left ventricle and the aorta
   c. right ventricle and the pulmonary artery
   d. left atrium and the left ventricle
   e. right ventricle and the pulmonary valve

6. The QRS complex represents which of the following?
   a. Atrial depolarization only
   b. Ventricular repolarization only
   c. Atrial repolarization only
   d. Ventricular depolarization only
   e. Both atrial and ventricular repolarization

7. The mean intraluminal pressure in the pulmonary capillaries is
   a. 5 mm Hg
   b. 10 mm Hg
   c. 15 mm Hg
   d. 20 mm Hg
   e. 25 mm Hg

8. An increase in which of the following suggests a bacterial infection?
   a. Lymphocytes
   b. Neutrophils
   c. Monocytes

    d. Eosinophils

    e. Basophils

9. The force the ventricles must work against to pump blood is called

    a. myocardial contractility

    b. ventricular afterload

    c. negative inotropism

    d. ventricular preload

    e. positive inotropism

10. Compared to the systemic circulation, the pressure in the pulmonary circulation is about

    a. 1/10 the pressure

    b. 1/4 the pressure

    c. 1/3 the pressure

    d. 1/2 the pressure

    e. the same pressure

11. The difference between the pressure in the lumen of a vessel and that of the pressure surrounding the vessel is called the

    a. driving pressure

    b. transmural pressure

    c. diastolic pressure

    d. intravascular pressure

    e. transpulmonary pressure

12. Which of the following cause(s) pulmonary vasoconstriction?

    I. Hypercapnia

    II. Hypoxia

    III. Acidemia

    IV. Increased H^+ concentration

      a. I only

      b. III only

      c. II and IV only

      d. II, III, and IV only

      e. I, II, III, and IV

13. The cardioinhibitor center of the medulla slows the heart by sending neural impulses by way of the

    I. tenth cranial nerve

    II. parasympathetic nervous system

    III. sympathetic nervous system

    IV. vagus nerve

      a. I only

      b. IV only

      c. III only

      d. I and IV only

      e. I, II, and IV only

14. Which of the following cause passive changes in the pulmonary vascular resistance?

    I. pH changes

    II. Transpulmonary pressure changes

III. P_{CO_2} changes

IV. Blood viscosity changes

    a. II only

    b. III only

    c. I and III only

    d. II and IV only

    e. I, III, and IV only

15. Which of the following cause blood clotting at a traumatized site?

    a. Thrombocytes

    b. Basophils

    c. Monocytes

    d. Eosinophils

    e. Neutrophils

6

HEMODYNAMIC MEASUREMENTS

OBJECTIVES

By the end of this chapter, the student should be able to:

1. List the abbreviations and normal ranges of the following hemodynamic values *directly* measured by means of the pulmonary artery catheter:
   —Central venous pressure
   —Right atrial pressure
   —Mean pulmonary artery pressure
   —Pulmonary capillary wedge pressure
   —Cardiac output
2. List the abbreviations and normal ranges of the following *computed* hemodynamic values:
   —Stroke volume
   —Stroke volume index
   —Cardiac index
   —Right ventricular stroke work index
   —Left ventricular stroke work index
   —Pulmonary vascular resistance
   —Systemic vascular resistance
3. List factors that increase and decrease the following:
   —Stroke volume
   —Stroke volume index
   —Cardiac output
   —Cardiac index
   —Right ventricular stroke work index
   —Left ventricular stroke work index
4. List the factors that increase and decrease the *pulmonary vascular resistance*.
5. List the factors that increase and decrease the *systemic vascular resistance*.
6. Complete the review questions at the end of this chapter.

HEMODYNAMIC MEASUREMENTS DIRECTLY OBTAINED BY MEANS OF THE PULMONARY ARTERY CATHETER

The term **hemodynamics** is defined as the study of the forces that influence the circulation of blood. With the advent of the pulmonary artery catheter (Figure 6–1, page 190), the hemodynamic status of the critically ill patient can be accurately de-

Figure 6–1. *Insertion of the pulmonary catheter. The insertion site of the pulmonary catheter may be the basilic, brachial, femoral, subclavian, or internal jugular veins. The latter two are the most common insertion sites. As the catheter advances, pressure readings and wave forms are monitored to determine the catheter's position as it moves through the right atrium (RA), right ventricle (RV), pulmonary artery (PA), and finally into a pulmonary capillary "wedge" pressure (PCWP) position. Immediately after a PCWP reading, the balloon is deflated to allow blood to flow past the tip of the catheter. When the balloon is deflated, the catheter continuously monitors the pulmonary artery pressure.*

termined at the bedside.* The pulmonary artery catheter has enabled the respiratory care practitioner to measure several hemodynamic parameters directly. These direct measurements, in turn, can be used to compute other important hemodynamic values. Table 6–1 lists the major hemodynamic values that can be directly measured.

*See Appendix V for a representative example of a cardiopulmonary profile sheet used to monitor the hemodynamic status of the critically ill patient.

TABLE 6–1.	Hemodynamic Values Directly Obtained by Means of the Pulmonary Artery Catheter	
HEMODYNAMIC VALUE	**ABBREVIATION**	**NORMAL RANGE**
Central venous pressure	CVP	0–8 mm Hg
Right atrial pressure	RAP	0–8 mm Hg
Mean pulmonary artery pressure	PA	9–18 mm Hg
Pulmonary capillary wedge pressure	PCWP	
(also called pulmonary artery	PAW	4–12 mm Hg
wedge; pulmonary artery occlusion)	PAO	
Cardiac output	CO	4–8 L/min

HEMODYNAMIC VALUES COMPUTED FROM DIRECT MEASUREMENTS

Table 6–2 lists the major hemodynamic values that can be calculated from the direct measurements listed in Table 6–1. Today, such calculations are obtained either from a programmed calculator or by using the specific hemodynamic formula and a simple hand-held calculator. It should be noted, moreover, that since the hemodynamic parameters vary with the size of an individual, some hemodynamic values are "indexed" by body surface area (BSA). Clinically, the BSA is obtained from a height–weight nomogram (see Appendix IV). The normal adult BSA is 1.5 to 2 m^2.

STROKE VOLUME

The stroke volume (SV) is the volume of blood ejected by the ventricles with each contraction. The preload, afterload, and myocardial contractility are the major de-

TABLE 6–2.	Computed Hemodynamic Values	
HEMODYNAMIC VALUE	**ABBREVIATION**	**NORMAL RANGE**
Stroke volume	SV	60–130 ml
Stroke volume index	SVI	30–65 ml/beat/m^2
Cardiac index	CI	2.5–4.2 L/min/m^2
Right ventricular stroke work index	RVSWI	7–12 g m/m^2
Left ventricular stroke work index	LVSWI	40–60 g m/m^2
Pulmonary vascular resistance	PVR	20–120 dynes $\times$ sec $\times$ cm^{-5}
Systemic vascular resistance	SVR	800–1500 dynes $\times$ sec $\times$ cm^{-5}

terminants of stroke volume. Stroke volume is derived by dividing the cardiac output (CO) by the heart rate (HR).

$$SV = \frac{CO}{HR}$$

For example, if an individual has a cardiac output of 4.5 L/min (4500 ml/min) and a heart rate of 75 beats/min, the stroke volume would be calculated as follows:

$$SV = \frac{CO}{HR}$$

$$= \frac{4500 \text{ ml/min}}{75 \text{ beats/min}}$$

$$= 60 \text{ ml/beat}$$

Table 6–3 lists factors that increase and decrease the stroke volume.

TABLE 6–3. Factors Increasing and Decreasing Stroke Volume (SV), Stroke Volume Index (SVI), Cardiac Output (CO), Cardiac Index (CI), Right Ventricular Stroke Work Index (RVSWI), and Left Ventricular Stroke Work Index (LVSWI)

INCREASES	DECREASES
Positive Inotropic Drugs (Increased Contractility)	**Negative Inotropic Drugs (Decreased Contractility)**
Dobutamine (Dobutrex®)	Propranolol (Inderal®)
Epinephrine (Adrenalin®)	Timolol (Blocadren®)
Dopamine (Intropin®)	Metoprolol (Lopressor®)
Isoproterenol (Isuprel®)	Atenolol (Tenormin®)
Digitalis	Nadolol (Corgard®)
Amrinone (Inocor®)	
	Abnormal Conditions
Abnormal Conditions	Septic shock (late stages)
Septic shock (early stages)	Congestive heart failure
Hyperthermia	Hypovolemia
Hypervolemia	Pulmonary emboli
Decreased vascular resistance	Increased vascular resistance
	Myocardial infarction
	Hyperinflation of Lungs
	Mechanical ventilation
	Continuous Positive Airway Pressure (CPAP)
	Positive End-Expiratory Pressure (PEEP)

STROKE VOLUME INDEX

The stroke volume index (SVI) (also known as stroke index) is derived by dividing the stroke volume (SV) by the body surface area (BSA).

$$SVI = \frac{SV}{BSA}$$

For example, if a patient has a stroke volume of 60 ml and a body surface area of 2 m^2, the stroke volume index would be determined as follows:

$$SVI = \frac{SV}{BSA}$$

$$= \frac{60 \text{ ml/beat}}{2 \text{ m}^2}$$

$$= 30 \text{ ml/beat/m}^2$$

Assuming that the heart rate remains the same, as the stroke volume index increases or decreases, the cardiac index also increases or decreases. The stroke volume index reflects the (1) contractility of the heart, (2) overall blood volume status, and (3) amount of venous return.

Table 6–3 lists factors that increase and decrease the stroke volume index.

CARDIAC INDEX

The cardiac index (CI) is calculated by dividing the cardiac output (CO) by the body's surface area (BSA).

$$CI = \frac{CO}{BSA}$$

For example, if a patient has a cardiac output of 5 liters per minute and a body surface area of 2 m^2, the cardiac index is computed as follows:

$$CI = \frac{CO}{BSA}$$

$$= \frac{5 \text{ L/min}}{2 \text{ m}^2}$$

$$= 2.5 \text{ L/min/m}^2$$

See Table 6–3 for a list of factors that increase and decrease the cardiac index.

RIGHT VENTRICULAR STROKE WORK INDEX

The right ventricular stroke work index (RVSWI) measures the amount of work required by the right ventricle to pump blood. The RVSWI is a reflection of the contractility of the right ventricle. In the presence of normal right ventricular contractility, increases in afterload (e.g., caused by pulmonary vascular constriction) cause the RVSWI to increase, until a pleateau is reached. When the contractility of the right ventricle is diminished by disease states, however, the RVSWI does not appropriately increase. The RVSWI is derived from the following formula:

$$RVSWI = SVI \times (PA - CVP) \times 0.0136 \text{ g/ml}$$

where SVI is stroke volume index, PA is mean pulmonary artery pressure, CVP is central venous pressure, and the density of mercury factor 0.0136 g/ml is needed to convert the equation to the proper units of measurement—i.e., gram meters/m^2 (g m/m^2).

For example, if a patient has an SVI of 35 ml, a PA of 20 mm Hg, and a CVP of 5 mm Hg, the patient's RVSWI is calculated as follows:

$$RVSWI = SVI \times (PA - CVP) \times 0.0136 \text{ g/ml}$$

$$= 35 \text{ ml/beat/m}^2 \times (20 \text{ mm Hg} - 5 \text{ mm Hg}) \times 0.0136 \text{ g/ml}$$

$$= 35 \text{ ml/beat/m}^2 \times 15 \text{ mm Hg} \times 0.0136 \text{ g/ml}$$

$$= 7.14 \text{ g m/m}^2$$

Factors that increase and decrease the right ventricular stroke work index are listed in Table 6–3.

LEFT VENTRICULAR STROKE WORK INDEX

The left ventricular stroke work index (LVSWI) measures the amount of work required by the left ventricle to pump blood. The LVSWI is a reflection of the contractility of the left ventricle. In the presence of normal left ventricular contractility, increases in afterload (e.g., caused by systemic vascular constriction) cause the LVSWI to increase until a plateau is reached. When the contractility of the left ventricle is diminished by disease states, however, the LVSWI does not increase appropriately. The following formula is used for determining this hemodynamic variable:

$$LVSWI = SVI \times (MAP - PCWP) \times 0.0136 \text{ g/ml}$$

where SVI is stroke volume index, MAP is mean arterial pressure, PCWP is pulmonary capillary wedge pressure, and the density of mercury factor 0.0136 g/ml is needed to convert the equation to the proper units of measurement—i.e., gram meters/m^2 (g m/m^2).

For example, if a patient has an SVI of 30 ml, an MAP of 100 mm Hg, and a PCWP of 5 mm Hg, then:

$$LVSWI = SVI \times (MAP - PCWP) \times 0.0136 \text{ g/ml}$$

$$= 30 \text{ ml/beat/m}^2 \times (100 \text{ mm Hg} - 5 \text{ mm Hg}) \times 0.0136 \text{ g/ml}$$

$$= 30 \text{ ml/beat/m}^2 \times (95 \text{ mm Hg}) \times 0.0136 \text{ g/ml}$$

$$= 38.76 \text{ g m/m}^2$$

Table 6–3 lists factors that increase and decrease the left ventricular stroke work index.

VASCULAR RESISTANCE

As blood flows through the pulmonary and the systemic vascular system there is resistance to flow. The pulmonary system is a *low resistance* system. The systemic vascular system is a *high resistance* system.

Pulmonary Vascular Resistance (PVR)

The PVR measurement reflects the afterload of the right ventricle. It is calculated by the following formula:

$$\text{PVR} = \frac{\text{PA} - \text{PCWP}}{\text{CO}} \times 80$$

where PA is the mean pulmonary artery pressure, PCWP is the pulmonary capillary wedge pressure, CO is the cardiac output, and 80 is a conversion factor for adjusting to the correct units of measurement (dyne $\times$ sec $\times$ cm^{-5}).

For example, to determine the PVR of a patient who has a PA of 15 mm Hg, a PCWP of 5 mm Hg, and a CO of 5 L/min:

$$\text{PVR} = \frac{\text{PA} - \text{PCWP}}{\text{CO}} \times 80$$

$$= \frac{15 \text{ mm Hg} - 5 \text{ mm Hg}}{5 \text{ L/min}} \times 80$$

$$= \frac{10 \text{ mm Hg}}{5 \text{ L/min}} \times 80$$

$$= 160 \text{ dynes} \times \text{sec} \times \text{cm}^{-5}$$

Table 6–4 (page 196) lists factors that increase the pulmonary vascular resistance. Factors that decrease the pulmonary vascular resistance are listed in Table 6–5 (page 196).

Systemic or Peripheral Vascular Resistance (SVR)

The SVR measurement reflects the afterload of the left ventricle. It is calculated by the following formula:

$$\text{SVR} = \frac{\text{MAP} - \text{CVP}}{\text{CO}} \times 80$$

where MAP is the mean arterial pressure, CVP is the central venous pressure, CO is the cardiac output, and 80 is a conversion factor for adjusting to the correct units of measurement (dyne $\times$ sec $\times$ cm^{-5}). (Note: The right atrial pressure (RAP) can be used in place of the CVP value.)

For example, if a patient has an MAP of 80 mm Hg, a CVP of 5 mm Hg, and a CO of 5 L/min, then:

$$\text{SVR} = \frac{\text{MAP} - \text{CVP}}{\text{CO}} \times 80$$

$$= \frac{80 \text{ mm Hg} - 5 \text{ mm Hg}}{5 \text{ L/min}} \times 80$$

$$= \frac{75 \text{ mm Hg} \times 80}{5 \text{ L/min}}$$

$$= 1200 \text{ dynes} \times \text{sec} \times \text{cm}^{-5}$$

Table 6–6 (page 197) lists factors that increase and decrease the systemic vascular resistance.

TABLE 6–4. Factors that Increase Pulmonary Vascular Resistance (PVR)

Chemical Stimuli
Decreased alveolar oxygenation
  (alveolar hypoxia)
Decreased pH (acidemia)
Increased P_{CO_2} (hypercapnia)

Pharmacologic Agents
Epinephrine (Adrenalin®)
Norepinephrine (Levophed®, Levarterenol®)
Dobutamine (Dobutrex®)
Dopamine (Intropin®)
Phenylephrine (Neo-Synephrine®)

Hyperinflation of Lungs
Mechanical ventilation
    Continuous Positive Airway Pressure (CPAP)
    Positive End-Expiratory Pressure (PEEP)

Pathologic Factors
Vascular blockage
    Pulmonary emboli
    Air bubble
    Tumor mass

Vascular wall disease
    Sclerosis
    Endarteritis
    Polyarteritis
    Scleroderma

Vascular destruction
    Emphysema
    Pulmonary interstitial fibrosis

Vascular compression
    Pneumothorax
    Hemothorax
    Tumor mass

Humoral Substances
Histamine
Angiotensin
Fibrinopeptides
Prostaglandin $F_{2\alpha}$
Serotonin

TABLE 6–5. Factors that Decrease Pulmonary Vascular Resistance (PVR)

PHARMACOLOGIC AGENTS	HUMORAL SUBSTANCES
Oxygen	Acetylcholine
Isoproterenol (Isuprel®)	Bradykinin
Aminophylline	Prostaglandin E
Calcium-blocking agent	Prostacyclin (prostaglandin I_2)

TABLE 6–6. **Factors that Increase and Decrease Systemic Vascular Resistance (SVR)**

INCREASES SVR	DECREASES SVR
Vasoconstricting Agents	**Vasodilating Agents**
Dopamine (Intropin®)	Nitroglycerin
Norepinephrine (Levarterenol®, Levophed®)	Nitroprusside (Nipride®)
Epinephrine (Adrenalin®)	Morphine
Phenylephrine (Neo-Synephrine®)	Amrinone (Inocor®)
	Hydralazine (Apresoline®)
Abnormal Conditions	Methyldopa (Aldomet®)
Hypovolemia	Diazoxide (Hyperstat®)
Septic shock (late stages)	
$\downarrow P_{CO_2}$	**Abnormal Conditions**
	Septic shock (early stages)
	$\uparrow P_{CO_2}$

$\uparrow$ = increased; $\downarrow$ = decreased.

CLINICAL APPLICATION 1

This 71-year-old female reported sudden chest pain to her husband while working in her garden at home. Moments later she collapsed; her husband called 911 immediately. Upon arrival, the paramedics charted these vital signs: blood pressure—64/35, heart rate—32 beats/min, and respiratory rate—4 breaths/min and shallow. Cardiopulmonary resuscitation (CPR) was instituted and the patient was transferred to the hospital. En route to the hospital an intravenous line was inserted and a bolus of epinephrine was administered.

In the emergency room, the patient's vital signs were: blood pressure—78/50, heart rate—42 beats/min, and a spontaneous respiratory rate of 16 breaths/min. Dopamine was administered and her heart rate increased to 60 beats per minute. Despite the improved heart rate, however, the patient's blood pressure remained low and her skin was cold and clammy. On 3 L/min oxygen via nasal cannula, the patient's arterial blood gas values were: pH 7.41, Pa_{CO_2} 25 mm Hg, HCO_3^- 23 mmol/L, Pa_{O_2} 62 mm Hg.

Her electrocardiogram (ECG) showed a complete heart block.* The patient was immediately transferred to the coronary care unit (CCU). At the bedside, a transvenous cardiac pacing wire was placed under fluoroscopy and the ventricles were paced at a rate of 80 beats per minute. A pulmonary catheter was then inserted *(continues)*

*The ventricles were contracting independently from the sinus atrial node rhythm.

(see Figure 6–1) and a hemodynamic profile was obtained (see Hemodynamic Profile No. 1).

HEMODYNAMIC PROFILE		
Parameter*	Profile No. 1	Profile No. 2
BP	88/54	91/55
HR	80 paced	80 paced
CVP	9	9
RAP	10	10
PA	18	16
PCWP	21	13
CI	1.1	1.8
SVR	2295	1670
Urine (ml/hr)	0	35

*BP = blood pressure; HR = heart rate; CVP = central venous pressure; RAP = right atrial pressure; PA = mean pulmonary artery pressure; PCWP = pulmonary capillary wedge pressure; CI = cardiac index; SVR = systemic vascular resistance. Normal ranges are given in Tables 6–1 and 6–2 on page 191.

After evaluating the first hemodynamic profile, the physician made the diagnosis of cardiogenic shock and prescribed nitroprusside for the patient. One hour later, while on an inspired oxygen concentration (FI_{O_2}) of 0.5, the patient's arterial blood gas values were: pH 7.43, Pa_{CO_2} 33 mm Hg, HCO_3^- 24 mmol/L, and Pa_{O_2} 108 mm Hg. Her urine output was 35 ml/hour. The patient's skin was warm and dry, and her respiratory rate was 12 breaths per minute. At this time, a second hemodynamic profile was obtained (see Hemodynamic Profile No. 2).

DISCUSSION

This case illustrates the adverse "ripple" effects of an elevated *afterload* (see Chapter Five, page 174) on a patient's hemodynamic parameters. The very high SVR and PCWP and low CI in Hemodynamic Profile No. 1 showed that the patient's afterload was elevated. Although dopamine is a good agent to increase the patient's CI (cardiac index), in larger doses it causes the SVR (peripheral vascular resistance) to increase. Because the SVR was already high, nitroprusside (a vasodilator) was used to reduce the patient's afterload.

After the administration of the nitroprusside, the patient's blood pressure essentially remained the same in the second hemodynamic profile while her PCWP, CI, SVR, and urine output all improved significantly. In short, as the patient's SVR decreased in response to the nitroprusside, the left ventricular afterload also decreased. This action in turn allowed blood to be more readily ejected from the left ventricle. The patient's cardiac pacemaker was permanently implanted and she progressively improved. On her seventh day of hospitalization, the patient was discharged.

CLINICAL APPLICATION

This 35-year-old male was found unconscious, face down, in about four inches of water at a local beach. He had fallen asleep on the beach at low tide while intoxicated. His pulse was weak and he was not breathing. Someone called 911 and the lifeguard started cardiopulmonary resuscitation (CPR). When the paramedics arrived, CPR was continued with an inspired oxygen concentration (FI_{O_2}) of 1.0, and the patient was transferred to the local hospital.

In the emergency room, the patient was semiconscious. Although he demonstrated a spontaneous respiratory rate of 8 breaths/min, his breathing was labored and shallow. He had a pulse of 115 beats/min and a blood pressure of 95/60. His chest x-ray showed a normal-sized heart, but patches of alveolar infiltrates (white areas) were visible throughout both lung fields. The laboratory report showed that the patient's alcohol level was 0.53, his complete blood count (CBC) was normal, and his hemoglobin level was normal, at 15 g% (see Chapter Seven). On an FI_{O_2} of 1.0, his arterial blood gas values were: pH 7.22, Pa_{CO_2} 52 mm Hg, HCO_3^- 20 mm Hg, and Pa_{O_2} 38 mm Hg.

The patient was intubated and transferred to the intensive care unit (ICU). At the time of intubation, sand and seaweed were suctioned from the patient's trachea. A pulmonary artery catheter and arterial line were inserted (see Figure 6–1). The patient was placed on a mechanical ventilator with the following settings: tidal volume 750 ml, respiratory rate 12, FI_{O_2} 1.0, and positive end-expiratory pressure (PEEP) 5 cm H_2O. The patient's arterial blood gas values on these settings were: pH 7.47, Pa_{CO_2} 28 mm Hg, HCO_3^- 22 mmol/L, Pa_{O_2} 57 mm Hg, and Sa_{O_2} 91 percent. At this time, a hemodynamic profile and arterial blood gas sample were obtained (see Hemodynamic Profile No. 1).

After reviewing the clinical data in the first hemodynamic profile, the physician had the res-

piratory therapist decrease the patient's tidal volume to 650 ml, to increase the patient's Pa_{CO_2}, which had been reduced too much by the first ventilator settings (the decreased Pa_{CO_2} was the cause of elevated pH). Because the patient's Pa_{O_2} was still very low on an FI_{O_2} of 1.0, the PEEP was increased to 10 cm H_2O. A second arterial blood gas sample showed the following values: pH 7.42, Pa_{CO_2} 36 mm Hg, HCO_3^- 23 mmol/L, Pa_{O_2} 61 mm Hg, and Sa_{O_2} 90 percent. A second hemodynamic profile was then obtained (see Hemodynamic Profile No. 2).

After reviewing the patient's second arterial blood gas sample and second hemodynamic profile, the physician had the respiratory therapist decrease the PEEP back to 5 cm H_2O. Fifteen minutes later a third arterial blood gas sample showed a pH of 7.42, Pa_{CO_2} 36 mm Hg, HCO_3^- 23 mmol/L, Pa_{O_2} 59 mm Hg, and Sa_{O_2} 90 percent. A third hemodynamic profile was then obtained (see Hemodynamic Profile No. 3). Despite the fact that the patient's Pa_{O_2} was less than satisfactory at this time, the physician asked the respiratory therapist to maintain the above treatment parameters.

DISCUSSION

This case illustrates that the best level of PEEP (commonly referred to as "Best PEEP") was the PEEP level that produced the least depression of cardiac output and the maximum total oxygen delivery. Inspection of the three hemodynamic profiles shows that 5 cm H_2O was the most effective by these criteria.[†] Despite the fact that the patient's clinical course was stormy, he was eventually weaned from the ventilator, sixteen days after his admission. Although he did regain consciousness, he was amnesic. He was also diagnosed to have moderate to severe mental and neuromuscular disorders. He was transferred to the rehabilitation unit where, at the time of this writing, progress was reported as slow.

HEMODYNAMIC PROFILE

Parameter*	Profile No. 1 PEEP 5 cm H_2O	Profile No. 2 PEEP 10 cm H_2O	Profile No. 3 PEEP 5 cm H_2O
BP	90/60	95/68	91/62
HR	107	105	98
CI	1.9	1.5	1.9
CO	3.83	3.1	3.82
SVI	36	31	37
SVR	1490	170	1493

*BP = blood pressure; HR = heart rate; CI = cardiac index; CO = cardiac output; SVI = stroke volume index; SVR = systemic vascular resistance.

[†]After the reader completes Chapter Seven, the patient's oxygen delivery for each level of PEEP can be calculated by using the Total Oxygen Delivery (D_{O_2}) formula. It is strongly recommended that the reader return to this case and calculate and compare the D_{O_2} when the patient was on 5 cm H_2O PEEP versus 10 cm H_2O PEEP. The D_{O_2} formula will show that even though the patient's Pa_{O_2} was less than desirable at 5 cm H_2O of PEEP, the cardiac output (and, therefore, the total oxygen delivery) was greater.

REVIEW QUESTIONS

Directions: On the line next to the hemodynamic parameters in Column A, match the normal range from Column B. Items in Column B can be used once, more than once, or not at all.

COLUMN A	COLUMN B
Hemodynamic Parameters	*Normal Range*

1. _____ Mean pulmonary artery pressure   a. 4–8 L/min
2. _____ Pulmonary vascular resistance   b. 800–1500 dynes $\times$ sec $\times$ cm^{-5}
3. _____ Cardiac output   c. 60–130 ml
4. _____ Left ventricular stroke work   d. 0–8 mm Hg
       index   e. 20–120 dynes $\times$ sec $\times$ cm^{-5}
5. _____ Central venous pressure   f. 9–18 mm Hg
6. _____ Stroke volume index   g. 30–65 ml/beat/m^2
7. _____ Pulmonary capillary wedge   h. 80 mm Hg
       pressure   i. 2.5–4.2 L/min/m^2
8. _____ Systemic vascular resistance   j. 4–12 mm Hg
9. _____ Right atrial pressure   k. 40–60 g m/m^2
10. _____ Cardiac index   l. 7–12 g m/m^2

1. Which of the following increases an individual's cardiac output?
    I. Epinephrine
   II. Hypovolemia
  III. Mechanical ventilation
  IV. Hyperthermia
     a. I only
     b. II only
     c. III only
     d. I and IV only
     e. I, II, and IV only

2. Pulmonary vascular resistance increases in response to:
    I. Acidemia
   II. Oxygen
  III. Mechanical ventilation
  IV. Epinephrine
     a. I only
     b. II only
     c. III only
     d. I and III only
     e. I, III, and IV only

3. An individual's systemic vascular resistance increases in response to:
    I. Morphrine
   II. Hypovolemia
  III. An increased P_{CO_2}
  IV. Epinephrine

    a. I only
    b. II only
    c. III only
    d. II and IV only
    e. I, III, and IV only

4. Which of the following decreases an individual's stroke volume index?
    I. Dobutamine
    II. Mechanical ventilation
    III. Propranolol
    IV. Congestive heart failure
       a. I only
       b. II only
       c. IV only
       d. I and III only
       e. II, III, and IV only

5. An individual's pulmonary vascular resistance decreases in response to:
    I. Bradykinin
    II. Emphysema
    III. Norepinephrine
    IV. Hypercapnia
       a. I only
       b. II only
       c. III only
       d. II and III only
       e. II, III, and IV only

CHAPTER SEVEN

OXYGEN TRANSPORT

OBJECTIVES

By the end of this chapter, the student should be able to:

1. Calculate the quantity of oxygen that *dissolves in the plasma* of the blood.
2. Describe the major features of *hemoglobin*, including:
   —Heme portion
   • Iron
   —Globin portion
   • Four amino acid chains
     ◦ Two alpha chains
     ◦ Two beta chains
   —Ferrous state vs. ferric state
   —Normal hemoglobin concentrations in the adult male and female and in the infant
3. Calculate the quantity of oxygen that *combines with hemoglobin*.
4. Calculate the *total amount* of oxygen in the blood.
5. Identify the abbreviations for the following:
   —Oxygen content of arterial blood
   —Oxygen content of mixed venous blood
   —Oxygen content of capillary blood
6. Describe how the following relate to the *oxygen dissociation curve:*
   —Oxygen pressure
   —Percentage of hemoglobin bound to oxygen
   —Oxygen content
7. Describe the clinical significance of the
   —flat portion of the oxygen dissociation curve
   —steep portion of the oxygen dissociation curve
   —P_{50}
8. Identify the factors that shift the oxygen dissociation curve to the right.
9. Identify the factors that shift the oxygen dissociation curve to the left.
10. Explain the clinical significance of a right or left shift of the oxygen dissociation curve in regard to the
    —loading of oxygen in the lungs
    —unloading of oxygen at the tissues
11. Calculate the following oxygen transport studies:
    —Total oxygen delivery
    —Arterial-venous oxygen content difference
    —Oxygen consumption
    —Oxygen extraction ratio
    —Mixed venous oxygen saturation
    —Pulmonary shunting
12. Identify the factors that increase and decrease the *oxygen transport* studies.
13. Differentiate between the following forms of *pulmonary shunting:*
    —Anatomic shunt

(continues)

—Capillary shunt
—Shunt-like effect
14. Explain the meaning of *venous admixture*.
15. Calculate the *shunt equation*.
16. Describe the clinical significance of intrapulmonary shunting.
17. Define the following four main types of tissue hypoxia:

—Hypoxic hypoxia
—Anemic hypoxia
—Circulatory hypoxia
—Histotoxic hypoxia
18. Explain the meaning of
—cyanosis
—polycythemia
19. Complete the review questions at the end of this chapter.

An understanding of oxygen transport is essential to the study of pulmonary physiology and to the clinical interpretation of arterial and venous blood gases. Table 7–1 lists the normal blood gas values.* To fully understand this subject, the student must understand (1) how oxygen is transported from the lungs to the tissues, (2) the oxygen dissociation curve and its clinical significance, (3) how various oxygen transport studies are used to identify the patient's cardiac and ventilatory status, and (4) the major forms of tissue hypoxia.

OXYGEN TRANSPORT

The transport of oxygen between the lungs and the cells of the body is a function of the blood and the heart. Oxygen is carried in the blood in two forms: (1) as dissolved oxygen in the blood plasma, and (2) chemically bound to the hemoglobin (Hb) that is encased in the erythrocytes, or red blood cells (RBCs).

OXYGEN DISSOLVED IN THE BLOOD PLASMA

As oxygen diffuses from the alveoli into the pulmonary capillary blood, it dissolves in the plasma of the blood. The term **dissolve** means that when a gas like oxygen enters the plasma, it maintains its precise molecular structure (in this case, O_2) and moves freely throughout the plasma in its normal gaseous state. Clinically, it is this portion of the oxygen that is measured to assess the patient's partial pressure of oxygen (P_{O_2}) (see Table 7–1).

The quantity of oxygen that dissolves in the plasma is a function of Henry's law, which states that the amount of gas that dissolves in a liquid (in this case,

---

*See Appendix V for a representative example of a cardiopulmonary profile sheet used to monitor the blood gas values of the critically ill patient.

TABLE 7–1.   **Normal Blood Gas Value Ranges**

BLOOD GAS VALUE*	ARTERIAL	VENOUS
pH	7.35–7.45	7.30–7.40
P_{CO_2}	35–45 mm Hg (Pa_{CO_2})	42–48 mm Hg (Pv_{CO_2})
HCO_3^-	22–28 mEq/L	24–30 mEq/L
P_{O_2}	80–100 mm Hg (Pa_{O_2})[†]	35–45 mm Hg (Pv_{O_2})

*Technically, only the oxygen (P_{O_2}) and carbon dioxide (P_{CO_2}) pressure readings are "true" blood gas values. The pH indicates the balance between the bases and acids in the blood. The bicarbonate (HCO_3^-) reading is an indirect measurement that is calculated from the pH and P_{CO_2} levels.

[†]For each year over 60 years, subtract 1 mm Hg from 80 mm Hg for the lower Pa_{O_2} limit. This and other effects of aging are discussed in Chapter Thirteen.

plasma) at a given temperature is proportional to the partial pressure of the gas. At normal body temperature, about 0.003 ml of oxygen will dissolve in 100 ml of blood for every 1 mm Hg of P_{O_2}. Thus, in the healthy individual with an arterial oxygen partial pressure (Pa_{O_2}) of 100 mm Hg, approximately 0.3 ml of oxygen is dissolved in every 100 ml of plasma (0.003×100 mm Hg = 0.3 ml). This is written as 0.3 volumes percent (vol%). Vol% represents the amount of O_2 in milliliters that is in 100 ml of blood (vol% = ml O_2/100 ml bd). For example, 10 vol% of O_2 means that there are 10 ml of O_2 in 100 ml of blood. In terms of total oxygen transport, a relatively small percentage of oxygen is transported in the form of dissolved oxygen.

OXYGEN BOUND WITH HEMOGLOBIN
Hemoglobin

Most of the oxygen that diffuses into the pulmonary capillary blood rapidly moves into the RBCs and chemically attaches to the hemoglobin. Each RBC contains approximately 280 million hemoglobin molecules, highly specialized to transport oxygen and carbon dioxide.

Normal adult hemoglobin, which is designated Hb A, consists of (1) four heme groups, which are the pigmented, iron-containing non-protein portions of the hemoglobin molecule, and (2) four amino acid chains (polypeptide chains) that collectively constitute globin (a protein) (Figure 7–1, page 206).

At the center of each heme group, the iron molecule can combine with one oxygen molecule in an easily reversible reaction to form oxyhemoglobin:

Hb	+	O_2	$\rightleftharpoons$	Hb_{O_2}
Reduced hemoglobin (uncombined or deoxygenated hemoglobin)		Oxygen		Oxyhemoglobin (combined or oxygenated hemoglobin)

Since there are four heme/iron groups in each Hb molecule, a total of four oxygen molecules can combine with each Hb molecule. When four oxygen molecules

Figure 7–1. *Schematic illustration of a hemoglobin molecule. The globin (protein) portion consists of two identical alpha (α) chains and two beta (β) chains. The four heme (iron-containing) portions are in the center of each globin molecule.*

are bound to one Hb molecule, the Hb is said to be 100-percent saturated with oxygen; a Hb molecule with three oxygen molecules is 75-percent saturated; and so forth. Hemoglobin bound with oxygen (Hb_{O_2}) is called **oxyhemoglobin**. Hemoglobin not bound with oxygen (Hb) is called **reduced hemoglobin** or **deoxyhemoglobin**. The amount of oxygen bound to Hb is directly related to the partial pressure of oxygen.

The globin portion of each Hb molecule consists of two identical alpha (α) chains, each with 141 amino acids, and two identical beta (β) chains, each with 146 amino acids ($\alpha_2\beta_2$). Normal fetal hemoglobin (Hb F) has two alpha (α) chains and two gamma (γ) chains ($\alpha_2\gamma_2$). This increases hemoglobin's attraction to oxygen and facilitates transfer of maternal oxygen across the placenta. Fetal hemoglobin is gradually replaced with Hb A over the first year of postnatal life.

When the precise number, sequence, or spatial arrangement of the globin amino acid chains is altered, the hemoglobin will be abnormal. For example, sickle cell hemoglobin (Hb S) has a different amino acid substituted into the β chain. This causes the deoxygenated hemoglobin molecule (hemoglobin not bound to oxygen) to change the RBC shape from biconcave to a crescent or "sickle" form that has a tendency to form thrombi (clots). Various drugs and chemicals, such as nitrites, can change the iron molecule in the heme from the *ferrous state* to the *ferric state*, eliminating the ability of hemoglobin to transport oxygen. This type of hemoglobin is known as *methemoglobin*.

The normal hemoglobin value for the adult male is 14 to 16 g/100 ml of blood. In other words, if all the hemoglobin were to be extracted from all the RBCs in 100 milliliters of blood, the hemoglobin would actually weigh between 14 and 16 grams. Clinically, the weight measurement of hemoglobin, in reference to 100 ml of blood, is referred to as either the *gram percent of hemoglobin* (g% Hb) or *grams per deciliter* (g/dl). The average adult female hemoglobin value is 12 to 15 g%. The average infant hemoglobin value is 14 to 20 g%. Hemoglobin constitutes about 33 percent of the RBC weight.

Quantity of Oyxgen Bound to Hemoglobin

Each g% of Hb is capable of carrying approximately 1.34 ml* of oxygen. Thus, if the hemoglobin level is 15 g%, and if the hemoglobin is fully saturated, about 20.1 vol% of oxygen will be bound to the hemoglobin. The figure 20.1 is calculated using the following formula:

$$O_2 \text{ bound to Hb} = 1.34 \text{ ml } O_2 \times 15 \text{ g\% Hb}$$
$$= 20.1 \text{ vol\% } O_2$$

At a normal arterial oxygen pressure (Pa_{O_2}) of 100 mm Hg, however, the hemoglobin saturation (Sa_{O_2}) is only about 97 percent because of these normal physiologic shunts:

- Thebesian venous drainage into the left atrium
- Bronchial venous drainage into the pulmonary veins
- Alveoli that are underventilated in proportion to pulmonary blood flow

Thus, the amount of arterial oxygen in the above equation must be adjusted to 97 percent. The equation is written as follows:

$$\begin{array}{r} 20.1 \text{ vol\% } O_2 \\ \times \quad .97 \\ \hline 19.5 \text{ vol\% } O_2 \end{array}$$

TOTAL OXYGEN CONTENT

To determine the total amount of oxygen in 100 ml of blood, the dissolved oxygen and the oxygen bound to hemoglobin must be added together. The following case example summarizes the calculations required to compute an individual's total oxygen content.

CASE STUDY: ANEMIC PATIENT

A 27-year-old woman with a long history of anemia (decreased hemoglobin concentration) is showing signs of respiratory distress. Her respiratory rate is 36 breaths per minute, her heart rate is 130 beats per minute, and her blood pressure is 155/90. Her hemoglobin concentration is 6 g%, and her Pa_{O_2} is 80 mm Hg (Sa_{O_2} 90%).

Based upon this information, the patient's total oxygen content is computed as follows:

1. Dissolved O_2:

$$\begin{array}{r} 80 \text{ } Pa_{O_2} \\ \times \quad 0.003 \text{ (dissolved } O_2 \text{ factor)} \\ \hline 0.24 \text{ vol\% } O_2 \end{array}$$

---

*The literature also reports the values 1.36, 1.38, and 1.39. The figure 1.34 is the commonly used factor and is used in this textbook.

2. Oxygen bound to hemoglobin:

$$\begin{array}{r} 6 \text{ g\% Hb} \\ \times \ 1.34 \ (O_2 \text{ bound to Hb factor}) \\ \hline 8.04 \text{ vol\% } O_2 \ (\text{at } Sa_{O_2} \text{ of } 100\%) \end{array}$$

$$\begin{array}{r} 8.04 \text{ vol\% } O_2 \\ \times \ \ .90 \ Sa_{O_2} \\ \hline 7.236 \text{ vol\% } O_2 \end{array}$$

3. Total Oxygen Content:

$$\begin{array}{r} 7.236 \text{ vol\% } O_2 \ (\text{bound to hemoglobin}) \\ + \ 0.24 \ \ \text{vol\% } O_2 \ (\text{dissolved } O_2) \\ \hline 7.476 \text{ vol\% } O_2 \ (\text{total amount of } O_2/100 \text{ ml of blood}) \end{array}$$

Note that the patient's total arterial oxygen content is less than 50 percent of normal. Her hemoglobin concentration, which is the primary mechanism for transporting oxygen, is very low. Once this problem is corrected, the clinical manifestations of respiratory distress should no longer be present.

The total oxygen content of the arterial blood (Ca_{O_2}), mixed venous blood (Cv_{O_2}), and pulmonary capillary blood (Cc_{O_2}) is calculated as follows:

Ca_{O_2}: Oxygen content of arterial blood
$(Hb \times 1.34 \times Sa_{O_2}) + (Pa_{O_2} \times 0.003)$

Cv_{O_2}: Oxygen content of mixed venous blood
$(Hb \times 1.34 \times Sv_{O_2}) + (Pv_{O_2} \times 0.003)$

Cc_{O_2}: Oxygen content of pulmonary capillary blood
$(Hb \times 1.34)^* + (PA_{O_2}{}^\dagger \times 0.003)$

It will be shown later in this chapter how various mathematical manipulations of the Ca_{O_2}, Cv_{O_2}, and Cc_{O_2} values are used in different oxygen transport studies to reflect important factors concerning the patient's cardiac and ventilatory status.

OXYGEN DISSOCIATION CURVE

As shown in Figure 7–2, the oxygen dissociation curve is part of a nomogram that graphically illustrates the *percentage of hemoglobin* (left-hand side of the graph) that is chemically bound to oxygen at each *oxygen pressure* (bottom portion of the graph). On the right-hand side of the graph, a second scale is included that gives the precise *oxygen content* that is carried by the hemoglobin at each oxygen pressure.

The curve is S-shaped with a steep slope between 10 and 60 mm Hg and a flat portion between 70 and 100 mm Hg. The steep portion of the curve shows that oxy-

---

*It is assumed that the hemoglobin saturation with oxygen in the pulmonary capillary blood (Sc_{O_2}) is 100 percent or 1.0.
†See Ideal Alveolar Gas Equation, Chapter Three.

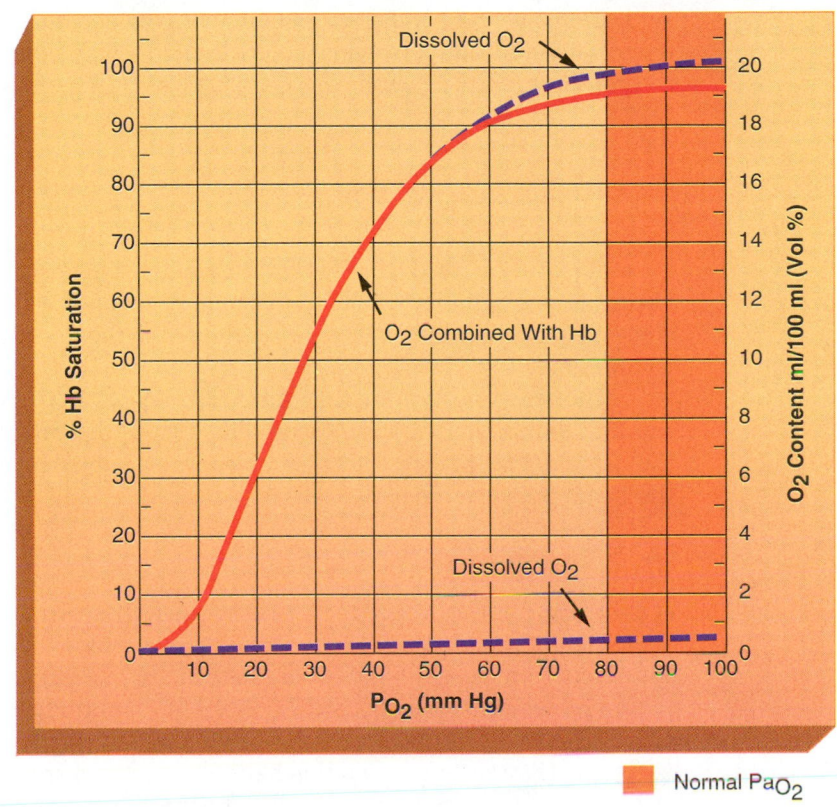

Figure 7–2. *Oxygen dissociation curve.*

gen rapidly combines with hemoglobin as the P_{O_2} increases. Beyond this point (60 mm Hg), a further increase in the P_{O_2} produces only a slight increase in oxygen/hemoglobin bonding. In fact, because the hemoglobin is already 90-percent saturated at a P_{O_2} of 60 mm Hg, an increase in the P_{O_2} from 60 to 100 mm Hg elevates the total saturation of the hemoglobin by only 7 percent (see Figure 7–2).

CLINICAL SIGNIFICANCE OF THE FLAT PORTION OF THE CURVE

The P_{O_2} can fall from 100 to 60 mm Hg and the hemoglobin will still be 90-percent saturated with oxygen. Thus, the upper curve plateau illustrates that hemoglobin has an excellent safety zone for the loading of oxygen in the lungs.

As the hemoglobin moves through the alveolar-capillary system to pick up oxygen, a significant partial pressure difference continues to exist between the alveolar gas and the blood even after most of the oxygen is transferred. This mechanism enhances the diffusion of oxygen during the transit time the hemoglobin is in the alveolar-capillary system.

The flat portion also means that increasing the P_{O_2} beyond 100 mm Hg adds very little additional oxygen to the blood. In fact, once the P_{O_2} increases enough to saturate 100 percent of the hemoglobin with oxygen, the hemoglobin will no longer accept any additional oxygen molecules. However, a small additional amount of oxygen continues to dissolve in the plasma as the P_{O_2} rises ($P_{O_2} \times 0.003 =$ dissolved O_2).

CLINICAL SIGNIFICANCE OF THE STEEP PORTION OF THE CURVE

P_{O_2} reductions below 60 mm Hg produce a rapid decrease in the amount of oxygen bound to hemoglobin. Clinically, therefore, when the P_{O_2} continues to fall below 60 mm Hg, the quantity of oxygen delivered to the tissue cells may be significantly reduced.

The steep portion of the curve also shows that as the hemoglobin moves through the capillaries of the tissue cells, a large amount of oxygen is released from the hemoglobin for only a small decrease in P_{O_2}. Thus, the diffusion of oxygen from the hemoglobin to the tissue cells is enhanced.

THE P_{50}

A common point of reference on the oxygen dissociation curve is the P_{50} (Figure 7–3). The P_{50} represents the partial pressure at which the hemoglobin is 50-percent saturated with oxygen—i.e., when there are two oxygen molecules on each hemoglobin molecule. Normally, the P_{50} is about 27 mm Hg. Clinically, however, there are a variety of abnormal conditions that can shift the oxygen dissociation curve to either the right or left. When this happens the P_{50} changes. For example, when the curve shifts to the right, the affinity of hemoglobin for oxygen decreases, causing the hemoglobin to be less saturated at a given P_{O_2}. Thus, *when the curve shifts to the right, the P_{50} increases.* On the other hand, when the curve moves to the left, the affinity of hemoglobin for oxygen increases, causing the hemoglobin to be more saturated at a given P_{O_2}. Thus, *when the curve shifts to the left, the P_{50} decreases* (see Figure 7–3).

FACTORS THAT SHIFT THE OXYGEN DISSOCIATION CURVE

pH

As the blood hydrogen-ion concentration increases (decreased pH), the oxygen dissociation curve shifts to the right. This mechanism enhances the unloading of oxygen at the cellular level, since the pH decreases in this area as carbon dioxide (the acidic end-product of cellular metabolism) moves into the blood. In contrast, as the blood hydrogen-ion (H^+) concentration decreases, the curve shifts to the left. This mechanism facilitates the loading of oxygen onto hemoglobin as blood passes through the lungs, since the pH increases as carbon dioxide moves out of the blood and into the alveoli.

Temperature

As the body temperature increases, the curve moves to the right. Thus, actively metabolizing tissue (e.g., exercise), which has an elevated temperature, enhances the release of oxygen as blood flows through the muscle capillaries. Conversely, as the

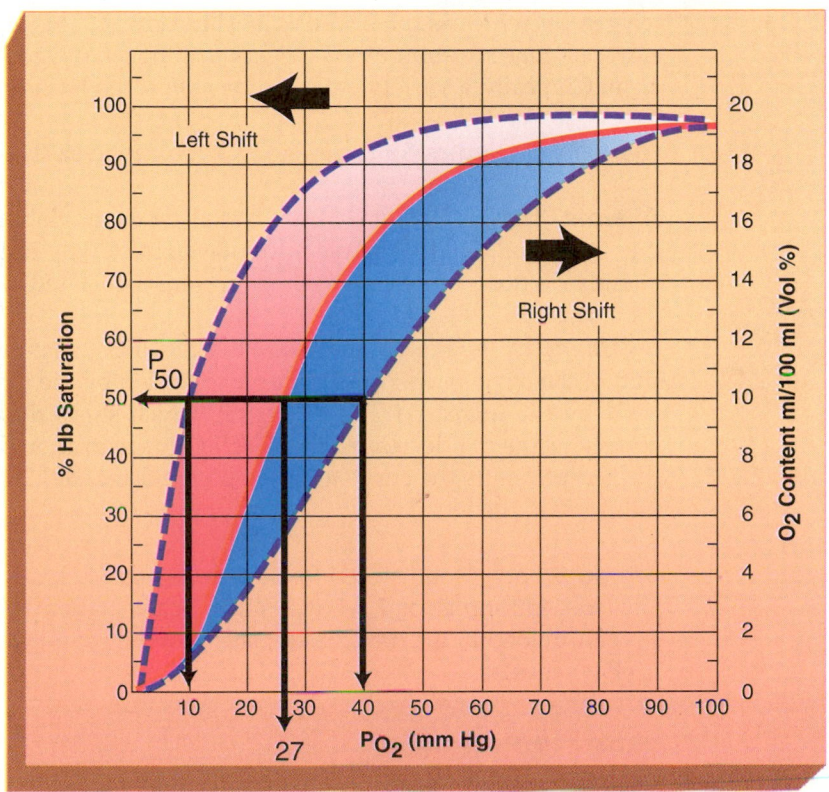

Figure 7–3. *The P_{50} represents the partial pressure at which hemoglobin is 50-percent saturated with oxygen. When the oxygen dissociation curve shifts to the right, the P_{50} increases. When the oxygen dissociation curve shifts to the left, the P_{50} decreases.*

body temperature decreases, the curve shifts to the left. This mechanism partly explains why an individual's lips, ears, and fingers appear blue while swimming in very cold water. That is, their Pa_{O_2} is normal, but oxygen is not readily released from the hemoglobin at the tissue sites.

Carbon Dioxide

As the P_{CO_2} level increases (increased H^+ concentration), the oxyhemoglobin saturation decreases, shifting the oxyhemoglobin dissociation curve to the right, whereas decreasing P_{CO_2} levels (decreased H^+ concentrations) shift the curve to the left. The effect of P_{CO_2} and pH on the oxyhemoglobin curve is known as the **Bohr effect**. The Bohr effect is most active in the capillaries of working muscles, particularly the myocardium.

2,3-Diphosphoglycerate

The red blood cells (RBCs) contain a large quantity (about 15 mol/g Hb) of the substance 2,3-diphosphoglycerate (2,3-DPG). 2,3-DPG is a metabolic intermediary that is formed by the RBCs during anaerobic glycolysis. Hemoglobin's affinity for oxygen decreases as the 2,3-DPG level increases. Thus, the physiologic effect of an elevated concentration of 2,3-DPG is to shift the oxygen dissociation curve to the right. Clinically, a variety of conditions affect the level of 2,3-DPG.

Hypoxia. Regardless of the etiology, hypoxia increases the 2,3-DPG level.

Anemia. The 2,3-DPG level increases as the hemoglobin concentration decreases. It is suggested that this mechanism may explain why individuals with anemia frequently do not manifest signs or symptoms associated with hypoxia.

pH Changes. As the pH increases, the 2,3-DPG concentration increases. Thus, the shift of the oxygen dissociation curve to the left by the increased pH is offset somewhat by the increased 2,3-DPG level, which shifts the curve to the right. Conversely, as the pH decreases, the 2,3-DPG concentration decreases. Thus, as the decreased pH shifts the curve to the right, the decreased 2,3-DPG level works to shift the curve to the left.

Stored Blood. Blood stored for as little as one week has been shown to have very low concentrations of 2,3-DPG. Thus, when patients receive stored blood, the oxygen unloading at their tissue sites may be reduced because of the decreased 2,3-DPG level.

Fetal Hemoglobin

Fetal hemoglobin (Hb F) is chemically different from adult hemoglobin (Hb A). Hb F has a greater affinity for oxygen and therefore shifts the oxygen dissociation curve to the left (reducing the P_{50}). During fetal development, the higher affinity of Hb F enhances the transfer of oxygen from maternal blood to fetal blood (see Chapter Eleven). After birth, Hb F progressively disappears and is completely absent after about one year.

Carbon Monoxide Hemoglobin

Carbon monoxide (CO) has about 210 times the affinity of oxygen for hemoglobin. Because of this, a small amount of CO can tie up a large amount of hemoglobin (CO_{Hb}) and, as a result, prevent oxygen molecules from bonding to hemoglobin. This mechanism can seriously reduce the amount of oxygen transferred to the tissue cells. In addition, when CO_{Hb} is present the affinity of hemoglobin for oxygen increases and shifts the oxygen dissociation curve to the left. Thus, the oxygen molecules that do manage to combine with hemoglobin are unable to unload easily at the tissues.

Figure 7–4 summarizes factors that shift the oxygen dissociation curve to the right and left and, additionally, how the P_{50} is affected by these shifts.

CLINICAL SIGNIFICANCE OF SHIFTS IN THE O_2 DISSOCIATION CURVE

When an individual's blood Pa_{O_2} is within normal limits (80–100 mm Hg), a shift of the oxygen dissociation curve to the right or left does not significantly affect the

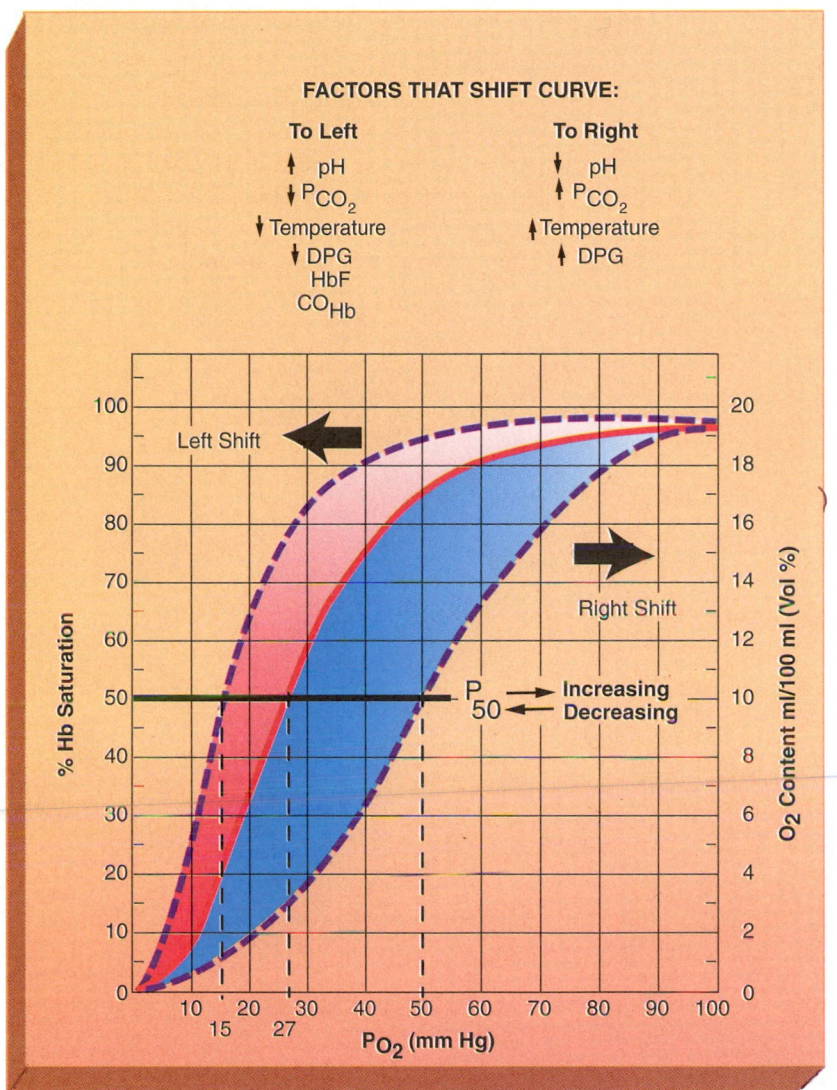

Figure 7–4. *Factors that shift the oxygen dissociation curve to the right and left. (DPG = 2,3-diphosphoglycerate for other abbreviations, see explanations in text.*

hemoglobin's ability to transport oxygen to the peripheral tissues. This is because shifts in this pressure range (80–100 mm Hg) occur on the flat portion of the curve. However, when an individual's blood Pa_{O_2} falls below the normal range, a shift to the right or left can have a remarkable effect on the hemoglobin's ability to pick up and release oxygen. This is because shifts below the normal pressure range occur on the steep portion of the curve. For example, consider the loading and unloading of oxygen during the following clinical conditions:

Right Shifts—Loading of Oxygen in the Lungs

Picture the loading of oxygen onto hemoglobin as blood passes through the alveo-lar-capillary system at a time when the alveolar oxygen tension ($P_{A_{O_2}}$) is moderately low—say, 60 mm Hg (caused, for example, by an acute asthmatic episode). Normally, when the $P_{A_{O_2}}$ is 60 mm Hg, the P_{O_2} of the pulmonary capillary blood (Pc_{O_2}) is also about 60 mm Hg. Thus, the hemoglobin is about 90-percent saturated with oxygen as it leaves the alveoli (Figure 7–5). If, however, the oxygen dissociation curve shifts to the right, as indicated in Figure 7–6 (caused by a pH of

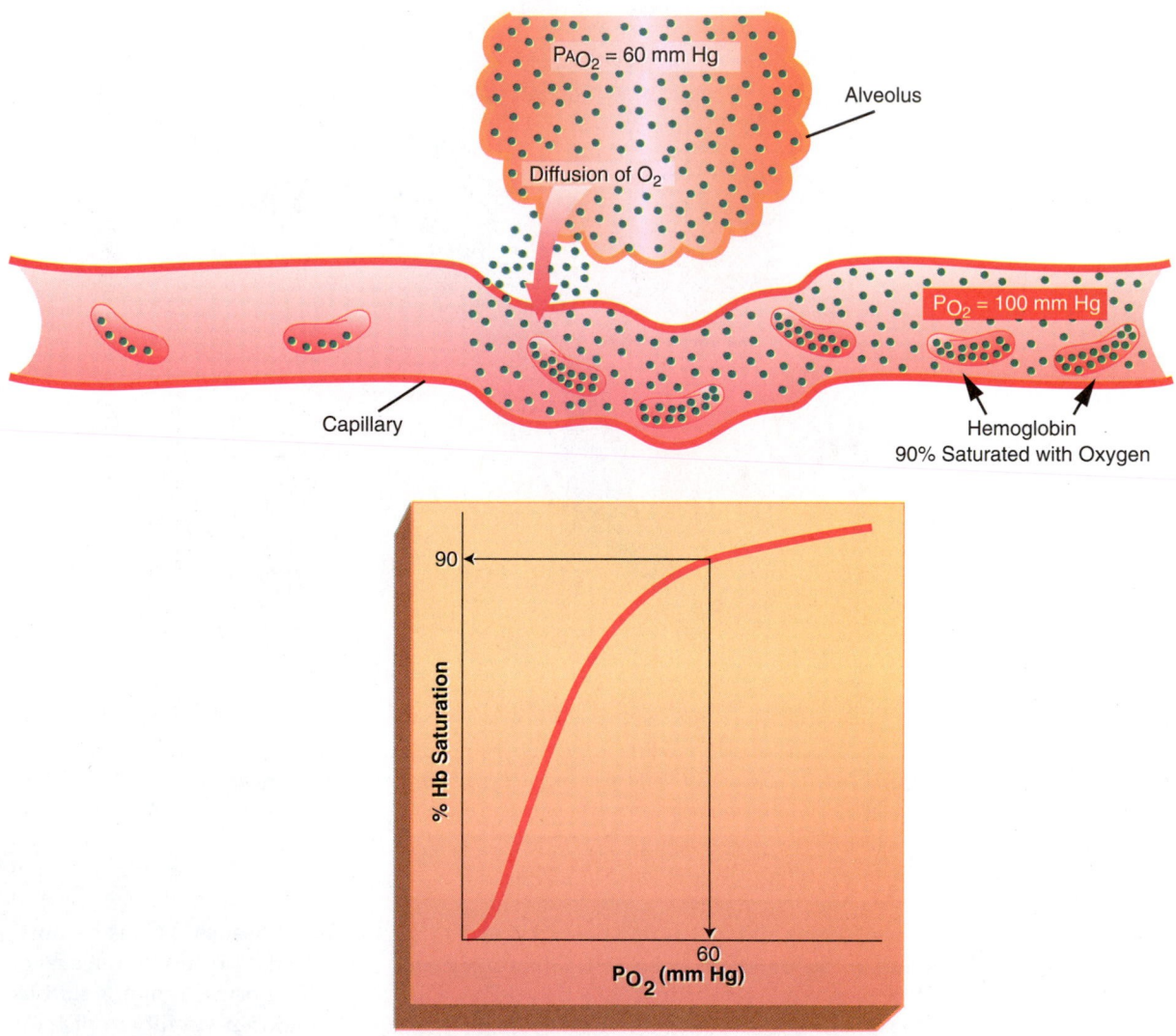

Figure 7–5. *Normally, when the $P_{A_{O_2}}$ is 60 mm Hg, the plasma P_{O_2} of the alveolar-capillary blood is also about 60 mm Hg and the hemoglobin is about 90-percent saturated with oxygen as it leaves the alveoli.*

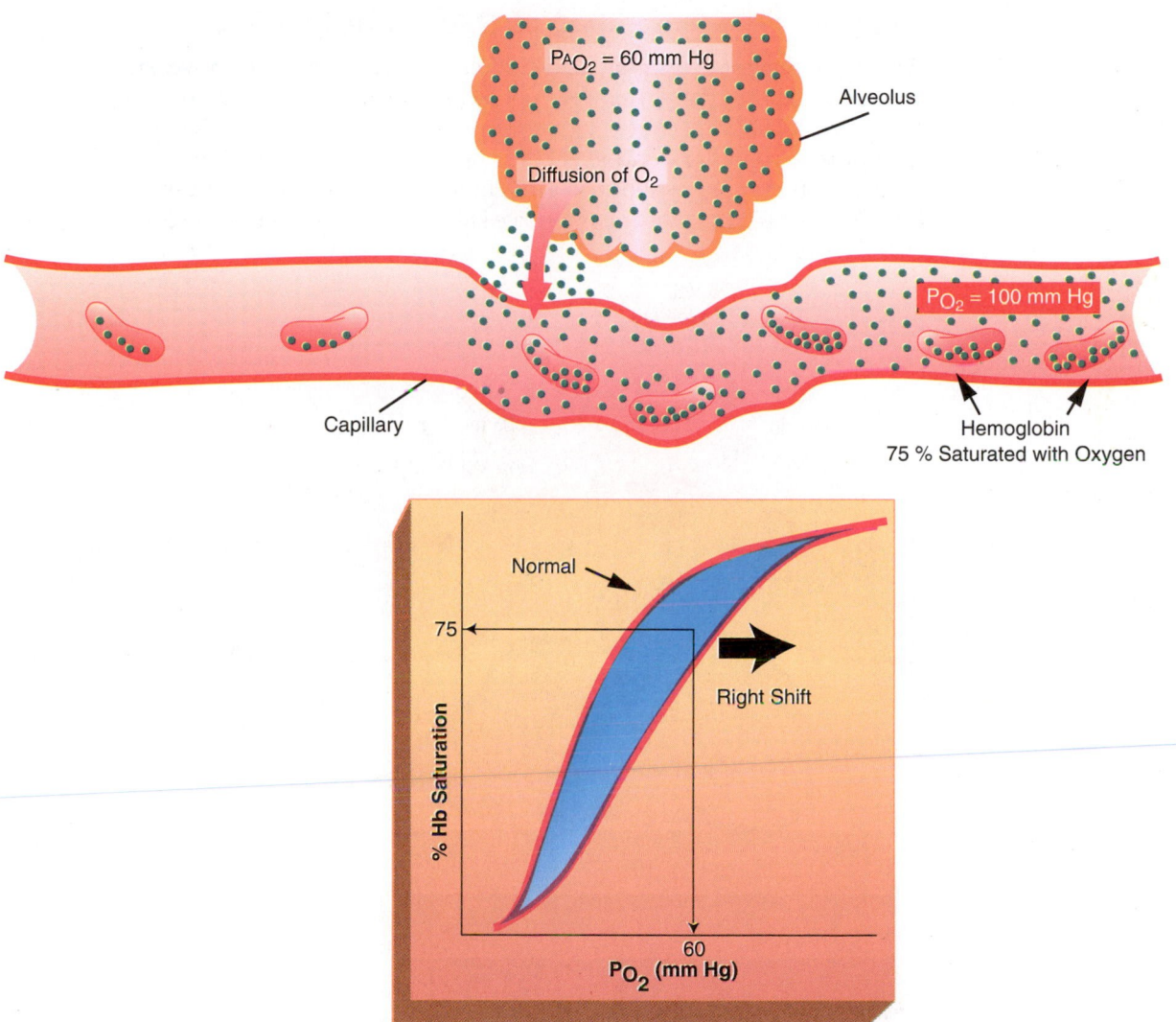

Figure 7–6. *When the PA_{O_2} is 60 mm Hg at a time when the oxygen dissociation curve has shifted to the right because of a pH of 7.1, the hemoglobin will only be about 75-percent saturated with oxygen as it leaves the alveoli.*

about 7.1), the hemoglobin will only be about 75-percent saturated with oxygen as it leaves the alveoli—in spite of the fact that the patient's plasma P_{O_2} is still 60 mm Hg.

In view of this gas transport phenomenon, therefore, it should be stressed that *the total oxygen delivery may be much lower than indicated by a particular Pa_{O_2} when the patient has some disease process that causes the oxygen dissociation curve to shift to the right* (see Figure 7–4). It should also be noted that when a right shift is accompanied by either a decreased cardiac output or a reduced level of hemoglobin, the patient's ability to transport oxygen will be jeopardized even more.

Right Shifts—Unloading of Oxygen at the Tissues

Although the total oxygen delivery may decrease in the above situation, the plasma P_{O_2} at the tissue sites does not have to fall as much to unload oxygen from the hemoglobin. For example, if the tissue cells metabolize 5 vol% oxygen at a time when the oxygen dissociation curve is in its normal position, the plasma P_{O_2} must fall from 60 mm Hg to about 35 mm Hg to free 5 vol% oxygen from the hemoglobin (Figure 7–7). If, however, the curve shifts to the right in response to a pH of 7.1,

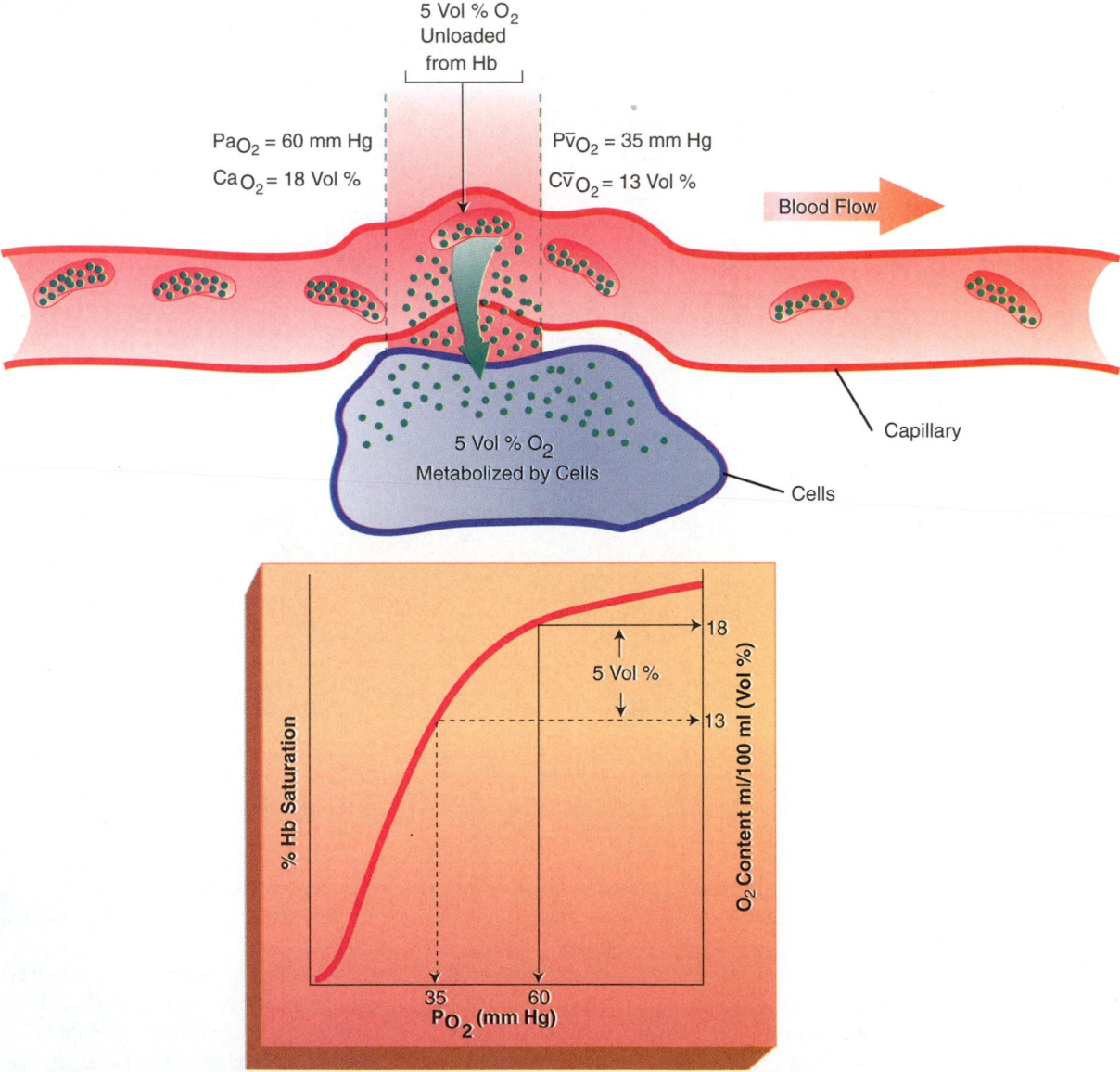

Figure 7–7. *Normally, when the plasma P_{O_2} is 60 mm Hg, the P_{O_2} must fall from 60 mm Hg to about 35 mm Hg to free 5 vol% oxygen from the hemoglobin for tissue metabolism.*

the plasma P_{O_2} at the tissue sites would only have to fall from 60 mm Hg to about 40 mm Hg to unload 5 vol% oxygen from the hemoglobin (Figure 7–8).

Left Shifts—Loading of Oxygen in the Lungs

If the oxygen dissociation curve shifts to the left, as indicated in Figure 7–9, page 218 (caused by a pH of about 7.6), at a time when the $P_{A_{O_2}}$ is 60 mm Hg, the

Figure 7–8. *When the Pa_{O_2} is 60 mm Hg at a time when the oxygen dissociation curve has shifted to the right because of a pH of 7.1, the plasma P_{O_2} at the tissue sites would only have to fall from 60 mm Hg to about 40 mm Hg to unload 5 vol% oxygen from the hemoglobin.*

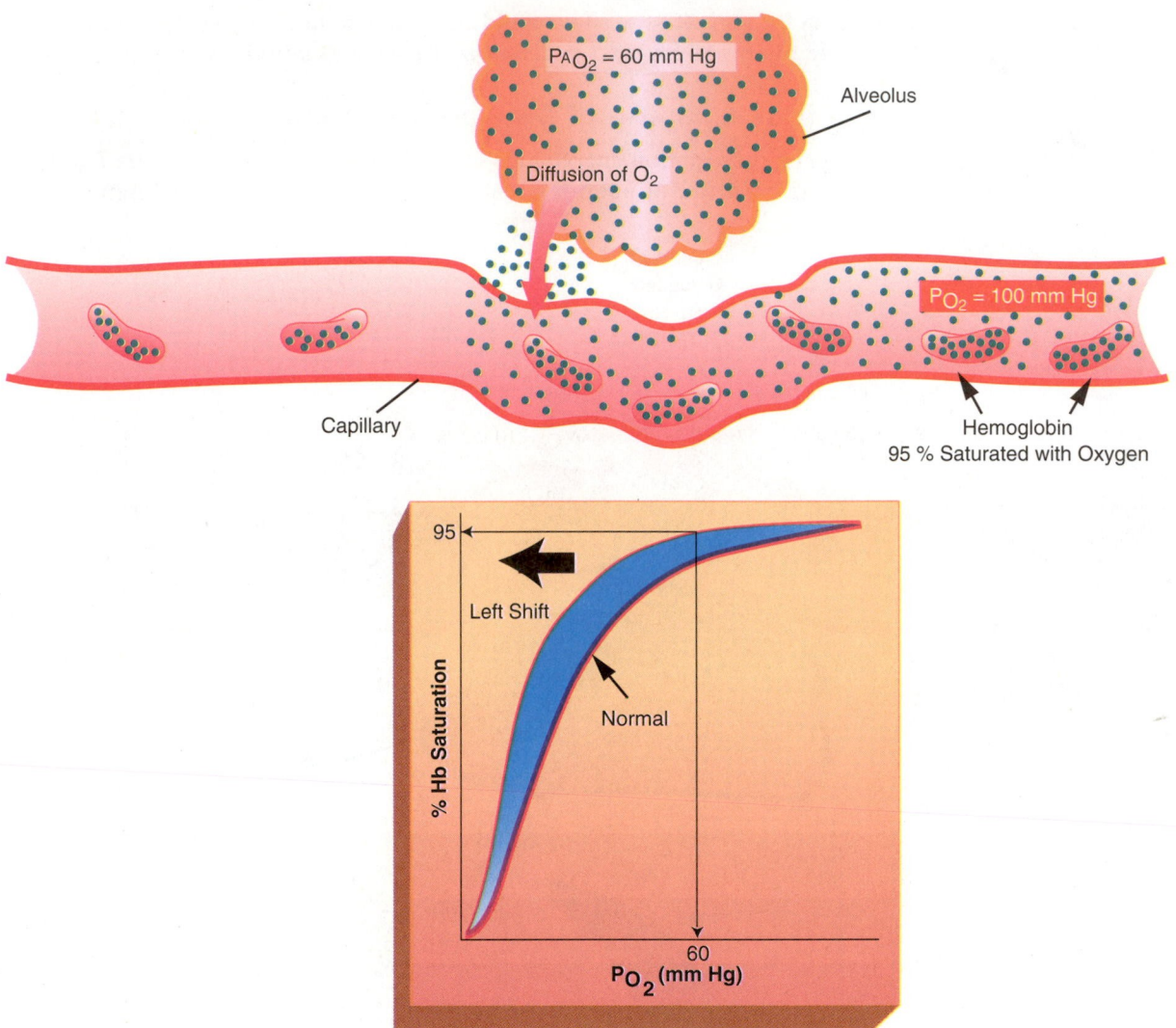

Figure 7–9.   *When the $P_{A_{O_2}}$ is 60 mm Hg at a time when the oxygen dissociation curve has shifted to the left because of a pH of 7.6, the hemoglobin will be about 95-percent saturated with oxygen as it leaves the alveoli.*

hemoglobin will be about 95-percent saturated with oxygen as it leaves the alveoli, even though the patient's plasma P_{O_2} is only 60 mm Hg.

Left Shifts—Unloading of Oxygen at the Tissues

Although the total oxygen delivery increases in the above situation, the plasma P_{O_2} at the tissue sites must decrease more than normal in order for oxygen to dissociate from the hemoglobin. For example, if the tissue cells require 5 vol% oxygen at a time when the oxygen dissociation curve is in its normal position, the plasma P_{O_2}

will fall from 60 mm Hg to about 35 mm Hg to free 5 vol% of oxygen from the hemoglobin (see Figure 7–7). If, however, the curve shifts to the left because of a pH of 7.6, the plasma P_{O_2} at the tissue sites would have to fall from 60 mm Hg to about 30 mm Hg in order to unload 5 vol% oxygen from the hemoglobin (Figure 7–10).

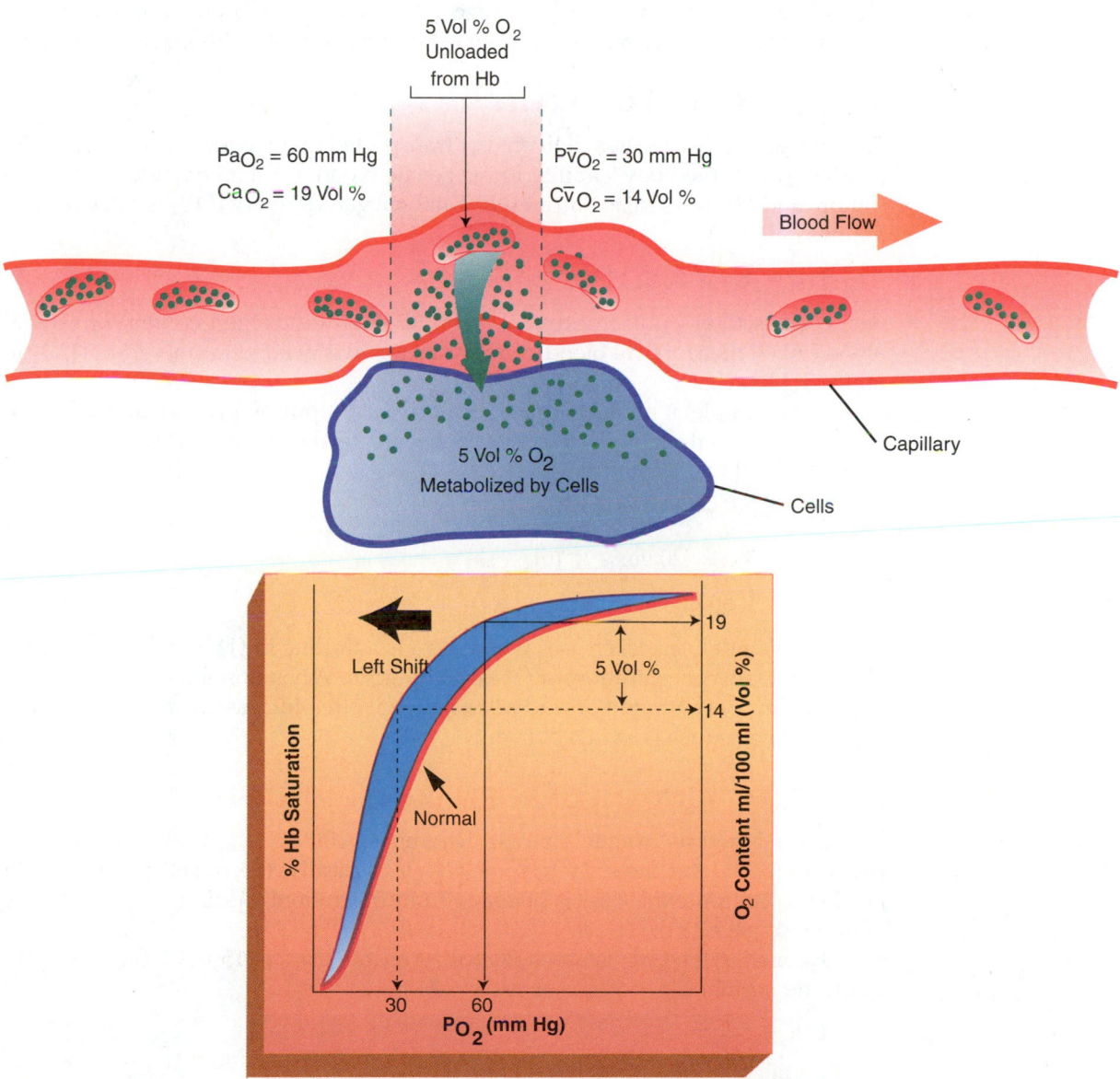

Figure 7–10. *When the Pa_{O_2} is 60 mm Hg at a time when the oxygen dissociation curve has shifted to the left because of a pH of 7.6, the plasma P_{O_2} at the tissue sites would have to fall from 60 mm Hg to about 30 mm Hg to unload 5 vol% oxygen from the hemoglobin.*

OXYGEN TRANSPORT STUDIES

Various mathematical manipulations of the Ca_{O_2}, Cv_{O_2}, and Cc_{O_2} values can serve as excellent indicators of an individual's cardiac and ventilatory status. Clinically, the most common oxygen transport studies performed are (1) total oxygen delivery, (2) arterial-venous oxygen content difference, (3) oxygen consumption, (4) oxygen extraction ratio, (5) mixed venous oxygen saturation, and (6) pulmonary shunting.*

TOTAL OXYGEN DELIVERY

The total amount of oxygen delivered or transported to the peripheral tissues is dependent on (1) the body's ability to oxygenate blood, (2) the hemoglobin concentration, and (3) the cardiac output ($\dot{Q}$). **Total oxygen delivery** (D_{O_2}) is calculated as follows:

$$D_{O_2} = \dot{Q}T \times (Ca_{O_2} \times 10)$$

where $\dot{Q}T$ is total cardiac output (L/min); Ca_{O_2} is the oxygen content of arterial blood (ml oxygen/100 ml blood); and the factor 10 is needed to convert the Ca_{O_2} to ml O_2/L blood.

For example, if an individual has a cardiac output of 5 L/min and a Ca_{O_2} of 20 vol%, the total amount of oxygen delivered to the peripheral tissues will be about 1000 ml O_2 per minute:

$$D_{O_2} = \dot{Q}T \times (Ca_{O_2} \times 10)$$
$$= 5\ L \times (20\ vol\% \times 10)$$
$$= 1000\ ml\ O_2/minute$$

Oxygen delivery decreases when there is a decline in (1) blood oxygenation, (2) hemoglobin concentration, or (3) cardiac output. When possible, an individual's hemoglobin concentration or cardiac output will often increase in an effort to compensate for a reduced oxygen delivery.

ARTERIAL-VENOUS OXYGEN CONTENT DIFFERENCE

The **arterial-venous oxygen content difference**, $C(a - v)_{O_2}$, is the difference between the Ca_{O_2} and the Cv_{O_2} ($Ca_{O_2} - Cv_{O_2}$). Clinically, the mixed venous blood needed to compute the Cv_{O_2} is obtained from the patient's pulmonary artery (see Figure 6–1, page 191).

Normally, the Ca_{O_2} is about 20 vol% and the Cv_{O_2} is 15 vol% (Figure 7–11). Thus, the normal $C(a - v)_{O_2}$ is about 5 vol%:

$$C(a - v)_{O_2} = Ca_{O_2} - Cv_{O_2}$$
$$= 20\ vol\% - 15\ vol\%$$
$$= 5\ vol\%$$

---

*See Appendix V for a representative example of a cardiopulmonary profile sheet used to monitor the oxygen transport status of the critically ill patient.

Figure 7–11.   *Oxygen dissociation curve. The normal oxygen content difference between arterial and venous blood is about 5 vol%. Note that both the right side and the left side of the graph illustrate that approximately 25 percent of the available oxygen is used for tissue metabolism, and therefore the hemoglobin returning to the lungs is normally about 75-percent saturated with oxygen.*

In other words, 5 ml of oxygen are extracted from each 100 ml of blood for tissue metabolism (50 ml O_2/L). Since the average individual has a cardiac output of about 5 liters per minute, and a $C(a - v)_{O_2}$ of about 5 vol%, approximately 250 ml of oxygen are extracted from the blood during the course of one minute (50 ml O_2/L × 5 L/min).

Clinically, the $C(a - v)_{O_2}$ can provide useful information regarding the patient's cardiopulmonary status, since oxygen changes in mixed venous blood can occur earlier than oxygen changes in an arterial blood gas. Table 7–2 (page 222) lists factors that can cause the $C(a - v)_{O_2}$ to increase. Factors that can cause the $C(a - v)_{O_2}$ to decrease are listed in Table 7–3 (page 222).

OXYGEN CONSUMPTION

The amount of oxygen extracted by the peripheral tissues during the period of one minute is called **oxygen consumption**, or *oxygen uptake* ($\dot{V}_{O_2}$). An individual's oxygen consumption is calculated by using this formula:

TABLE 7–2.   **Factors that Increase the C(a − v)$_{O_2}$**

Decreased cardiac output
Periods of increased oxygen consumption
   Exercise
   Seizures
   Shivering in postoperative patient
   Hyperthermia

$$\dot{V}_{O_2} = \dot{Q}\text{T} \, [C(a - v)_{O_2} \times 10]$$

where $\dot{Q}\text{T}$ is the total cardiac output (L/min); $C(a - v)_{O_2}$ is the arterial-venous oxygen content difference ($Ca_{O_2} - Cv_{O_2}$); and the factor 10 is needed to convert the $C(a - v)_{O_2}$ to ml O_2/L.

For example, if an individual has a cardiac output of 5 L/min, and a $C(a - v)_{O_2}$ of 5 vol%, the total amount of oxygen metabolized by the tissues in one minute will be 250 ml:

$$\dot{V}_{O_2} = \dot{Q}\text{T} \, [C(a - v)_{O_2} \times 10]$$

$$= 5 \text{ L/min} \times 5 \text{ vol\%} \times 10$$

$$= 250 \text{ ml } O_2/\text{min}$$

Clinically, the oxygen consumption is commonly indexed by the patient's body surface area (BSA) (see Appendix IV), since the amount of oxygen extracted by the peripheral cells varies with the height and weight of an individual. The patient's oxygen consumption index is derived by dividing the $\dot{V}_{O_2}$ by the BSA. The average oxygen consumption index ranges between 125 to 165 ml O_2/m^2.

Factors that cause an increase in oxygen consumption are listed in Table 7–4. Table 7–5 lists factors that cause a decrease in oxygen consumption.

OXYGEN EXTRACTION RATIO

The oxygen extraction ratio (O_2ER) is the amount of oxygen extracted by the peripheral tissues divided by the amount of oxygen delivered to the peripheral

---

TABLE 7–3.   **Factors that Decrease the C(a − v)$_{O_2}$**

Increased cardiac output
Skeletal relaxation (e.g., induced by drugs)
Peripheral shunting (e.g., sepsis, trauma)
Certain poisons (e.g., cyanide prevents cellular metabolism)
Hypothermia

TABLE 7–4.	Factors that Increase Oxygen Consumption

Exercise
Seizures
Shivering in postoperative patient
Hyperthermia

cells. The O_2ER is also known as the *oxygen coefficient ratio* or the *oxygen utilization ratio*.

The O_2ER is easily calculated by dividing the $C(a - v)_{O_2}$ by the Ca_{O_2}. In considering the normal Ca_{O_2} of 20 vol%, and the normal Cv_{O_2} of 15 vol% (see Figure 7–11), the O_2ER ratio of the healthy individual is about 25 percent:

$$O_2ER = \frac{Ca_{O_2} - Cv_{O_2}}{Ca_{O_2}}$$

$$= \frac{20 \text{ vol\%} - 15 \text{ vol\%}}{20 \text{ vol\%}}$$

$$= \frac{5 \text{ vol\%}}{20 \text{ vol\%}}$$

$$= .25$$

Under normal circumstances, therefore, an individual's hemoglobin returns to the alveoli approximately 75-percent saturated with oxygen (see Figure 7–11). In an individual with a total oxygen delivery of 1000 ml/minute, an extraction ratio of 25 percent would mean that during the course of one minute, 250 ml of oxygen are metabolized by the tissues and 750 ml of oxygen are returned to the lungs.

Factors that can cause the O_2ER to increase are listed in Table 7–6 (page 224). Table 7–7 (page 224) lists factors that can cause the O_2ER to decrease.

The O_2ER provides an important view of an individual's oxygen transport status that is not readily available from other oxygen transport measurements. For example, in an individual with normal Ca_{O_2} and normal Cv_{O_2}:

$$\begin{array}{ll} Ca_{O_2}: & 20 \text{ vol\%} \\ - Cv_{O_2}: & 15 \text{ vol\%} \\ \hline C(a - v)_{O_2} = & 5 \text{ vol\%} \end{array}$$

TABLE 7–5.	Factors that Decrease Oxygen Consumption

Skeletal relaxation (e.g., induced by drugs)
Peripheral shunting (e.g., sepsis, trauma)
Certain poisons (e.g., cyanide prevents cellular metabolism)
Hypothermia

TABLE 7–6. **Factors that Increase the O$_2$ER**

Decreased cardiac output
Periods of increased oxygen consumption
   Exercise
   Seizures
   Shivering in postoperative patient
   Hyperthermia
Anemia
Decreased arterial oxygenation

the $C(a - v)_{O_2}$ is 5 vol% and the O$_2$ER is 25 percent (normal). In an individual, however, with reduced Ca_{O_2} and reduced Cv_{O_2}:

$$
\begin{array}{ll}
Ca_{O_2}: & 10 \text{ vol\%} \\
- Cv_{O_2}: & 5 \text{ vol\%} \\
\hline
C(a - v)_{O_2} = & 5 \text{ vol\%}
\end{array}
$$

the $C(a - v)_{O_2}$ is still 5 vol% (assuming O$_2$ consumption remains constant), but the extraction ratio (O$_2$ER) is now 50 percent—clinically, a potentially dangerous oxygen transport status.

MIXED VENOUS OXYGEN SATURATION

In the presence of a normal arterial oxygen saturation level (Sa_{O_2}) and hemoglobin concentration, the continuous monitoring of mixed venous oxygen saturation (Sv_{O_2}) is often used in the clinical setting as an early indicator of changes in the patient's $C(a - v)_{O_2}$, $\dot{V}_{O_2}$, and O$_2$ER. Normally, the Sv_{O_2} is about 75 percent (see Figure 7–11). Clinically, an Sv_{O_2} of about 65 percent is acceptable.

Factors that can cause the Sv_{O_2} to decrease are listed in Table 7–8. Table 7–9 lists factors that can cause the Sv_{O_2} to increase.

Continuous Sv_{O_2} monitoring can signal changes in the patient's $C(a - v)_{O_2}$, $\dot{V}_{O_2}$, and O$_2$ER earlier than routine arterial blood gas monitoring, since the Pa_{O_2} and Sa_{O_2} levels are of-

TABLE 7–7. **Factors that Decrease the O$_2$ER**

Increased cardiac output
Skeletal relaxation (e.g., induced by drugs)
Peripheral shunting (e.g., sepsis, trauma)
Certain poisons (e.g., cyanide prevents cellular metabolism)
Hypothermia (slows cellular metabolism)
Increased hemoglobin concentration
Increased arterial oxygenation

TABLE 7–8. **Factors that Decrease the Sv_{O_2}**

Decreased cardiac output
Periods of increased oxygen consumption
  Exercise
  Seizures
  Shivering in postoperative patient
  Hyperthermia

NOTE: A decreased Sv_{O_2} indicates that the $C(a-v)_{O_2}$, $\dot{V}_{O_2}$, and O_2ER are increasing.

ten normal during early $C(a-v)_{O_2}$, $\dot{V}_{O_2}$, and O_2ER changes. Table 7–10 summarizes how various clinical factors will likely alter an individual's D_{O_2}, $\dot{V}_{O_2}$, $C(a-v)_{O_2}$, O_2ER, and Sv_{O_2}.

MECHANISMS OF PULMONARY SHUNTING

Pulmonary shunting is defined as that portion of the cardiac output that enters the left side of the heart without exchanging gases with alveolar gases (*true shunt*) or as blood that does exchange gases with alveolar gases but does not obtain a P_{O_2} that equals that of a normal alveolus (*shunt-like effect*). Because the physiologic effect of pulmonary shunting is **hypoxemia** (decreased arterial oxygen tensions), it is important to understand clinical conditions that produce (1) true shunt, and (2) shunt-like effect.

True Shunt

Clinical conditions that cause true shunt can be grouped under two major categories: **anatomic shunts** and **capillary shunts**.

Anatomic Shunts. An anatomic shunt exists when blood flows from the right side of the heart to the left side without coming in contact with an alveolus for gas exchange (see Figures 7–12A and 7–12B, page 227). Normally this is calculated to be about 2 to 5 percent of the cardiac output. This normal shunted blood comes from the bronchial, pleural, and Thebesian veins, which are systemic veins that

TABLE 7–9. **Factors that Increase the Sv_{O_2}**

Increased cardiac output
Skeletal relaxation (e.g., induced by drugs)
Peripheral shunting (e.g., sepsis, trauma)
Certain poisons (e.g., cyanide prevents cellular metabolism)
Hypothermia

NOTE: A increased Sv_{O_2} indicates that the $C(a-v)_{O_2}$, $\dot{V}_{O_2}$, and O_2ER are decreasing.

TABLE 7–10.   Clinical Factors Affecting Various Oxygen Transport Study Values

CLINICAL FACTORS	OXYGEN TRANSPORT STUDIES				
	D_{O_2} (1000 ml O_2/min)	$\dot{V}_{O_2}$ (250 ml O_2/min)	$C(a-v)_{O_2}$ (5 vol%)	O_2ER (25%)	Sv_{O_2} (75%)
↑O_2 Consumption	Same	↑	↑	↑	↓
↓O_2 Consumption	Same	↓	↓	↓	↑
↓Cardiac Output	↓	Same	↑	↑	↓
↑Cardiac Output	↑	Same	↓	↓	↑
↓Pa_{O_2}	↓	Same	Same	↑	↓
↑Pa_{O_2}	↑	Same	Same	↓	↑
↓Hb	↓	Same	Same	↑	↓
↑Hb	↑	Same	Same	↓	↑
Peripheral Shunting	Same	↓	↓	↓	↑

↑ = increased; ↓ = decreased.

empty into the pulmonary venous system. The following are common abnormalities that cause anatomic shunting:

- Congenital heart disease
- Intrapulmonary fistula
- Vascular lung tumors

Congenital Heart Disease. Certain congenital defects permit blood to flow from the right side of the heart to the left side without going through the alveolar-capillary system for gas exchange (e.g., defect of the ventricular septum).

Intrapulmonary Fistula. In this type of anatomic shunting, a right-to-left flow of pulmonary blood does not pass through the alveolar-capillary system. It may be caused by chest trauma or disease. For example, a penetrating chest wound that damages both the arteries and veins of the lung can leave an arterial-venous shunt as a result of the healing process.

Vascular Lung Tumors. Some lung tumors can become very vascular. Some permit pulmonary arterial blood to move through the tumor mass and into the pulmonary veins without passing through the alveolar-capillary system.

Capillary Shunts. Capillary shunting is commonly caused by (1) alveolar collapse or atelectasis, (2) alveolar fluid accumulation, or (3) alveolar consolidation (see Figure 7–12C).

The sum of the anatomic and capillary shunts is referred to as true, or absolute shunt. Absolute shunting is *refractory* to oxygen therapy. That is, the hypoxemia produced by this form of pulmonary shunting cannot be treated by simply increasing the concentration of inspired oxygen, since (1) the alveoli are unable to accommodate any form of ventilation, and (2) the blood that passes by functioning

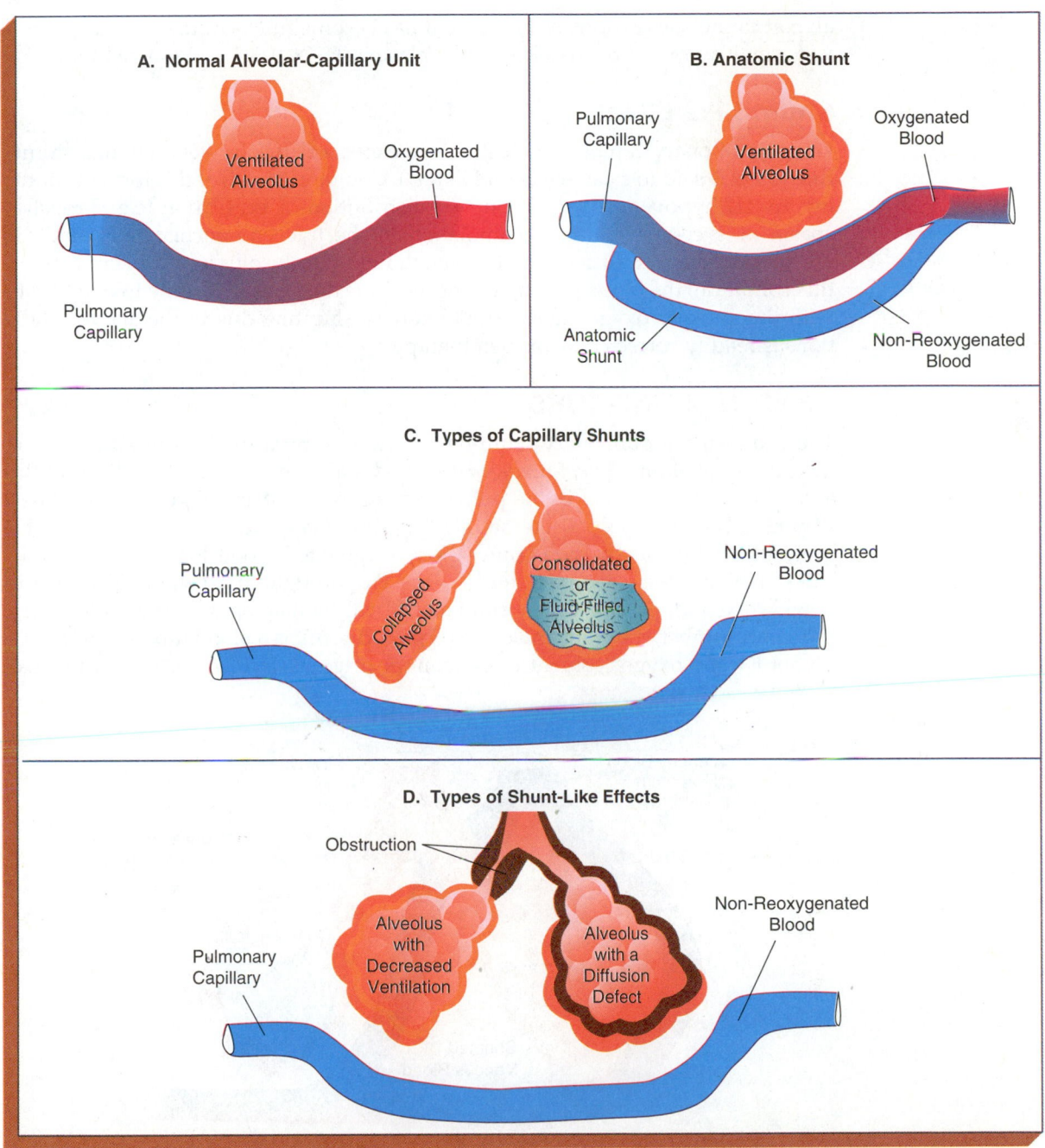

Figure 7–12. *Pulmonary shunting. A) Normal alveolar-capillary unit; B) anatomic shunt; C) types of capillary shunts; D) types of shunt-like effects.*

alveoli cannot carry more oxygen once it has become fully saturated—except for a very small amount that dissolves in the plasma ($P_{O_2} \times 0.003$ = dissolved O_2).

Shunt-Like Effect

When pulmonary capillary perfusion is in excess of alveolar ventilation, a **shunt-like effect** is said to exist (see Figure 7–12D). Common causes of this form of shunting are (1) hypoventilation, (2) uneven distribution of ventilation (e.g., bronchospasm or excessive mucus accumulation in the tracheobronchial tree), and (3) alveolar-capillary diffusion defects (even though the alveolus may be ventilated in this condition, the blood passing by the alveolus does not have time to equilibrate with the alveolar oxygen tension). Pulmonary shunting due to the above conditions is readily corrected by oxygen therapy.

VENOUS ADMIXTURE

The end result of pulmonary shunting is **venous admixture**. Venous admixture is the mixing of shunted, *non-reoxygenated blood* with *reoxygenated blood* distal to the alveoli (i.e., downstream in the pulmonary venous system) (Figure 7–13). When venous admixture occurs, the shunted, non-reoxygenated blood gains oxygen molecules while, at the same time, the reoxygenated blood loses oxygen molecules. This process continues until (1) the P_{O_2} throughout all the plasma of the newly mixed blood is in equilibrium and (2) all the hemoglobin molecules carry the same number of oxygen molecules. The end result is a blood mixture that has a higher P_{O_2} and oxygen content value than the original shunted, non-reoxygenated

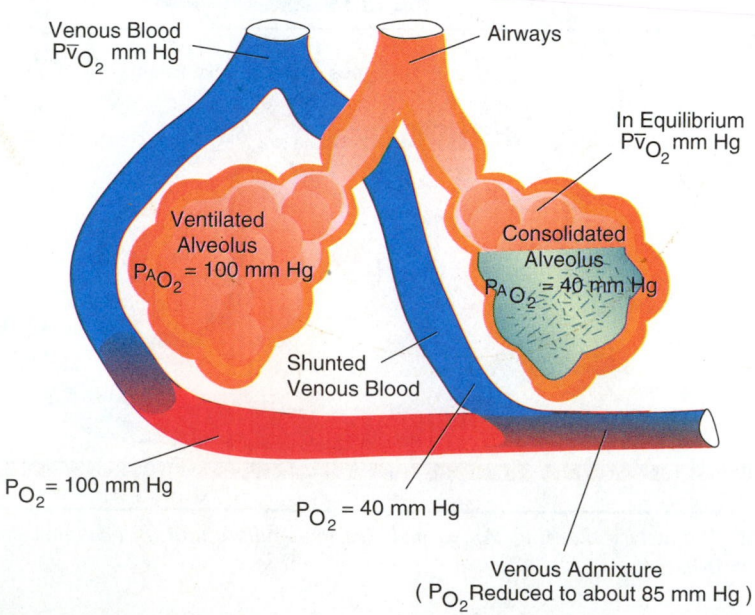

Figure 7–13. *Venous admixture occurs when reoxygenated blood mixes with non-reoxygenated blood distal to the alveoli.*

blood, but a lower P_{O_2} and oxygen content than the original reoxygenated blood. Clinically, it is this blood mixture that is evaluated downstream (e.g., from the radial artery) to determine an individual's arterial blood gas measurements (see Table 7–1).

SHUNT EQUATION

Because pulmonary shunting and venous admixture are common complications in respiratory disorders, knowledge of the degree of shunting is often desirable when developing patient care plans. The amount of intrapulmonary shunting can be calculated by using the classic shunt equation, which is written as follows:

$$\frac{\dot{Q}s}{\dot{Q}T} = \frac{Cc_{O_2} - Ca_{O_2}}{Cc_{O_2} - Cv_{O_2}}$$

where $\dot{Q}s$ is cardiac output that is shunted, $\dot{Q}T$ is total cardiac output, Cc_{O_2} is oxygen content of capillary blood, Ca_{O_2} is oxygen content of arterial blood, and Cv_{O_2} is oxygen content of mixed venous blood.

In order to obtain the data necessary to calculate the degree of pulmonary shunting, the following clinical information must be gathered:

- P_B (barometric pressure)
- Pa_{O_2} (partial pressure of arterial oxygen)
- Pa_{CO_2} (partial pressure of arterial carbon dioxide)
- Pv_{O_2} (partial pressure of mixed venous oxygen)
- Hb (hemoglobin concentration)
- PA_{O_2} (partial pressure of alveolar oxygen)*
- FI_{O_2} (fractional concentration of inspired oxygen)

CASE STUDY: MOTORCYCLE ACCIDENT VICTIM

A 38-year-old man is on a volume-cycled mechanical ventilator on a day when the barometric pressure is 750 mm Hg. The patient is receiving an FI_{O_2} of .70. The following clinical data are obtained:

Hb:	13 g%
Pa_{O_2}:	50 mm Hg (Sa_{O_2} = 85%)
Pa_{CO_2}:	43 mm Hg
Pv_{O_2}:	37 mm Hg (Sv_{O_2} = 65%)

With this information, the patient's PA_{O_2}, Cc_{O_2}, Ca_{O_2}, and Cv_{O_2} can now be calculated. (Remember: P_{H_2O} represents alveolar water vapor pressure and is always considered 47 mm Hg.)

1. $PA_{O_2} = (P_B - P_{H_2O})FI_{O_2} - Pa_{CO_2} (1.25)$
   $= (750 - 47).70 - 43(1.25)$
   $= (703).70 - 53.75$
   $= 492.1 - 53.75$
   $= 438.35$ mm Hg

---

*See Ideal Alveolar Gas Equation, Chapter Three.

2. $Cc_{O_2} = (Hb \times 1.34)* + (P_{A_{O_2}}{}^\dagger \times 0.003)$
   $= (13 \times 1.34) + (438.35 \times 0.003)$
   $= 17.42 + 1.315$
   $= 18.735 (vol\% \ O_2)$

3. $Ca_{O_2} = (Hb \times 1.34 \times Sa_{O_2}) + (Pa_{O_2} \times 0.003)$
   $= (13 \times 1.34 \times .85) + (50 \times 0.003)$
   $= 14.807 + 0.15$
   $= 14.957 (vol\% \ O_2)$

4. $Cv_{O^2} = (Hb \times 1.34 \times Sv_{O_2}) + (Pv_{O_2} \times 0.003)$
   $= (13 \times 1.34 \times .65) + (37 \times 0.003)$
   $= 11.323 + 0.111$
   $= 11.434 (vol\% \ O_2)$

Based upon the above calculations, the patient's degree of pulmonary shunting can now be calculated:

$$\frac{\dot{Q}s}{\dot{Q}T} = \frac{Cc_{O_2} - Ca_{O_2}}{Cc_{O_2} - Cv_{O_2}}$$

$$= \frac{18.735 - 14.957}{18.735 - 11.434}$$

$$= \frac{3.778}{7.301}$$

$$= \ .517$$

Thus, in this case 51.7 percent of the patient's pulmonary blood flow is perfusing lung tissue that is not being ventilated.

Today, most critical care units have programmed the oxygen transport calculations into inexpensive personal computers. What was once a time-consuming, error-prone task is now quickly and accurately performed.

THE CLINICAL SIGNIFICANCE OF PULMONARY SHUNTING

Pulmonary shunting below 10 percent reflects normal lung status.

A shunt between 10 and 20 percent is indicative of an intrapulmonary abnormality, but is seldom of clinical significance.

Pulmonary shunting between 20 and 30 percent denotes significant intrapulmonary disease, and may be life-threatening in patients with limited cardiovascular or central nervous system function.

When the pulmonary shunting is greater than 30 percent, a potentially life-threatening situation exists and aggressive cardiopulmonary supportive measures are almost always necessary.

---

*It is assumed that the hemoglobin saturation with oxygen in the pulmonary capillary blood is 100 percent or 1.0.
†See Ideal Alveolar Gas Equation, Chapter Three.

Calculating the degree of pulmonary shunting is not reliable in patients who demonstrate (1) a questionable perfusion status, (2) a decreased myocardial reserve, or (3) an unstable oxygen consumption demand. This is because these conditions directly affect a patient's Ca_{O_2} and Cv_{O_2} values—two major components of the shunt equation.

TISSUE HYPOXIA

Tissue hypoxia means that the amount of oxygen available for cellular metabolism is inadequate. There are four main types of hypoxia: (1) hypoxic hypoxia, (2) anemic hypoxia, (3) circulatory hypoxia, and (4) histotoxic hypoxia. When hypoxia exists, alternate anaerobic mechanisms are activated in the tissues that produce dangerous metabolites (such as lactate and hydrogen ions) as waste products. These ions form a nonvolatile acid known as lactic acid and cause the blood pH to decrease.

HYPOXIC HYPOXIA

Hypoxic hypoxia (also called hypoxemic hypoxia) refers to the condition in which the Pa_{O_2} and Ca_{O_2} are abnormally low. Clinically, this form of hypoxia is better known as *hypoxemia* (low oxygen concentration in the blood). This form of hypoxia can develop from pulmonary shunting and from the following conditions:

Low Alveolar P_{O_2} (i.e., Decreased PA_{O_2})

Because the arterial P_{O_2} (Pa_{O_2}) is determined by the alveolar P_{O_2} (PA_{O_2}), conditions that decrease the PA_{O_2} will lead to reductions in the Pa_{O_2} and Ca_{O_2} levels. A low PA_{O_2} can develop from such conditions as (1) hypoventilation from any cause (e.g., chronic obstructive pulmonary disease, drug overdose, or neuromuscular diseases that affect the respiratory muscles, such as myasthenia gravis), (2) ascent to high altitudes, and (3) the breathing of gas mixtures that contain less than 21 percent oxygen (e.g., suffocation).

Diffusion Impairment

In the presence of certain pulmonary diseases, the time available for oxygen equilibrium across the alveolar-capillary membrane may not be adequate. Such conditions include interstitial fibrosis, alveolar consolidation, and interstitital or alveolar edema (see Figure 3–6, page 117).

Ventilation/Perfusion ($\dot{V}/\dot{Q}$ Ratio) Mismatch

When the pulmonary capillary blood flow is in excess of the alveolar ventilation, a decreased $\dot{V}/\dot{Q}$ ratio is said to exist. This condition can cause a shunt-like effect, which in turn causes the Pa_{O_2} and Ca_{O_2} to decrease (the effects of different ventilation/perfusion relationships are discussed in greater detail in Chapter Nine).

While the presence of hypoxemia strongly suggests the possibility of tissue hypoxia, it does not necessarily indicate the absolute existence of cellular hypoxia. The reduced level of oxygen in the arterial blood may be offset by an increased cardiac output.

ANEMIC HYPOXIA

In this type of hypoxia, the oxygen tension in the arterial blood is normal, but the oxygen-carrying capacity of the blood is inadequate. This form of hypoxia can develop from (1) a low amount of hemoglobin in the blood or (2) a deficiency in the ability of hemoglobin to carry oxygen, as occurs in carbon monoxide poisoning or methemoglobinemia.

Anemic hypoxia develops in carbon monoxide poisoning because the affinity of carbon monoxide for hemoglobin is about 210 times greater than that of oxygen. As carbon monoxide combines with hemoglobin, the ability of hemoglobin to carry oxygen diminishes and tissue hypoxia may ensue. In methemoglobinemia, iron atoms in the hemoglobin are oxidized to the ferric state which in turn eliminates the hemoglobin's ability to carry oxygen. Increased cardiac output is the main compensatory mechanism for anemic hypoxia.

CIRCULATORY HYPOXIA

In circulatory hypoxia, the arterial blood that reaches the tissue cells may have a normal oxygen tension and content, but the amount of blood—and therefore the amount of oxygen—is not adequate to meet tissue needs. The two main causes of circulating hypoxia are (1) stagnant hypoxia and (2) arterial-venous shunting.

Stagnant hypoxia can occur when the peripheral capillary blood flow is slow or stagnant (*pooling*). This condition can be caused by a decreased cardiac output, vascular insufficiency, or neurochemical abnormalities. When blood flow through the tissue capillaries is sluggish, the time needed for oxygen exchange increases while, at the same time, the oxygen supply decreases. Because tissue metabolism continues at a steady rate, the oxygen pressure gradient between the blood and the tissue cells can become insufficient, causing tissue hypoxia. Stagnant hypoxia is primarily associated with cardiovascular disorders and often occurs in the absence of arterial hypoxemia. It is commonly associated with a decreased Sv_{O_2}.

When arterial blood completely bypasses the tissue cells and moves into the venous system, an **arterial-venous shunt** is said to exist. This condition can also cause tissue hypoxia, since arterial blood is prevented from delivering oxygen to the tissue cells. Localized arterial or venous obstruction can cause a similar form of tissue hypoxia, since the flow of blood in or out of the tissue capillaries is impeded. A circulatory hypoxia can also develop when the tissues' need for oxygen exceeds the available oxygen supply from the blood.

HISTOTOXIC HYPOXIA

Histotoxic hypoxia develops in any condition that impairs the ability of tissue cells to utilize oxygen. Cyanide poisoning produces this form of hypoxia. Clinically, the Pa_{O_2} and Ca_{O_2} in the blood are normal, but the tissue cells are extremely hypoxic. The Pv_{O_2}, Cv_{O_2}, and Sv_{O_2} are elevated because oxygen is not utilized.

CYANOSIS

When hypoxemia is severe, signs of cyanosis may develop. Cyanosis is the term used to describe the blue-gray or purplish discoloration seen on the mucous membranes, fingertips, and toes whenever the blood in these areas contains at least 5 g% of reduced hemoglobin per dl (100 ml). When the normal 14 to 15 g% of hemoglobin is fully saturated, the Pa_{O_2} will be about 97 to 100 mm Hg and there will be about 20 vol% of oxygen in the blood. In a cyanotic patient with one-third (5 g%) of the hemoglobin reduced, the Pa_{O_2} will be about 30 mm Hg and there will be about 13 vol% of oxygen in the blood (Figure 7–14). In the patient with polycythemia, however, cyanosis may be present at a Pa_{O_2} well above 30 mm Hg, since the amount of reduced hemoglobin is often greater than 5 g% in these patients—even when their total oxygen transport is within normal limits (about 20 vol% of O_2).

The detection and interpretation of cyanosis is difficult and there is wide individual variation between observers. The recognition of cyanosis depends on the acuity of the observer, on the lighting conditions in the examining room, and the pigmentation of the patient. Cyanosis of the nail beds is also influenced by the temperature, since vasoconstriction induced by cold may slow circulation to the point where the blood becomes bluish in the surface capillaries even though the arterial blood in the major vessels is not oxygen-poor.

Figure 7–14. *Cyanosis will likely appear whenever the blood contains at least 5 g% (g/dl) of reduced hemoglobin. In the normal individual with 15 g% hemoglobin, a Pa_{O_2} of about 30 mm Hg will produce 5 g% of reduced hemoglobin. Overall, however, the hemoglobin is still about 60-percent saturated with oxygen.*

POLYCYTHEMIA

When pulmonary disorders produce chronic hypoxemia, the hormone **erythropoietin** responds by stimulating the bone marrow to increase red blood cell (RBC) production. RBC production is known as **erythropoiesis**. An increased level of RBCs is called **polycythemia**. The polycythemia that results from hypoxemia is an adaptive mechanism designed to increase the oxygen-carrying capacity of the blood.

Unfortunately, the advantage of the increased oxygen-carrying capacity in polycythemia is offset by the increased viscosity of the blood when the hematocrit reaches about 55 to 60 percent. Because of the increased viscosity of the blood, a greater driving pressure is needed to maintain a given flow. The work of the right and left ventricles must increase in order to generate the pressure needed to overcome the increased viscosity. This can ultimately lead to left ventricular hypertrophy and failure and to right ventricular hypertrophy, or *cor pulmonale*.

CLINICAL APPLICATION

This 12-year-old female was a victim of a "drive-by" shooting. She was standing in line outside a movie theater with some friends when a car passed by and someone inside began shooting at three boys standing nearby. Two of the boys died immediately, one was shot in the shoulder and lower jaw, and she was shot in the upper anterior chest. Although she was breathing spontaneously through a non-rebreathing oxygen mask when she was brought to the emergency room twenty-five minutes later, she was unconscious and had obviously lost a lot of blood. Her clothes were completely soaked with blood.

The patient's skin, lips, and nail beds all were blue. Her skin felt cool and clammy. A small bullet hole could be seen over her left anterior chest between the second and third rib at the midclavicular line. No exit bullet hole could be seen. Her vital signs were: blood pressure—55/35, heart rate—120 beats/min, and respiratory rate 22 breaths/min. Auscultation of her chest revealed normal breath sounds. A portable chest x-ray showed that the bullet passed through the upper portion of her aorta and lodged near her spine. Her lungs were not damaged by the bullet.

Her hematocrit was 15 percent and her hemoglobin was 4 g%. A unit of blood was started immediately, and a pulmonary catheter and arterial line were inserted (see Figure 6–1, page 191). Her cardiac output was 6 liters per minute (L/min). Her arterial blood gas values (on a non-rebreathing oxygen mask) were: pH 7.47, Pa_{CO_2} 31 mm Hg, H_{CO_3} 23 mmol/L, and Pa_{O_2} 503 mm Hg. Her Sa_{O_2} was 98 percent. At this time, her oxygen indices were assessed (see Oxygen Transport Studies, Study No. 1):

The patient was rushed to surgery to repair her damaged aorta. Three hours later she was transferred to the surgical intensive care unit (ICU) and placed on a mechanical ventilator. The surgery was considered a success, and the patient's parents were relieved to learn that it was expected that she should fully recover. The patient was conscious and appeared comfortable and her skin felt warm and dry. Her vital signs were: blood pressure—125/83, heart rate—76 beats/min, respiratory rate—12 breaths/min (i.e., the ventilator rate was set at 12), and temperature 37°C. Auscultation revealed normal bronchovesicular breath sounds.

OXYGEN TRANSPORT STUDIES

D_{O_2}	$\dot{V}_{O_2}$	$C(a-\bar{v})_{O_2}$	O_2ER	$S\bar{v}_{O_2}$	$\dot{Q}s \div \dot{Q}T$
Study No. 1					
316 ml	214 ml	3.58 vol%	68%	32%	3%
Study No. 2					
935 ml	245 ml	5 vol%	25%	75%	3%

D_{O_2} = total oxygen delivery; $\dot{V}_{O_2}$ = oxygen consumption, or uptake; $C(a-v)_{O_2}$ = the arterial-venous oxygen content difference; O_2ER = oxygen extraction ratio; Sv_{O_2} = mixed venous oxygen saturation; $\dot{Q}s \div \dot{Q}T$ = the amount of intrapulmonary shunting.

A portable chest x-ray showed no remarkable cardiopulmonary problems. Laboratory blood work showed a hematocrit of 41 percent and her hemoglobin was 12 g%. Her arterial blood gas values (while on the mechanical ventilation and on an inspired oxygen concentration [FI_{O_2}] of 0.4) were: pH 7.43, Pa_{CO_2} 38 mm Hg, HCO_3 24 mmol/L, and Pa_{O_2} 109 mm Hg. Her Sa_{O_2} was 97 percent. A second oxygen transport study showed significant improvement (see Oxygen Transport Study No. 2 above). Over the next four days, the patient was weaned from the ventilator and transferred from the surgical intensive care unit (ICU) to the medical ward. A week later the patient was discharged from the hospital.

DISCUSSION

This case illustrates the importance of *hemoglobin* in the oxygen transport system. As a result of the gunshot wound to the chest, the patient lost a great deal of blood. Because of the excessive blood loss, the patient was unconscious, cyanotic, and hypotensive, and her skin was cool and damp to the touch. Despite the fact the patient that the patient had an elevated Pa_{O_2} of 503 mm Hg (normal is 80–100 mm Hg) and an Sa_{O_2} of 98 percent in the emergency room, her tissue oxygenation was seriously impaired. In fact, the patient's Pa_{O_2} and Sa_{O_2} in this case were very misleading. Clinically, this was verified by the oxygen transport studies. For example, her D_{O_2} was only 316 ml (normal is about 1000 ml).*

Furthermore, it should be noted that because the patient's $\dot{V}_{O_2}$ was 214 ml/min and her O_2ER was 68 percent (the normal extraction ratio is 25 percent). In other words, the patient was consuming 68 percent of the D_{O_2} (214 ml of oxygen out of a possible 316 ml of oxygen per minute). Her oxygen reserve was only about 30 percent. If this condition had not been treated immediately, she would not have survived much longer. It should be stressed that the patient's Pa_{O_2} of 503 mm Hg and Sa_{O_2} of 98 percent were very misleading—and dangerous.

$$* \; D_{O_2} = \dot{Q}T \times (Ca_{O_2}{}^{\dagger} \times 10)$$
$$= 6 \times (5.265 \times 10)$$
$$= 316 \text{ ml}$$

$$^{\dagger} Ca_{O_2} = (1.34 \times 4 \text{ g% Hb} \times .98\%) + (503 \text{ mm Hg} \times .003) = 5.265$$

CLINICAL APPLICATION

This 18-year-old female presented in the emergency room at 0630 in severe respiratory distress. She was well known to the respiratory care team. She had suffered from asthma all of her life. Over the years, she had been admitted to the hospital on numerous occasions, averaging about three admissions per year. Five separate asthmatic episodes had required mechanical ventilation. Although she was usually weaned from the ventilator within 48 hours, on

(continues)

one occasion she was on the ventilator for seven days. At the time of this admission, it had been over four years since she was last placed on mechanical ventilation.

Upon observation, the patient appeared fatigued and cyanotic, and she was using her accessory muscles of inspiration (see Figure 1–39, page 47). She was in obvious respiratory distress. Her vital signs were: blood pressure—177/110, heart rate—160 beats/min, and respiratory rate—32 breaths/min and shallow. Her breath sounds were diminished and wheezing could be heard bilaterally. A portable chest x-ray showed that her lungs were hyperinflated and her diaphragm was depressed. Her arterial blood gas values on 4 L/min oxygen by cannula were: pH 7.25, Pa_{CO_2} 71, HCO_3^- 27, Pa_{O_2} 27 mm Hg, and Sa_{O_2} 42 percent.

Because she was in acute ventilatory failure with severe hypoxemia, and was clearly fatigued, the patient was immediately transferred to the intensive care unit (ICU), intubated, and placed on mechanical ventilation at a rate of 3 breaths per minute. A pulmonary catheter and arterial line were inserted. An intravenous (IV) infusion was started and medications to treat her bronchoconstriction were administered. A hemodynamic study showed that her cardiac output ($\dot{Q}T$) was 6.5 liters per minute. Her hemoglobin was 13 g%. An oxygen transport study was performed at this time (see Oxygen Transport Studies, Study No. 1):

OXYGEN TRANSPORT STUDIES

D_{O_2}	$\dot{V}_{O_2}$	$C(a-\bar{v})_{O_2}$	O_2ER	$S\bar{v}_{O_2}$	$\dot{Q}s \div \dot{Q}T$
Study No. 1					
523 ml	314 ml	4.83 vol%	58%	24%	47%
Study No. 2					
990 ml	255 ml	5 vol%	24%	75%	3%

D_{O_2} = total oxygen delivery; $\dot{V}_{O_2}$ = oxygen consumption, or uptake; $C(a-v)_{O_2}$ = the arterial-venous oxygen content difference; O_2ER = oxygen extraction ratio; Sv_{O_2} = mixed venous oxygen saturation; $\dot{Q}s \div \dot{Q}T$ = the amount of intrapulmonary shunting.

Although the patient's first day in the ICU was a stormy one, her asthma progressively improved over the second day. On the morning of the third day, her skin was pink and dry and she was resting comfortably on the mechanical ventilator. Although she was receiving three mechanical breaths per minute, the patient was breathing primarily on her own. Her vital signs were: blood pressure—125/76, heart rate—70 beats/min, and respiratory rate—10 breaths/min (10 spontaneous breaths in between the 3 mechanical ventilations per minute). Auscultation revealed normal bronchovesicular breath sounds, and her portable chest x-ray no longer showed hyperinflated lungs or a flattened diaphragm. Her arterial blood gas values on an inspired oxygen concentration (FI_{O_2}) of 0.25 were: pH 7.42, Pa_{CO_2} 37, HCO_3^- 24, Pa_{O_2} 115 mm Hg, and Sa_{O_2} 97 percent. An oxygen transport study was performed at this time (see Oxygen Transport Study No. 2). The patient was weaned from the ventilator and was discharged from the hospital the next day.

DISCUSSION

This case illustrates the clinical significance of a *right shift* in the *oxygen dissociation curve* on (1) the loading of oxygen on hemoglobin in the lungs, and (2) the patient's total oxygen delivery (D_{O_2}). As a result of the asthmatic episode (i.e., bronchial smooth muscle constriction), the patient's alveolar ventilation was very poor in the emergency room. Clinically, this was verified by the chest x-ray showing alveolar hyperinflation and a flattened diaphragm and by the arterial blood gases and the oxygen indices.

It should be noted here that alveolar "hyperinflation" does not mean the lungs are being excessively ventilated. In fact, they are being underventilated. The lungs become hyperinflated during a severe asthmatic episode because gas is unable to leave the lungs during exhalation. As a result, "fresh" ventilation is impeded on subsequent inspirations. This condition causes the alveolar oxygen (PA_{O_2}) to decrease and the alveolar carbon dioxide ($P_{A_{CO_2}}$) to increase (see Figure 2–35, page 97). As the $P_{A_{O_2}}$ declined, the patient's intrapulmonary shunting ($\dot{Q}s \div \dot{Q}T$) and oxygen extraction ratio (O_2ER) increased and total oxygen delivery (DO_2) decreased (see Oxygen Transport Study No. 1)

In addition, as shown in the first arterial blood gas analysis, her condition was further compromised by the presence of a decreased pH (7.25) and an increased Pa_{CO_2} (72 mm Hg), which caused the patient's oxygen dissociation curve to shift to the right. A right shift of the oxygen dissociation curve reduces the ability of oxygen to move across the alveolar-capillary membrane and bond to hemoglobin (see Figure 7–8). Because of this condition, the patient's hemoglobin saturation was lower than expected for a particular Pa_{O_2} level. In this case, the patient's Sa_{O_2} was only 42 percent at a time when the Pa_{O_2} was 27 mm Hg. Normally, when the Pa_{O_2} is 27 mm Hg, the hemoglobin saturation is 50 percent (see Figure 7–4). Thus, it should be emphasized that when additional clinical indicators are present that shift the oxygen dissociation curve to the right or left, the respiratory practitioner should consider these factors in the final analysis of the patient's total oxygenation status.

REVIEW QUESTIONS

1. If a patient has a 14 g% Hb level, and a Pa_{O_2} of 55 mm Hg (85-percent saturated with oxygen), approximately how much oxygen is transported to the peripheral tissues in each 100 ml of blood?
   a. 16 vol%
   b. 17 vol%
   c. 18 vol%
   d. 19 vol%
   e. 20 vol%
2. When the blood pH decreases, the oxygen dissociation curve shifts to the
   a. right and the P_{50} decreases
   b. left and the P_{50} increases
   c. right and the P_{50} increases
   d. left and the P_{50} decreases
   e. right and the P_{50} remains the same
3. When shunted, non-reoxygenated blood mixes with reoxygenated blood distal to the alveoli (*venous admixture*), the
   I. P_{O_2} of the non-reoxygenated blood increases
   II. Ca_{O_2} of the reoxygenated blood decreases
   III. P_{O_2} of the reoxygenated blood increases
   IV. Ca_{O_2} of the non-reoxygenated blood decreases
       a. I only
       b. IV only
       c. I and II only
       d. III and IV only
       e. II and III only

4. The lowest acceptable Pa_{O_2} for a 75-year-old patient is about
   a. 60 mm Hg
   b. 65 mm Hg
   c. 70 mm Hg
   d. 75 mm Hg
   e. 80 mm Hg

5. The normal calculated anatomic shunt is about
   a. 0.5–1%
   b. 2–5%
   c. 6–9%
   d. 10–12%
   e. 13–20%

6. In which of the following types of hypoxia is the oxygen pressure of the arterial blood (Pa_{O_2}) usually normal?
   I. Hypoxic hypoxia
   II. Anemic hypoxia
   III. Circulatory hypoxia
   IV. Histotoxic hypoxia
      a. I only
      b. II only
      c. III only
      d. III and IV only
      e. II, III, and IV only

7. If a patient normally has a 12 g% Hb, cyanosis will likely appear when
   a. 11 g% Hb is saturated with oxygen
   b. 10 g% Hb is saturated with oxygen
   c. 9 g% Hb is saturated with oxygen
   d. 8 g% Hb is saturated with oxygen
   e. 7 g% Hb is saturated with oxygen

8. The advantages of polycythemia begin to be offset by the increased blood viscosity when the hematocrit reaches about
   a. 30–40%
   b. 40–50%
   c. 55–60%
   d. 60–70%
   e. 70–80%

9. Assuming everything else remains the same, when an individual's cardiac output decreases, the
   I. $C(a - v)_{O_2}$ increases
   II. O_2ER decreases
   III. $\dot{V}_{O_2}$ increases
   IV. Sv_{O_2} decreases
      a. I only
      b. IV only
      c. II and III only
      d. I and IV only
      e. I, II, and IV only

10. Under normal conditions, the O_2ER is about
    a. 5%
    b. 10%
    c. 15%
    d. 20%
    e. 25%

11. Case Study: Automobile Accident Victim
    A 37-year-old woman is on a volume-cycled mechanical ventilator on a day when the barometric pressure is 745 mm Hg. The patient is receiving an $F_{I_{O_2}}$ of 0.50. The following clinical data are obtained:

    Hb: 11 g% Hb
    Pa_{O_2}:   60 mm Hg (Sa_{O_2} = 90%)
    Pv_{O_2}:   35 mm Hg (Sv_{O_2} = 65%)
    Pa_{CO_2}:   38 mm Hg
    Cardiac Output: 6 L/minute

    Based on the above information, calculate the patient's
    a. total oxygen delivery

        Answer: _____

    b. arterial-venous oxygen content difference

        Answer: _____

    c. intrapulmonary shunting

        Answer: _____

    d. oxygen consumption

        Answer: _____

    e. oxygen extraction ratio

        Answer: _____

CHAPTER EIGHT

CARBON DIOXIDE TRANSPORT AND ACID-BASE BALANCE

O B J E C T I V E S

By the end of this chapter, the student should be able to:

1. List the three ways in which carbon dioxide is transported in the *plasma*.
2. List the three ways in which carbon dioxide is transported in the *red blood cells*.
3. Describe how carbon dioxide is converted to HCO_3^- at the tissue sites and then transported in the plasma to the lungs.
4. Explain how carbon dioxide is eliminated at the lungs.
5. Describe how the *carbon dioxide dissociation curve* differs from the *oxygen dissociation* curve.
6. Explain how the *Haldane effect* relates to the carbon dioxide dissociation curve.
7. Define the meaning of
   —Electrolytes
   —Buffer
   —Strong acid
   —Weak acid
   —Weak base
   —Strong base
   —Dissociation constant
   —pH
8. List the three major mechanisms that maintain the narrow pH range.
9. Describe the components of the *Henderson-Hasselbalch equation*.
10. Explain how the P_{CO_2}, HCO_3^-, and pH levels change in the following respiratory acid-base imbalances:
    —Acute ventilatory failure
    —Chronic ventilatory failure and renal compensation
    —Acute alveolar hyperventilation
    —Chronic alveolar hyperventilation and renal compensation
11. Describe how the P_{CO_2}, HCO_3^-, and pH levels change in the following metabolic acid-base imbalances:
    —Metabolic acidosis
    • Lactic acidosis
    • Ketoacidosis
    • Renal failure
    —Chronic metabolic acidosis and respiratory compensation
    —Metabolic alkalosis
    • Hypokalemia
    • Hypochloremia
    • Gastric suction or vomiting
    • Excessive administration of steroids
    • Excessive administration of sodium bicarbonate
    —Chronic metabolic alkalosis and respiratory compensation
12. Complete the review questions at the end of this chapter.

In addition to understanding oxygen transport, an understanding of carbon dioxide (CO_2) transport is also essential to the study of pulmonary physiology and to the clinical interpretation of arterial blood gases (see Table 7–1, page 205). To fully comprehend this subject, a basic understanding of (1) how carbon dioxide is transported from the tissues to the lungs, (2) acid-base balance, (3) the $P_{CO_2}/HCO_3^-/pH$ relationship in respiratory acid-base imbalances, and (4) the $P_{CO_2}/HCO_3^-/pH$ relationship in metabolic acid-base imbalances is necessary.

CARBON DIOXIDE TRANSPORT

At rest, the metabolizing tissue cells consume about 250 ml of oxygen and produce about 200 ml of carbon dioxide each minute. The newly formed carbon dioxide is transported from the tissue cells to the lungs by six different mechanisms—three mechanisms in the plasma and three mechanisms in the red blood cells (RBCs) (Figure 8–1).

IN PLASMA

- Carbamino Compound (bound to protein)
- Bicarbonate
- Dissolved CO_2

Although relatively insignificant, about 1 percent of the CO_2 that dissolves in the plasma chemically combines with free amino groups of protein molecules and forms a **carbamino compound** (see Figure 8–1).

Approximately 5 percent of the CO_2 that dissolves in the plasma ionizes as **bicarbonate** (HCO_3^-). Initially, CO_2 combines with water in a process called *hydrolysis*. The hydrolysis of CO_2 and water forms carbonic acid (H_2CO_3), which in turn rapidly ionizes into HCO_3^- and H^+ ions.

$$CO_2 + H_2O \rightleftharpoons H_2CO_3 \rightleftharpoons HCO_3^- + H^+$$

The resulting H^+ ions are buffered by the plasma proteins. The rate of this hydrolysis reaction in the plasma is very slow and, therefore, the amount of HCO_3^- and H^+ ions that form by this mechanism is small.

Dissolved carbon dioxide (CO_2) in the plasma accounts for about 5 percent of the total CO_2 released at the lungs. Clinically, it is this portion of the carbon dioxide transport system in the venous blood that is measured to assess the patient's partial pressure of carbon dioxide (P_{CO_2}) (see Table 7–1).

It should also be noted that the concentration of H_2CO_3 that forms in the plasma is about 1/1000 that of the physically dissolved carbon dioxide (P_{CO_2}) and, therefore, is proportional to the partial pressure of the CO_2. The H_2CO_3 concentration can be determined by multiplying the partial pressure of carbon dioxide by the factor 0.03. For example, a P_{CO_2} of 40 mm Hg generates a H_2CO_3 concentration of 1.2 mEq/L ($0.03 \times 40 = 1.2$) (see Figure 8–1).

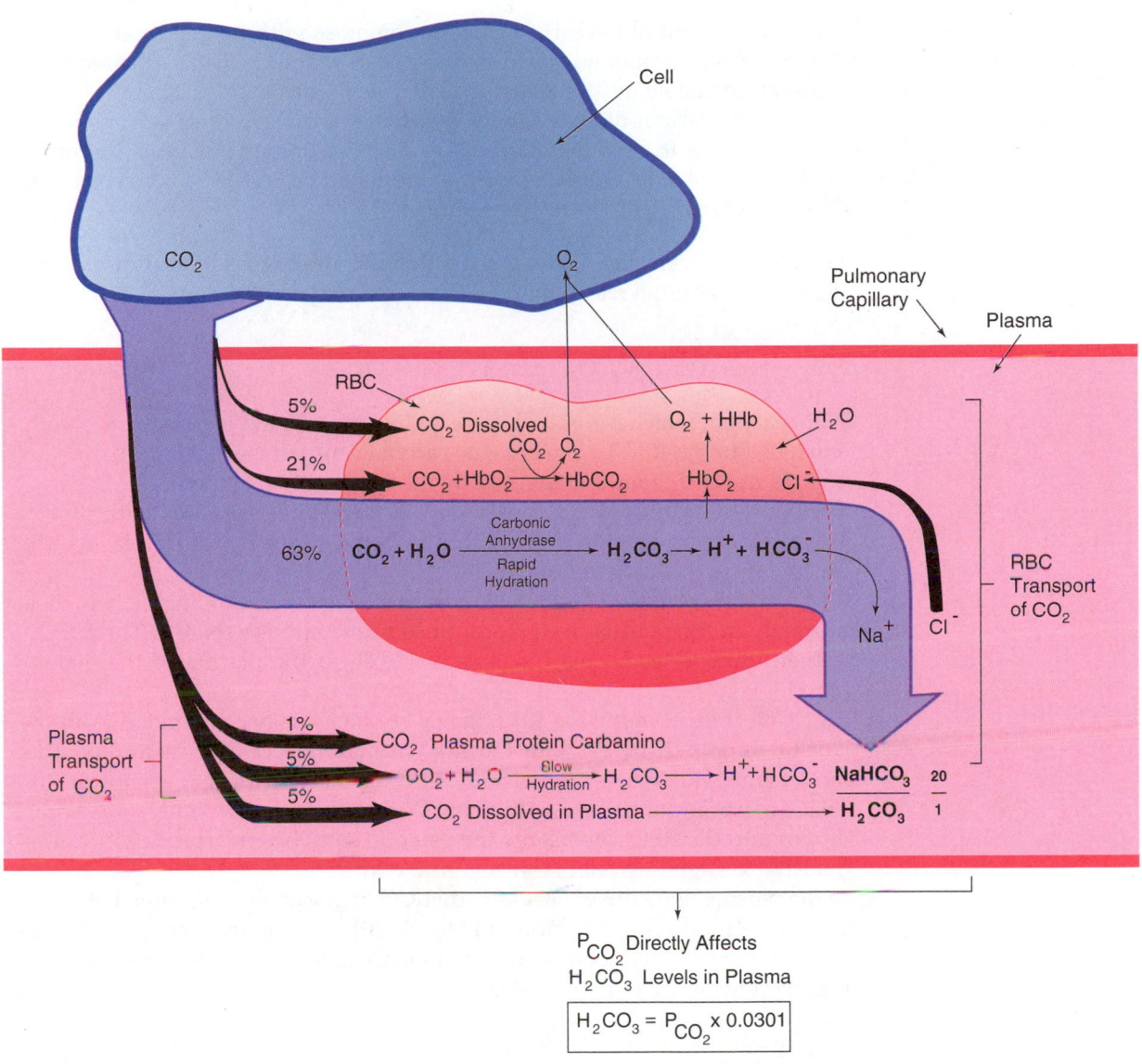

Figure 8–1. *How CO_2 is converted to HCO_3^- at the tissue sites. Most of the CO_2 that is produced at the tissue cells is carried to the lungs in the form of HCO_3^-.*

IN RED BLOOD CELLS

- Dissolved CO_2
- Carbamino-Hb
- Bicarbonate

Dissolved carbon dioxide (CO_2) in the intracellular fluid of the red blood cells accounts for about 5 percent of the total CO_2 released at the lungs (see Figure 8–1).

About 21 percent of the carbon dioxide combines with the red blood cell hemoglobin to form a compound called **carbamino-Hb**. The O_2 that is released from this reaction is available for tissue metabolism (see Figure 8–1).

Most of the carbon dioxide (about two-thirds, or 63 percent) is transported from the tissue cells to the lungs in the form of **bicarbonate** (HCO_3^-). The major portion of the dissolved CO_2 that enters the red blood cells (RBCs) is converted to HCO_3^- by the following reactions (see Figure 8–1):

1. The bulk of dissolved CO_2 that enters the RBC undergoes hydrolysis according to the following reaction (CA = carbonic anhydrase):

$$CO_2 + H_2O \overset{CA}{\rightleftharpoons} H_2CO_3 \rightleftharpoons H^+ + HCO_3^-$$

   This reaction, which is normally a very slow process in the plasma, is greatly enhanced in the RBC by the enzyme carbonic anhydrase (CA).

2. The resulting H^+ ions are buffered by the reduced hemoglobin.

3. The rapid hydrolysis of CO_2 causes the RBC to become saturated with HCO_3^-. To maintain a concentration equilibrium between the RBC and plasma, the excess HCO_3^- diffuses out of the RBC.

4. Once in the plasma, the HCO_3^- combines with sodium (Na^+), which is normally in the plasma in the form of sodium/chloride (NaCl). The HCO_3^- is then transported to the lungs as $NaHCO_3$ in the plasma of the venous blood.

5. As HCO_3^- moves out of the RBC, the Cl^- (which has been liberated from the NaCl compound) moves into the RBC to maintain electric neutrality. This movement is known as the **chloride shift**, or the **Hamburger phenomenon**, or as an **anionic shift to equilibrium**. During the chloride shift, some water moves into the RBC to preserve the osmotic equilibrium. This action causes the RBC to slightly swell in the venous blood.

6. In the plasma, the ratio of HCO_3^- and H_2CO_3 is normally maintained at 20 : 1. This 20 : 1 ratio keeps the blood pH level within the normal range of 7.35 to 7.45. The pH of the blood becomes more alkaline as the ratio increases and less alkaline as the ratio decreases.

CARBON DIOXIDE ELIMINATION AT THE LUNGS

As shown in Figure 8–2, as the venous blood enters the alveolar capillaries, the chemical reactions occurring at the tissue level are reversed. These chemical processes continue until the CO_2 pressure is equal throughout the entire system. Table 8–1 summarizes the percentage and quantity of the total carbon dioxide that is transported from the tissue cells to the lungs by the six carbon dioxide mechanisms each minute.

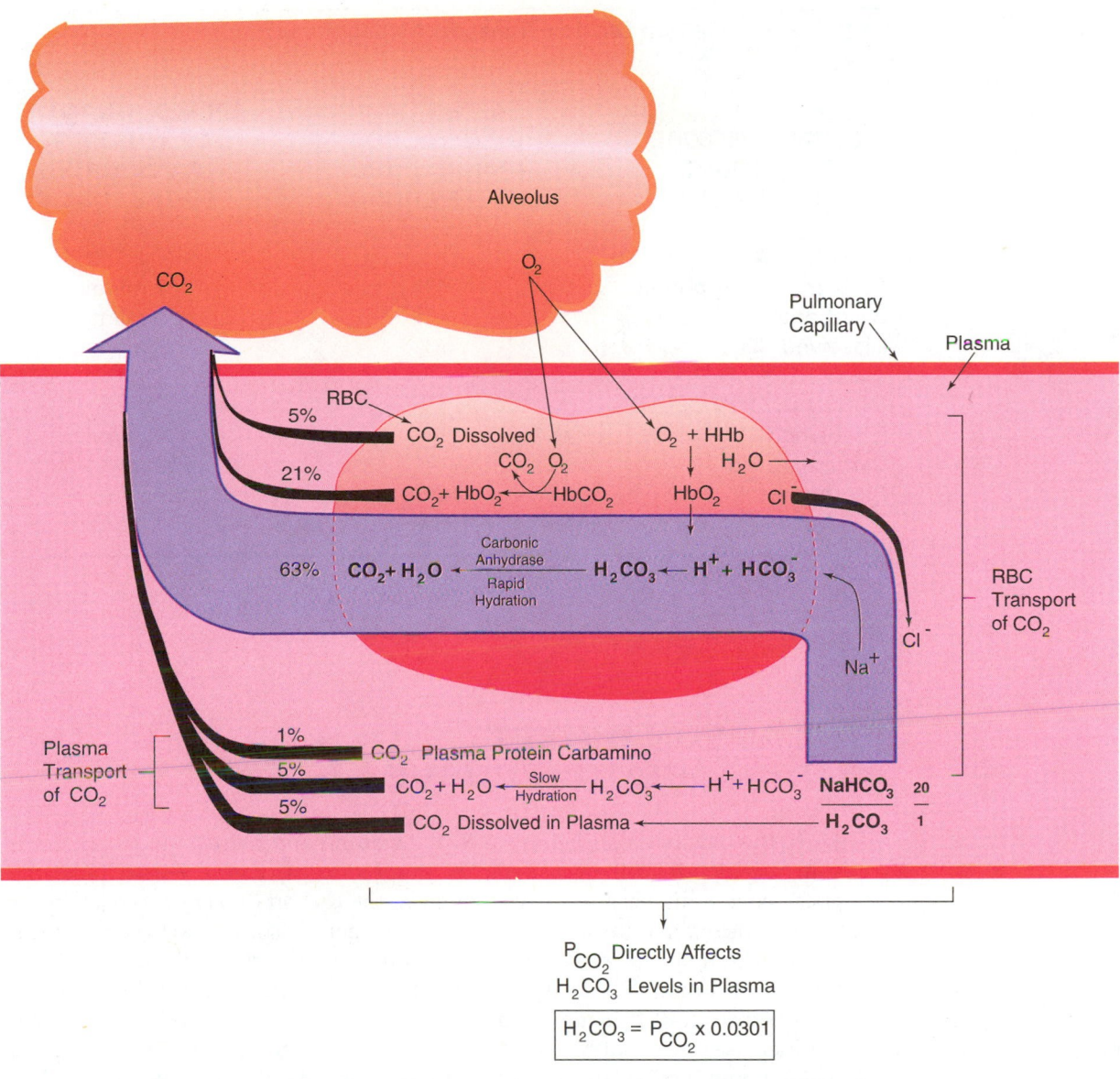

Figure 8–2. *How HCO_3^- is transformed back into CO_2 and eliminated in the alveoli.*

TABLE 8–1.	Carbon Dioxide Transport Mechanisms	
CARBON DIOXIDE TRANSPORT MECHANISMS	**APPROX. % OF TOTAL CO$_2$ TRANSPORTED TO THE LUNGS**	**APPROX. QUANTITY OF TOTAL CO$_2$ TRANSPORTED TO THE LUNGS**
IN PLASMA		
Carbamino Compound	1%	2 ml/min
Bicarbonate	5%	10 ml/min
Dissolved CO$_2$	5%	10 ml/min
IN RED BLOOD CELLS		
Dissolved CO$_2$	5%	10 ml/min
Carbamino-Hb	21%	42 ml/min
Bicarbonate	63%	126 ml/min
Total	100% Total	200 ml/min

CARBON DIOXIDE DISSOCIATION CURVE

Similar to the oxygen dissociation curve, the loading and unloading of carbon dioxide in the blood can be illustrated in graphic form (Figure 8–3). Unlike the S-shaped oxygen dissociation curve, however, the carbon dioxide curve is almost linear. This means that in comparison to the oxygen dissociation curve there is a more direct relationship between the partial pressure of carbon dioxide (P_{CO_2}) and the amount of carbon dioxide (CO$_2$ content) in the blood. For example, when the P_{CO_2} increases from 40 to 46 mm Hg between the arterial and venous blood, the CO$_2$ content increases by about 5 vol% (Figure 8–4). The same partial pressure change of oxygen would increase the oxygen content only by about 2 vol% (see Figure 7–2, page 209).

The level of saturation of hemoglobin with oxygen (e.g., Sa_{O_2} or Sv_{O_2}) also affects the carbon dioxide dissociation curve. When the hemoglobin is 97-percent saturated with oxygen, for example, there is less CO$_2$ content for any given P_{CO_2} than if the hemoglobin is, say, 75-percent saturated with oxygen (Figure 8–5, page 248). The fact that deoxygenated blood enhances the loading of carbon dioxide is called the Haldane effect. It should also be noted that the Haldane effect works the other way—that is, the oxygenation of blood enhances the unloading of CO$_2$.

Figure 8–6 (page 248) compares both the oxygen and the carbon dioxide dissociation curves in terms of partial pressure, content, and shape.

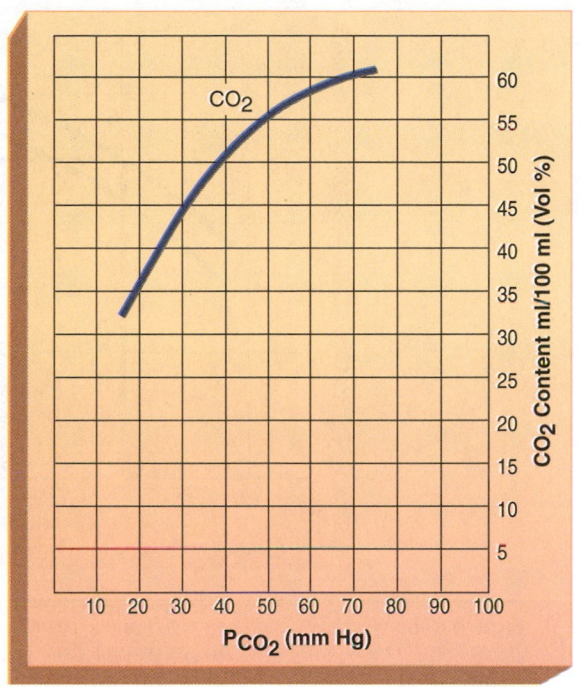

Figure 8–3.   *Carbon dioxide dissociation curve.*

Figure 8–4.   *Carbon dioxide dissociation curve. An increase in the P_{CO_2} from 40 mm Hg to 46 mm Hg raises the CO_2 content by about 5 vol%. P_{CO_2} changes have a greater effect on CO_2 content levels than P_{O_2} changes have on O_2 levels.*

Figure 8–5. *Carbon dioxide dissociation curve at two different oxygen/hemoglobin saturation levels (Sa_{O_2} of 97 percent and 75 percent). When the saturation of O_2 increases in the blood, the CO_2 content decreases at any given P_{CO_2}. This is known as the Haldane effect.*

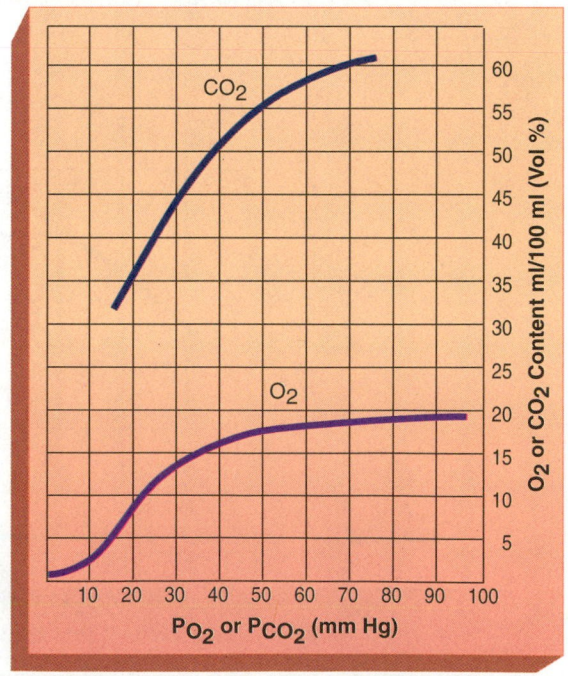

Figure 8–6. *Comparison of the oxygen and carbon dioxide dissociation curves in terms of partial pressure, content, and shape.*

ACID-BASE BALANCE

To fully understand acid-base balance, a working definition of the following terms and phrases is essential.

Electrolytes: Charged species (ions) that can conduct a current in solution.
Buffer: A substance that is capable of neutralizing both acids and bases without causing an appreciable change in the original pH.
Strong acid: An acid that dissociates completely into hydrogen ions (H^+) and an anion (an acid is a hydrogen ion donor).
Weak acid: An acid that dissociates only partially into ions.
Strong base: A base that dissociates completely.
Weak base: A base that reacts with water to form OH^- in an equilibrium; partial dissociation.
Dissociation constant: Refers to weak acid or base systems that have an equilibrium between the molecular form and its ions. For example,

$$HA \xrightleftharpoons{} [H^+] + [A^-]$$
$$\text{(molecule)} \qquad \text{(ions)}$$

$$K_a = \frac{[H^+][A^-]}{[HA]}$$

where K_a is the concentration of all species at equilibrium, [ ] means concentration in terms of molarity (M), H^+ is the hydrogen ion, A^- is the anion, and HA is the molecular weak acid.

HA is said to be in the *un-ionized* (undissociated) state. $[H^+]$ and $[A^-]$ are said to be in the *ionized* (dissociated) state.

THE pH SCALE

Because the transport of carbon dioxide can affect the hydrogen ion concentration $[H^+]$, and because hydrogen ion activity can significantly affect the metabolic function of the cells, it is important to understand the quantitative measurement of the hydrogen ion concentration. Clinically, the pH scale is used. A pH of 7 is neutral, a pH of less than 7 is acidic, and a pH greater than 7 is basic.

In chemistry, the pH is defined as the *negative logarithm, to the base 10, of the hydrogen ion concentration*:

$$pH = -\log_{10}[H^+]$$

Thus, a pH of 7 (e.g., pure water) is equal to 10^{-7} mole/L (0.0000001 mole/L) of hydrogen ions. The normal pH range in the human body is 7.35 to 7.45. An **acid** is a substance that donates $[H^+]$ and therefore increases the hydrogen ion concentration of a solution and causes the numerical value of the pH to decrease. A **base** is a substance that accepts $[H^+]$ and therefore decreases the hydrogen ion concentration and causes the pH value to increase.

The narrow pH range is maintained by (1) the buffer systems of the blood and tissues, (2) the respiratory system's ability to regulate the elimination of CO_2 (see

Chapter Ten), and (3) the renal system's ability to regulate the excretion of hydrogen and the reabsorption of bicarbonate ions (see Chapter Twelve).

THE BUFFER SYSTEMS

The ability of an acid-base mixture to resist large changes in pH is called its buffer action. There are numerous acid-base combinations, or buffer combinations, in the body that can do this. The following are buffers of special interest to the respiratory care practitioner:

- Plasma
  - Carbonic acid/sodium bicarbonate (H_2CO_3/$NaHCO_3$)
  - Sodium acid phosphate/sodium alkaline phosphate (NaH_2PO_4/$NaHPO_4$)
  - Acid proteinate/sodium proteinate (H_{prot}/Na_{prot})
- Erythrocytes
  - Acid hemoglobin/potassium hemoglobin (HHb/KHb)
  - Potassium acid phosphate/potassium alkaline phosphate (KH_2PO_4/K_2HPO_4)

In regard to the above buffer examples, the carbonic acid/sodium bicarbonate combination (H_2CO_3/$NaHCO_3$) is the most important and, therefore, is used in the following discussion.

When a strong acid like hydrochloric acid (HCl) is added to the H_2CO_3/$NaHCO_3$, the following chain of events occurs:

$$HCl + NaHCO_3^- \rightleftharpoons H_2CO_3 + NaCl$$

As shown, this reaction reduces the strong acid into a weak acid (H_2CO_3) and a neutral salt (NaCl). Because of this chemical process, the pH movement toward the acidic range is minimal.

In contrast, when a strong base like sodium hydroxide (NaOH) is added to a H_2CO_3/$NaHCO_3$ system, the following reaction occurs:

$$NaOH + H_2CO_3 \rightleftharpoons NaHCO_3 + H_2O$$

As can be seen, this reaction causes the formation of sodium bicarbonate and the loss of H_2CO_3. Because the carbonic acid (H_2CO_3) is a weak acid, the increase in pH is small.

THE HENDERSON-HASSELBALCH EQUATION

The Henderson-Hasselbalch equation uses the components of the H_2CO_3/HCO_3^- system in the following way:

$$pH = pK + \log \frac{[HCO_3^-]}{[H_2CO_3]}$$

pK is derived from the dissociation constant of the acid portion of the buffer combination. Normally, the pK is 6.1.

Under normal conditions, when the HCO_3^- is 24 mEq/L and the H_2CO_3 is 1.2 mEq/L, use of the Henderson-Hasselbalch equation allows us to calculate a pH of 7.4 as follows:

$$pH = pK + \log \frac{[HCO_3^-]}{[H_2CO_3]}$$

$$= 6.1 + \log \frac{24 \text{ mEq/L}}{1.2 \text{ mEq/L}}$$

$$= 6.1 + \log \frac{20}{1}$$

$$= 6.1 + 1.3$$

$$= 7.4$$

As the above equation illustrates, the major component of the Henderson-Hasselbalch formula is the ratio of HCO_3^- to H_2CO_3, which is normally $20:1$.

Thus, when the HCO_3^- to H_2CO_3 ratio changes, the pH will also change: for example, when the ratio increases to, say, $25:1$, the pH increases as follows:

$$pH = 6.1 + \log \frac{25}{1}$$

$$= 6.1 + 1.4$$

$$= 7.5$$

In contrast, when the HCO_3^- to H_2CO_3 ratio decreases to, say, $15:1$, the pH decreases as follows:

$$pH = 6.1 + \log \frac{15}{1}$$

$$= 6.1 + 1.18$$

$$= 7.29$$

THE ROLE OF THE P_{CO_2}/HCO_3^-/pH RELATIONSHIP IN ACID-BASE BALANCE

RESPIRATORY ACID-BASE IMBALANCES

The bulk of CO_2 is transported from the tissues to the lungs as HCO_3^-. As the CO_2 level increases, the plasma P_{CO_2}, HCO_3^-, and H_2CO_3 increase. The converse is also true: as the level of CO_2 decreases, the plasma P_{CO_2}, HCO_3^-, and H_2CO_3 decrease.

Because the blood pH is dependent on the ratio between the plasma HCO_3^- (base) and the plasma H_2CO_3 (acid), acute ventilatory changes will immediately alter the pH. The normal HCO_3^- to H_2CO_3 ratio is $20:1$. It should be noted that even though both plasma HCO_3^- and plasma H_2CO_3 move in the same direction during acute ventilatory changes, acute changes in the H_2CO_3 level play a much more powerful role in altering the pH status than acute changes in the HCO_3^- level. This is due to the $20:1$ ratio between HCO_3^- to H_2CO_3. *In other words, for every H_2CO_3 molecule increase or decrease, twenty HCO_3^- molecules must also increase or decrease,*

Figure 8–7. *Alveolar hypoventilation causes the $P_{A_{CO_2}}$ and the plasma P_{CO_2}, H_2CO_3, and HCO_3^- to increase. This action decreases the HCO_3^-/H_2CO_3 ratio, which in turn decreases the blood pH.*

respectively, in order to maintain a 20 : 1 ratio between HCO_3^- and H_2CO_3 (the normal pH status).

Acute Ventilatory Failure

During **acute ventilatory failure** (e.g., acute hypoventilation caused by an overdose of narcotics or barbiturates), the $P_{A_{CO_2}}$ progressively increases. This action necessarily increases the blood P_{CO_2}, H_2CO_3, and HCO_3^- levels (Figure 8–7). Because acute changes in H_2CO_3 levels are more significant than acute changes in HCO_3^- levels, a decreased HCO_3^- to H_2CO_3 ratio develops (a ratio less than 20 : 1). This action causes the patient's blood pH to decrease, or become less alkaline. The *normal buffer line* on the $P_{CO_2}/HCO_3^-/pH$ nomogram in Figure 8–8 illustrates the expected HCO_3^- and pH changes that develop as a result of CO_2 changes only.

Chronic Ventilatory Failure and Kidney Compensation

If the patient hypoventilates for a long period of time (e.g., more than 24 to 48 hours), the kidneys will work to correct the decreased pH by retaining HCO_3^- in the blood. Renal compensation in the presence of chronic hypoventilation can be verified when the calculated HCO_3^- and pH readings are higher than expected for a particular P_{CO_2} level. For example, in terms of the absolute $P_{CO_2}/HCO_3^-/pH$ relationship, when the P_{CO_2} is about 80 mm Hg, the pH level should be less than 7.2, and the HCO_3^- level should be about 30 mEq/L, according to the normal blood buffer line (Figure 8–9, page 254). If the HCO_3^- and pH levels are greater than these values (i.e., the pH and HCO_3^- readings cross the P_{CO_2} *isobar** above the normal blood buffer line in the upper left-hand corner of the nomogram), renal retention

---

*The isobars on the $P_{CO_2}/HCO_3^-/pH$ nomogram illustrate the pH changes that develop in the blood as a result of (1) metabolic changes (i.e., HCO_3^- changes), or (2) a combination of metabolic and respiratory (CO_2) changes.

Figure 8–8. *Nomogram of $P_{CO_2}/HCO_3^-/pH$ relationship.*

of HCO_3^- (**partial renal compensation**) has likely occurred. When the HCO_3^- level increases enough to return the acidic pH to normal, **complete renal compensation** is said to have occurred (see Figure 8–9).

Acute Alveolar Hyperventilation

During **acute alveolar hyperventilation** (e.g., hyperventilation due to pain and/or anxiety), the $P_{A_{CO_2}}$ will decrease and allow more CO_2 molecules to leave the pulmonary blood. This action necessarily decreases the blood P_{CO_2}, H_2CO_3, and HCO_3^- levels (Figure 8–10, page 254). Because acute changes in H_2CO_3 levels are more significant than acute changes in HCO_3^- levels, an increased HCO_3^- to H_2CO_3 ratio develops (a ratio greater than 20 : 1). This action causes the patient's blood pH to increase, or become more alkaline. The normal buffer line on the $P_{CO_2}/HCO_3^-/pH$ nomogram illustrates this relationship (see Figure 8–8).

Chronic Alveolar Hyperventilation and Renal Compensation

If the patient hyperventilates for a long period of time (e.g., a patient who has been mechanically hyperventilated for more than 24 to 48 hours), the kidneys will attempt to correct the increased pH by excreting excess HCO_3^- in the urine. Renal compensation in the presence of chronic hyperventilation can be verified when the calculated

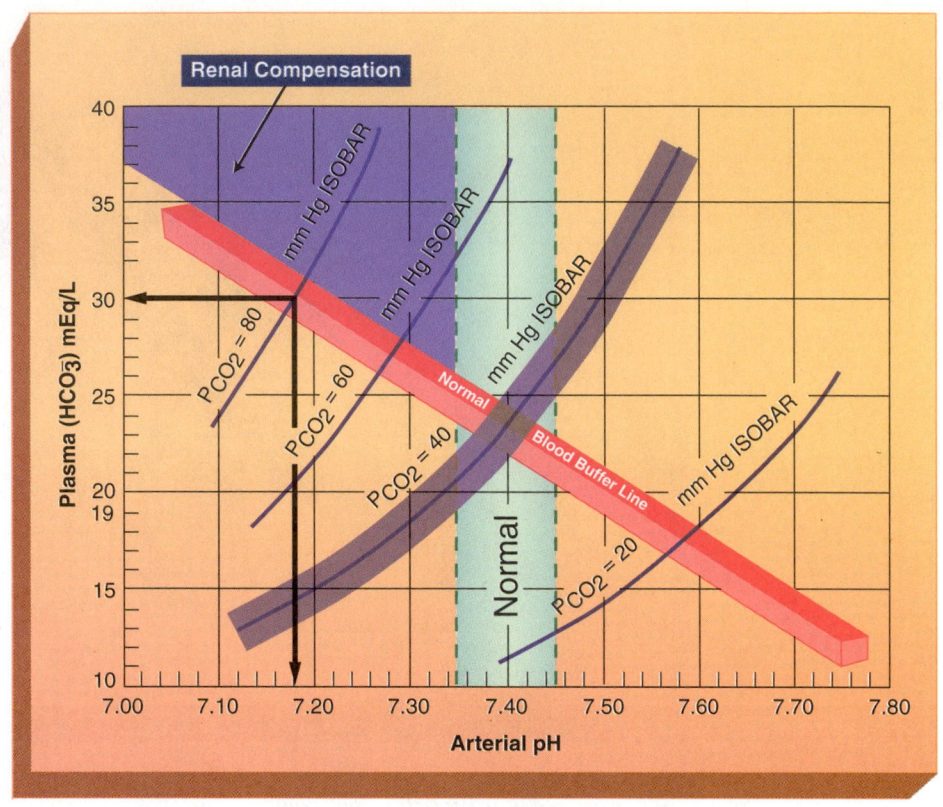

Figure 8–9. *The expected pH and HCO_3^- levels when the P_{CO_2} is about 80 mm Hg. When the HCO_3^- and pH lines cross an isobar in the shaded area, renal compensation is present.*

Figure 8–10. *Alveolar hyperventilation causes the PA_{CO_2} and the plasma P_{CO_2}, H_2CO_3, and HCO_3^- to decrease. This action increases the HCO_3^-/H_2CO_3 ratio, which in turn increases the blood pH.*

HCO_3^- and pH readings are lower than expected for a particular P_{CO_2} level. For example, in terms of the absolute $P_{CO_2}/HCO_3^-/pH$ relationship, when the P_{CO_2} is about 25 mm Hg, the pH level should be greater than 7.5, and the HCO_3^- level should be about 19 mEq/L. If the HCO_3^- and pH levels are lower than these values (i.e., the pH and HCO_3^- readings cross a P_{CO_2} isobar below the normal blood buffer line in the lower right-hand corner), renal excretion of HCO_3^- (**partial renal compensation**) has likely occurred. When the HCO_3^- level decreases enough to return the alkalotic pH to normal, **complete renal compensation** is said to have occurred (Figure 8–11).

As a general rule, the kidneys do not overcompensate for an abnormal pH. That is, if the patient's blood pH becomes acidic for a long period of time due to hypoventilation, the kidneys will not retain enough HCO_3^- for the pH to climb higher than 7.4. The opposite is also true: should the patient's blood pH become alkalotic for a long period of time due to hyperventilation, the kidneys will not excrete enough HCO_3^- for the pH to fall below 7.4.

There is one important exception to this rule. In persons chronically hypoventilating for a long period of time (e.g., in chronic obstructive pulmonary disease), it is not uncommon to find a pH greater than 7.4. This is believed to be due to water and chloride ion shifts between the intercellular and extracellular spaces that occur when the renal system works to compensate for a decreased blood pH.

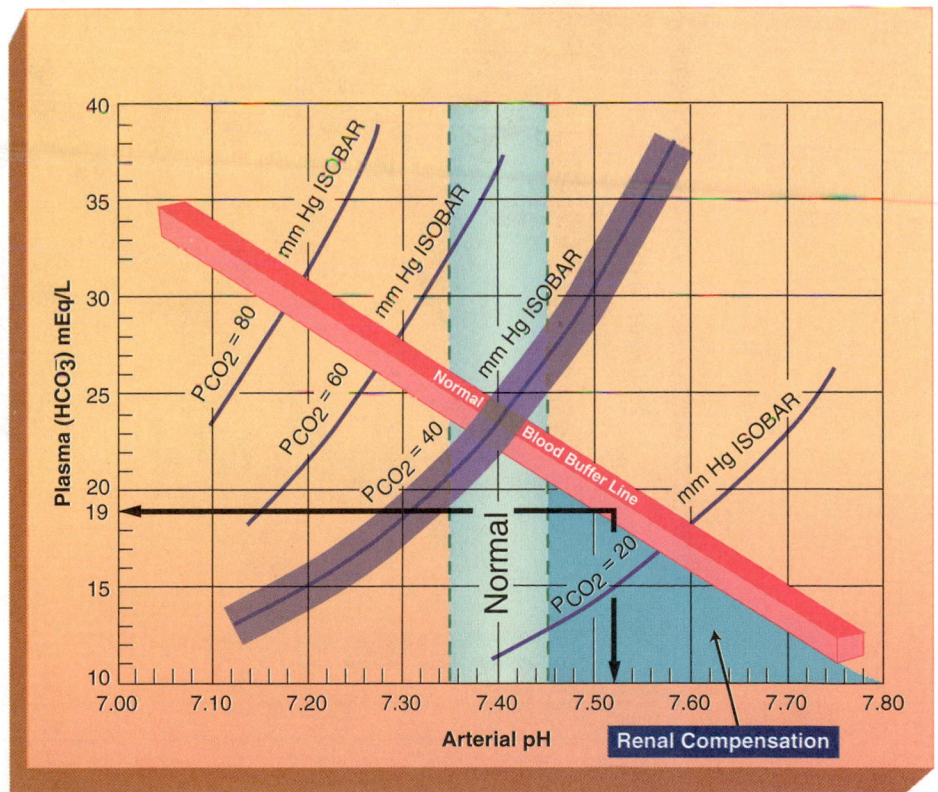

Figure 8–11. *The expected pH and HCO_3^- levels when the P_{CO_2} is about 25 mm Hg. When the HCO_3^- and pH lines cross an isobar in the shaded area, renal compensation is present.*

To summarize: the lungs play an important role in maintaining the P_{CO_2}, HCO_3^-, and pH levels on a moment-to-moment basis. The kidneys, on the other hand, play an important role in balancing the HCO_3^- and pH levels during long periods of hyperventilation or hypoventilation.

METABOLIC ACID-BASE IMBALANCES

Metabolic Acidosis

By using the isobars of the $P_{CO_2}/HCO_3^-/pH$ nomogram, the presence of other acids, not related to an increased P_{CO_2} level or to renal compensation, can be identified. This condition is referred to as **metabolic acidosis**.

When metabolic acidosis is present, the calculated HCO_3^- reading and pH will both be lower than expected for a particular P_{CO_2} level in terms of the absolute $P_{CO_2}/HCO_3^-/pH$ relationship. For example, a HCO_3^- reading of 17 mEq/L and a pH of 7.25 would both be less than expected in a patient who has a P_{CO_2} of 40 mm Hg, according to the normal blood buffer line (Figure 8–12).

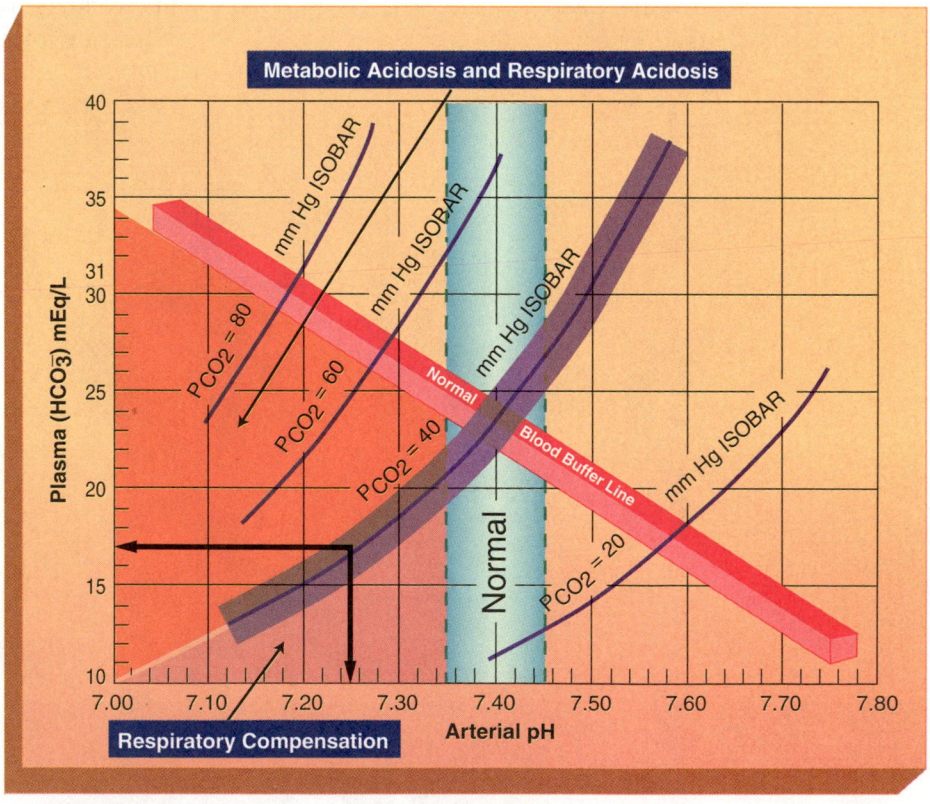

Figure 8–12. *When the HCO_3^- and pH lines cross an isobar in the darker shaded area, both metabolic and respiratory acidosis are present. When the HCO_3^- and pH lines cross an isobar in the lighter shaded area, the metabolic acidosis is partially corrected by means of respiratory compensation (hyperventilation).*

Common Causes of Metabolic Acidosis

- **Lactic Acidosis**. When the oxygen level is inadequate to meet tissue needs, alternate biochemical reactions are activated that do not utilize oxygen. This is known as **anaerobic metabolism** (non-oxygen-utilizing). Lactic acid is the end-product of this process. When these ions move into the blood, and a patient has both a reduced oxygen level and a decreased pH level, lactic acidosis is present.
- **Ketoacidosis**. When blood insulin is low in the diabetic patient, serum glucose cannot easily enter the tissue cells for metabolism. This condition activates alternate metabolic processes that produce **ketones** as metabolites. Ketone accumulation in the blood causes ketoacidosis. The absence of glucose because of starvation can also cause ketoacidosis. Ketoacidosis may also be seen in patients with excessive alcohol intake.
- **Renal Failure**. During renal failure, an accumulation of hydrogen ions can cause metabolic acidosis.

Chronic Metabolic Acidosis and Respiratory Compensation

Normally, the immediate compensatory response for metabolic acidosis is an increased ventilatory rate (respiratory compensation) that causes the patient's Pa_{CO_2} to decline. This process causes the hydrogen ion concentration to decrease and therefore works to offset the metabolic acidosis. When the Pa_{CO_2} decreases enough to move the acidic pH back to normal, **complete respiratory compensation** is said to have occurred (see Figure 8–12).

When the pH is acidic and the HCO_3^- reading is below the normal blood buffer line while, at the same time, the P_{CO_2} level is above 40 mm Hg, both metabolic acidosis and respiratory acidosis are present (see Figure 8–12).

Metabolic Alkalosis

The presence of other bases, not related to either a decreased P_{CO_2} level or to renal compensation, can also be identified by using the isobars of a nomogram illustrating the $P_{CO_2}/HCO_3^-/pH$ relationship (Figure 8–13). This condition is known as metabolic alkalosis.

When metabolic alkalosis is present, the calculated HCO_3^- reading and pH reading will both be higher than expected for a particular P_{CO_2} level in terms of the absolute $P_{CO_2}/HCO_3^-/pH$ relationship. For example, a HCO_3^- reading of 31 mEq/L and a pH level of 7.5 would both be higher than expected in a patient who has a P_{CO_2} of 40 mm Hg, according to the normal blood buffer line (see Figure 8–13, page 258).

Common Causes of Metabolic Alkalosis

- **Hypokalemia**. The depletion of total body potassium can occur from (1) several days of intravenous therapy without adequate replacement of potassium, (2) diuretic therapy, and (3) diarrhea.

  Whenever the potassium level is low, the normal kidney attempts to save potassium by excreting hydrogen ions. This mechanism causes the blood base to increase. In addition, as the potassium level in the blood

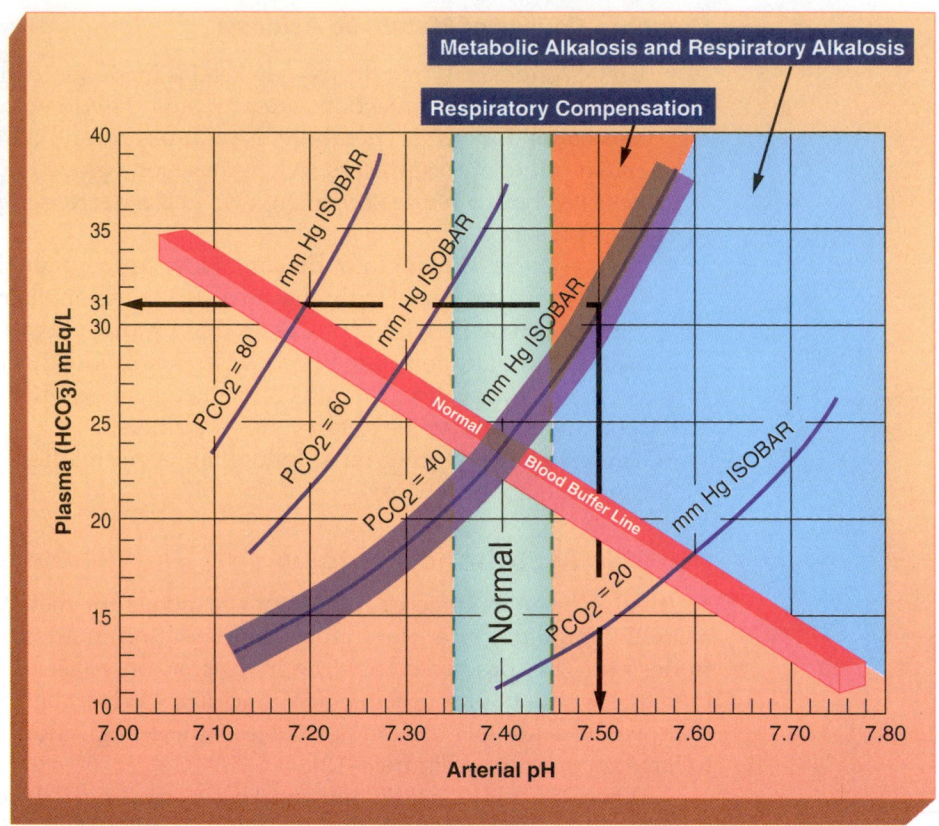

Figure 8–13. *When the HCO$_3^-$ and pH lines cross an isobar in the darker shaded area, both metabolic and respiratory alkalosis are present. When the HCO$_3^-$ and pH lines cross an isobar in the lighter shaded area, the metabolic acidosis is partially corrected by means of repiratory compensation (hypoventilation).*

decreases, intracellular potassium moves into the extracellular space in an effort to offset the reduced potassium level in the blood serum. As the potassium cation (K$^+$) leaves the cell, however, a hydrogen cation (H$^+$) enters the cell. This mechanism causes the blood serum to become more alkalotic.

Patients with hypokalemia frequently demonstrate the clinical triad of (1) metabolic alkalosis, (2) muscular weakness, and (3) cardiac dysrhythmias.

- **Hypochloremia**. When the chloride ion (Cl$^-$) concentration decreases, bicarbonate ions increase in an attempt to maintain a normal cation balance in the blood serum. As the bicarbonate ion increases, the patient's blood serum becomes alkalotic. The kidneys, moreoever, usually excrete potassium ions when chloride ions are unavailable which, as described above, will also contribute to the patient's metabolic alkalosis.
- **Gastric Suction or Vomiting**. Excessive gastric suction or vomiting causes a loss of hydrochloric acid (HCl) and the result is an increase in blood base; i.e., metabolic alkalosis.

- **Excessive Administration of Steroids**. Large doses of sodium-retaining steroids can cause the kidneys to accelerate the excretion of hydrogen ions and potassium. Excessive excretion of either one or both of these ions will cause metabolic alkalosis.
- **Excessive Administration of Sodium Bicarbonate**. If an excessive amount of sodium bicarbonate is administered, metabolic alkalosis will occur. This used to happen frequently during cardiopulmonary resuscitation.

Chronic Metabolic Alkalosis and Respiratory Compensation

Normally, the immediate compensatory response to metabolic alkalosis is a decreased ventilatory rate (*respiratory compensation*) which causes the patient's Pa_{CO_2} to increase. The excess hydrogen ions produced by the elevated blood Pa_{CO_2} work to offset the patient's metabolic alkalosis. When the Pa_{CO_2} increases enough to move the alkalotic pH back to normal, *complete respiratory compensation* is said to have occurred (see Figure 8–13).

When the pH is alkalotic and the HCO_3^- reading is above the normal blood buffer line, while at the same time the P_{CO_2} level is below 40 mm Hg, both metabolic alkalosis and respiratory alkalosis are present (see Figure 8–13).

BASE EXCESS/DEFICIT

Clinically, the $P_{CO_2}/HCO_3^-/pH$ nomogram also serves as an excellent tool to calculate the patient's total **base excess/deficit**. By knowing the base excess/deficit, non-respiratory acid-base imbalances can be quantified and managed. The base excess/deficit is reported in milliequivalents per liter (mEq/L) of base above or below the normal buffer base line of the $P_{CO_2}/HCO_3^-/pH$ nomogram.

For example, if the patient has a pH of 7.25 and a HCO_3^- of 17 mEq/L, the $P_{CO_2}/HCO_3^-/pH$ nomogram will confirm that the patient has (1) metabolic acidosis and (2) a base excess of −7 (more properly called a *base deficit* of 7) (see Figure 8–12). Metabolic acidosis may be treated by the careful intravenous infusion of sodium bicarbonate ($NaHCO_3$).

In contrast, if the patient has a pH of 7.5 and a HCO_3^- of 31 mEq/L, the $P_{CO_2}/HCO_3^-/pH$ nomogram will verify that the patient has (1) metabolic alkalosis and (2) a base excess of 7 mEq/L (see Figure 8–13). Metabolic alkalosis is commonly treated by (1) correcting the underlying electrolyte problem (e.g., hypokalemia or hypochloremia), or (2) administering ammonium chloride (NH_4Cl).

EXAMPLE OF CLINICAL USE OF $P_{CO_2}/HCO_3^-/pH$ NOMOGRAM

It has been shown that the $P_{CO_2}/HCO_3^-/pH$ nomogram is an excellent clinical tool to confirm the presence of (1) respiratory acid-base imbalances, (2) metabolic acid-base imbalances, or (3) a combination of a respiratory and metabolic acid-base imbalance. To demonstrate the clinical usefulness of the $P_{CO_2}/HCO_3^-/pH$ nomogram consider the following case:

CLINICAL APPLICATION

This 36-year-old man, who had been working on his car in the garage while the motor was running, suddenly experienced confusion, disorientation, and nausea. A few minutes later he started to vomit. Concerned, he called out to his wife, who was nearby. Moments later he collapsed and lost consciousness. His wife called 911. Eleven minutes later, the emergency medical team (EMT) arrived, quickly assessed the patient's condition, placed a non-rebreathing oxygen mask on the patient's face, and then transported him to the ambulance. In route to the hospital, the EMT reported that the patient continued to vomit intermittently. Because of this, the patient was frequently suctioned orally to prevent aspiration.

In the emergency room, the patient's skin was cherry red. Although he was still unconscious, he was breathing on his own through a non-rebreathing oxygen mask. A medical student assigned to the emergency room stated that it appeared that the patient was being overoxygenated—since his skin appeared cherry red—and that perhaps the oxygen mask should be discontinued. The respiratory therapist working with the patient strongly disagreed.

The patient's vital signs were: blood pressure—165/105, heart rate—122 beats/min, and respiratory rate—36 breaths/min. His arterial blood gas values on the non-rebreathing oxygen mask were: pH 7.52, Pa_{CO_2} 25mm Hg, HCO_3^- 19 mmol/L, and Pa_{O_2} 539 mm Hg. His carboxyhemoglobin level (CO_{Hb}) was 55 percent.

The patient was transferred to the intensive care unit (ICU), where he continued to be monitored closely. Although the patient never required mechanical ventilation, he continued to receive high concentrations of oxygen for the first 48 hours. By the end of the third day he was breathing room air and was conscious and able to talk with his family and the medical staff. His vital signs were: blood pressure—117/77, heart rate—68 beats/min, and respiratory rate—12 breaths/min. His arterial blood gas values were: pH 7.4, Pa_{CO_2} 40 mm Hg, HCO_3^- 24 mmol/L, and Pa_{O_2} 97 mm Hg. His carboxyhemoglobin level (CO_{Hb}) was 3 percent. Four days after his admission, the patient was discharged.

DISCUSSION

This case illustrates (1) how clinical signs and symptoms can sometimes be very misleading, and (2) how the $P_{CO_2}/HCO_3^-/pH$ nomogram can be used to objectively determine the cause of certain arterial blood gas findings. Even though the patient's Pa_{O_2} was very high (because of the non-rebreathing oxygen mask), the CO_{Hb} level of 55 percent had seriously impaired the patient's hemoglobin's ability to carry oxygen (see Figure 3–9, page 122). In addition, any oxygen that was being carried by the hemoglobin was unable to detach itself easily from the hemoglobin. This was because CO_{Hb} causes the oxygen dissociation curve to shift to the left (see Figure 7–4, page 213).

Thus, despite the fact that the patient's Pa_{O_2} was very high (539 mm Hg) in the emergency room, the patient's oxygen delivery system—and tissue oxygenation—was in fact very low and seriously compromised. The "cherry red" skin color noted in the emergency room by the medical student was a classic sign of carbon monoxide poisoning, not a sign of good skin color and oxygenation. The increased blood pressure, heart rate, and respiratory rate seen in the emergency room were compensatory mechanisms activated to counteract the decreased arterial oxygenation, i.e., these mechanisms increased the total oxygen delivery (see D_{O_2} in Table 7–10, page 226).

Because it was reported that the patient had vomited excessively prior to the arterial blood gas sample obtained in the emergency room, it was not readily apparent whether the high pH was a result of (1) the low Pa_{CO_2} caused by the acute alveolar hyperventilation (which was caused by the low oxygen delivery), or (2) a combination of both the acute alveolar hyperventilation and low Pa_{CO_2} and the loss of stomach acids (caused by the vomiting). Clinically, the answer to this question can be obtained by using the $P_{CO_2}/HCO_3^-/pH$ nomogram. In this case, when the pH, Pa_{CO_2}, and HCO_3^- values of this patient are applied to the $P_{CO_2}/HCO_3^-/pH$ nomogram, it can be seen that the elevated pH was due solely to the decreased Pa_{CO_2} level, since all three variables cross through the normal buffer line (see Figure 8–11).*

*See Appendix VI for a credit-card size $P_{CO_2}/HCO_3^-/pH$ nomogram that can be copied and laminated for use as a handy clinical reference tool.

CLINICAL APPLICATION

During a routine physical examination, this 67-year-old man had a cardiac arrest while performing a stress test in the pulmonary rehabilitation department. The patient had a long history of chronic bronchitis and emphysema. Although the patient had been in reasonably good health for the past three years, he had recently complained to his family physician of shortness of breath and heart palpitations. Concerned, his physician ordered a full diagnostic evaluation of the patient, which included a complete pulmonary function study and stress test.

During the interview, the patient reported that he had not performed any form of exercise in years. In fact, he jokingly stated that whenever he would start to feel as if he should start to exercise, he would quickly sit down and the feeling would go away. During the stress test, the patient was about 35 pounds overweight and appeared moderately ashen and diaphoretic. When the patient collapsed, a "Code Blue" was called and cardiopulmonary resuscitation (CPR) was started immediately by one of the practitioners working with the patient during the stress test. When the Code Blue Team arrived, the patient had an oral airway in place and was being manually ventilated, with room air only, with a face mask and bag.

An intravenous infusion was started and the patient's heart activity was monitored with an electrocardiogram (ECG). An arterial blood gas sample was obtained and showed a pH of 7.11, Pa_{CO_2} 80 mm Hg, HCO_3^- 25 mmol/L, Pa_{O_2} 38 mm Hg, and Sa_{O_2} 53 percent. Upon seeing these arterial blood gas analysis results, the physician reevaluated the patient's chest and breath sounds. It was quickly established that the patient's head was not hyperextended appropriately (which, as a result, impeded air flow through the oral and laryngeal airways). The patient's breath sounds were very diminished, and it was also noted that the patient's chest did not rise appropriately during each manual resuscitation. Immediately, the patient was intubated and manually ventilated with a bag and mask with an inspired oxygen concentration ($F_{I_{O_2}}$) of 1.0. Despite the fact the patient's pH was only 7.11 at this time, no sodium bicarbonate was administered.

Immediately after the patient was intubated, breath sounds could be heard bilaterally. Additionally, the patient's chest could been seen to move upward during each manual ventilation, and his skin started to turn pink. Another arterial blood gas sample was then drawn. While waiting for the arterial blood gas analysis results, epinephrine and norepinephrine were

(continues)

administered. Moments later, normal ventricular activity was seen. The arterial blood gas values from the second sample were: pH 7.44, Pa_{CO_2} 35 mm Hg, HCO_3^- 24 mmol/L, Pa_{O_2} 360 mm Hg, and Sa_{O_2} 98 percent. Thirty minutes later, the patient was breathing spontaneously on an FI_{O_2} of 0.4, and he was conscious and alert. Two hours later, it was determined that the patient would not require mechanical ventilation and he was extubated. Four days later the patient was discharged from the hospital.

DISCUSSION

This case illustrates how the $P_{CO_2}/HCO_3^-/pH$ nomogram can be used to (1) confirm both a respiratory and metabolic acidosis, and (2) prevent the unnecessary administration of sodium bicarbonate during an emergency situation. As a result of the cardiopulmonary arrest, the patient's Pa_{CO_2} rapidly increased while, at the same time, his pH and Pa_{O_2} decreased. Because the patient's head was not positioned correctly, the lungs were not ventilated adequately. As a result, the Pa_{CO_2}, pH, and Pa_{O_2} continued to deteriorate. Fortunately, this was discovered when the first arterial blood gas values were seen.

The fact that the initial pH (7.11) and HCO_3^- (25 mmol/L) were both lower than expected for an acute increase in the Pa_{CO_2} (80 mm Hg) suggested that there were additional acids present in the patient's blood (i.e., acids other than those produced by the increased Pa_{CO_2}). According to the $P_{CO_2}/HCO_3^-/pH$ nomogram, an acute increase in the patient's Pa_{CO_2} to 80 mm Hg should have caused the pH to fall to about 7.18 and the HCO_3^- level should have increased to about 29 mmol/L (Figure 8–9). In this case, both the pH and HCO_3^- were lower than expected. According to the $P_{CO_2}/HCO_3^-/pH$ nomogram, the patient had both a respiratory and metabolic acidosis (see Figure 8–12). In this case, the most likely cause of the metabolic acidosis was the low Pa_{O_2} (38 mm Hg), which produces lactic acids (see causes of metabolic acidosis in this chapter).

The fact that the $P_{CO_2}/HCO_3^-/pH$ nomogram confirmed that the cause of the patient's lower than expected pH and HCO_3^- levels were solely due to the poor ventilation eliminated the need to administer sodium bicarbonate. In other words, because the patient's head was not positioned correctly, the patient's lungs were not being ventilated. This condition, in turn, caused the patient's Pa_{CO_2} to increase (which caused the pH to fall) and the Pa_{O_2} to decrease (which produced lactic acids and caused the pH to fall even further). In this case, therefore, the treatment of choice was to correct the cause of the respiratory and metabolic acidosis. Because the cause of the respiratory and metabolic acidosis was inadequate ventilation, the treatment of choice was aggressive ventilation.

Finally, as shown by the second arterial blood gas sample, the patient's arterial blood gases were rapidly corrected when the endotracheal tube was inserted. In fact, the patient's Pa_{O_2} was overly corrected (360 mm Hg). The patient's inspired oxygen concentration (FI_{O_2}) was subsequently reduced. If sodium bicarbonate had been administered to correct the patient's pH of 7.11 before the patient was appropriately ventilated, his pH and HCO_3^- readings would have been higher than his normal after his Pa_{CO_2} was ventilated down from 80 mm Hg to his normal level of about 40 mm Hg.

REVIEW QUESTIONS

1. During acute alveolar hypoventilation, the blood
   I. H_2CO_3 increases
   II. pH increases

   III. HCO_3^- increases

   IV. P_{CO_2} increases

     a. II only

     b. IV only

     c. II and III only

     d. I and IV only

     e. I, III, and IV only

2. The bulk of the CO_2 produced in the cells is transported to the lungs as

   a. H_2CO_3

   b. HCO_3^-

   c. CO_2 and H_2O

   d. Carbonic anhydrase

   e. HHb

3. During acute alveolar hyperventilation, the blood

   I. P_{CO_2} increases

   II. H_2CO_3 decreases

   III. HCO_3^- increases

   IV. pH decreases

     a. II only

     b. IV only

     c. I and III only

     d. II and IV only

     e. II, III, and IV only

4. In chronic hypoventilation, renal compensation has likely occurred when the

   I. HCO_3^- is higher than expected for a particular P_{CO_2}

   II. pH is lower than expected for a particular P_{CO_2}

   III. HCO_3^- is lower than expected for a particular P_{CO_2}

   IV. pH is higher than expected for a particular P_{CO_2}

     a. I only

     b. II only

     c. I and IV only

     d. III and IV only

     e. I and II only

5. When metabolic acidosis is present, the patient's blood

   I. HCO_3^- is higher than expected for a particular P_{CO_2}

   II. pH is lower than expected for a particular P_{CO_2}

   III. HCO_3^- is lower than expected for a particular P_{CO_2}

   IV. pH is higher than expected for a particular P_{CO_2}

     a. I only

     b. II only

     c. I and IV only

     d. III and IV only

     e. II and III only

6. Ketoacidosis can develop from

   I. an inadequate oxygen level

   II. renal failure

     III. an inadequate insulin level

     IV. anerobic metabolism

     V. an inadequate glucose level

       a. I only

       b. II and III only

       c. IV and V only

       d. III and V only

       e. II, III, and V only

7. Metabolic alkalosis can develop from

     I. hyperchloremia

     II. hypokalemia

     III. hypochloremia

     IV. hyperkalemia

       a. I only

       b. IV only

       c. I and III only

       d. I and IV only

       e. II and III only

8. Which of the following HCO_3^- to H_2CO_3 ratios represent an acidic pH?

     I. 18 : 1

     II. 28 : 1

     III. 12 : 1

     IV. 22 : 1

       a. I only

       b. II only

       c. III only

       d. II and III only

       e. I and III only

9. If a patient has a P_{CO_2} level of 70 mm Hg, what is the H_2CO_3 concentration?

     a. 0.7 mEq/L

     b. 1.3 mEq/L

     c. 1.5 mEq/L

     d. 1.7 mEq/L

     e. 2.1 mEq/L

10. The value of the pK in the Henderson-Hasselbalch equation is

     a. 1.0

     b. 6.1

     c. 7.4

     d. 20.1

     e. 24

CHAPTER NINE

VENTILATION-PERFUSION RELATIONSHIPS

O B J E C T I V E S

By the end of this chapter, the student should be able to:

1. Define *ventilation-perfusion ratio*.
2. Describe the overall ventilation-perfusion ratio in the normal upright lung.
3. Explain how the ventilation-perfusion ratio progressively changes from the upper to the lower lung regions in the normal, upright lung.
4. Describe how an increased and decreased ventilation-perfusion ratio affects the *alveolar gases*.
5. Describe how the ventilation-perfusion ratio affects the *end-capillary gases* and the *pH level*.
6. Define
   —respiratory quotient
   —respiratory exchange ratio
7. Identify respiratory disorders that *increase* the ventilation-perfusion ratio.
8. Identify respiratory disorders that *decrease* the ventilation-perfusion ratio.
9. Complete the review questions at the end of this chapter.

VENTILATION-PERFUSION RATIO

Ideally, each alveolus in the lungs should receive the same amount of ventilation and pulmonary capillary blood flow. In reality, however, this is not the case. Overall, alveolar ventilation is normally about 4 L/min and pulmonary capillary blood flow is about 5 L/min, making the average overall ratio of ventilation to blood flow 4 : 5, or 0.8. This relationship is called the **ventilation-perfusion ratio** ($\dot{V}/\dot{Q}$ ratio) (Figure 9–1, page 266).

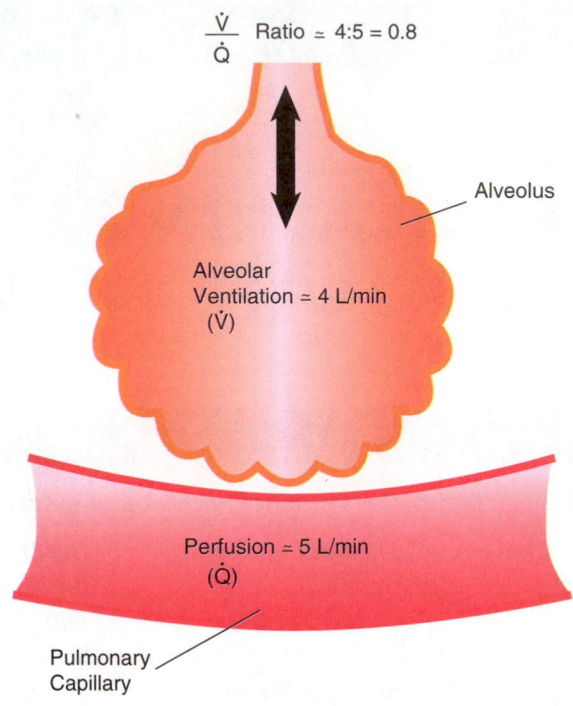

$$\frac{\dot{V}}{\dot{Q}} \text{ Ratio} \simeq 4{:}5 = 0.8$$

Alveolus

Alveolar
Ventilation ≃ 4 L/min
($\dot{V}$)

Perfusion ≃ 5 L/min
($\dot{Q}$)

Pulmonary
Capillary

Figure 9–1. *The normal ventilation-perfusion ratio ($\dot{V}/\dot{Q}$ ratio) is about 0.8.*

Although the overall $\dot{V}/\dot{Q}$ ratio is about 0.8, the ratio varies remarkably throughout the lung. For example, in the normal individual in the upright position, the alveoli in the upper portions of the lungs (apices) receive a moderate amount of ventilation and little blood flow. As a result, the $\dot{V}/\dot{Q}$ ratio in the upper lung region is higher than 0.8.

In the lower regions of the lung, however, alveolar ventilation is moderately increased and blood flow is greatly increased, since blood flow is gravity dependent. As a result, the $\dot{V}/\dot{Q}$ ratio is lower than 0.8. In summary, the $\dot{V}/\dot{Q}$ ratio progressively decreases from top to bottom in the upright lung, and the average $\dot{V}/\dot{Q}$ ratio is about 0.8 (Figure 9–2).

HOW THE VENTILATION-PERFUSION RATIO AFFECTS THE ALVEOLAR GASES

The $\dot{V}/\dot{Q}$ ratio profoundly affects the oxygen and carbon dioxide pressures in the alveoli ($P_{A_{O_2}}$ and $P_{A_{CO_2}}$). Although the normal $P_{A_{O_2}}$ and $P_{A_{CO_2}}$ are typically about 100 mm Hg and 40 mm Hg, respectively, this is not the case throughout most of the alveolar units. These figures merely represent an average.

The $P_{A_{O_2}}$ is determined by the balance between (1) the amount of oxygen entering into the alveoli and (2) its removal by capillary blood flow. The $P_{A_{CO_2}}$, on the other hand, is determined by the balance between (1) the amount of carbon diox-

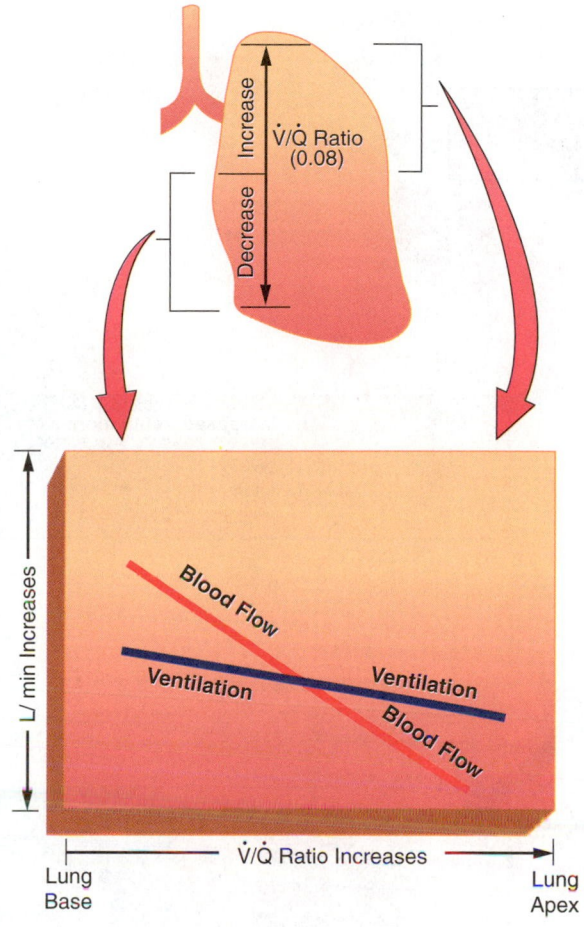

Figure 9–2. *In the upright lung, the* $\dot{V}/\dot{Q}$ *ratio progressively decreases from the apex to the base.*

ide that diffuses into the alveoli from the capillary blood and (2) its removal out of the alveoli by means of ventilation. Thus, changing $\dot{V}/\dot{Q}$ ratios alter the $P_{A_{O_2}}$ and $P_{A_{CO_2}}$ levels for the reasons discussed below.

Increased $\dot{V}/\dot{Q}$ Ratio

When the $\dot{V}/\dot{Q}$ ratio increases, the $P_{A_{O_2}}$ rises and the $P_{A_{CO_2}}$ falls. The $P_{A_{CO_2}}$ decreases because it washes out of the alveoli faster than it is replaced by the venous blood. The $P_{A_{O_2}}$ increases because it does not diffuse into the blood* as fast as it enters (or is ventilated into) the alveolus (Figure 9–3, page 268). The $P_{A_{O_2}}$ also increases because the $P_{A_{CO_2}}$ decreases and therefore allows the $P_{A_{O_2}}$ to move closer to the partial pressure of atmospheric oxygen, which is about 159 mm Hg at sea level (see

---

*See how oxygen can be classified as either perfusion or diffusion limited, in Chapter Three.

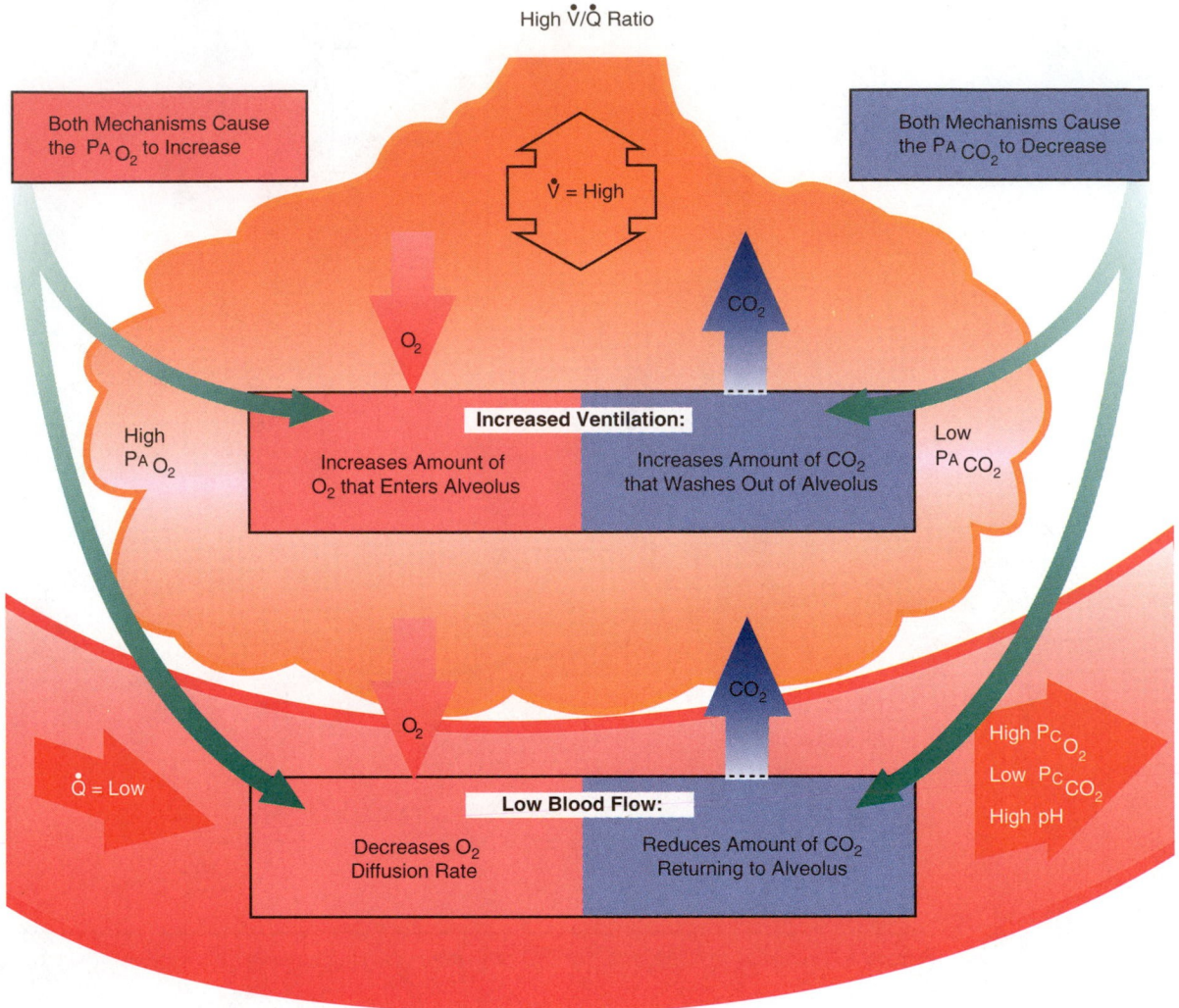

Figure 9–3.   *When the $\dot{V}/\dot{Q}$ ratio is high, the alveolar oxygen pressure ($P_{A_{O_2}}$) increases and the alveolar carbon dioxide pressure ($P_{A_{CO_2}}$) decreases.*

Table 3–2, page 111).[†] This $\dot{V}/\dot{Q}$ relationship is present in the upper segments of the upright lung (see Figure 9–2).

Decreased $\dot{V}/\dot{Q}$ Ratio

When the $\dot{V}/\dot{Q}$ ratio decreases, the $P_{A_{O_2}}$ falls and the $P_{A_{CO_2}}$ rises. The $P_{A_{O_2}}$ decreases because oxygen moves out of the alveolus and into the pulmonary capillary blood faster than it is replenished by ventilation. The $P_{A_{CO_2}}$ increases because it moves out of the capillary blood and into the alveolus faster than it is washed out of the alve-

[†]See The Ideal Alveolar Gas Equation, Chapter Three.

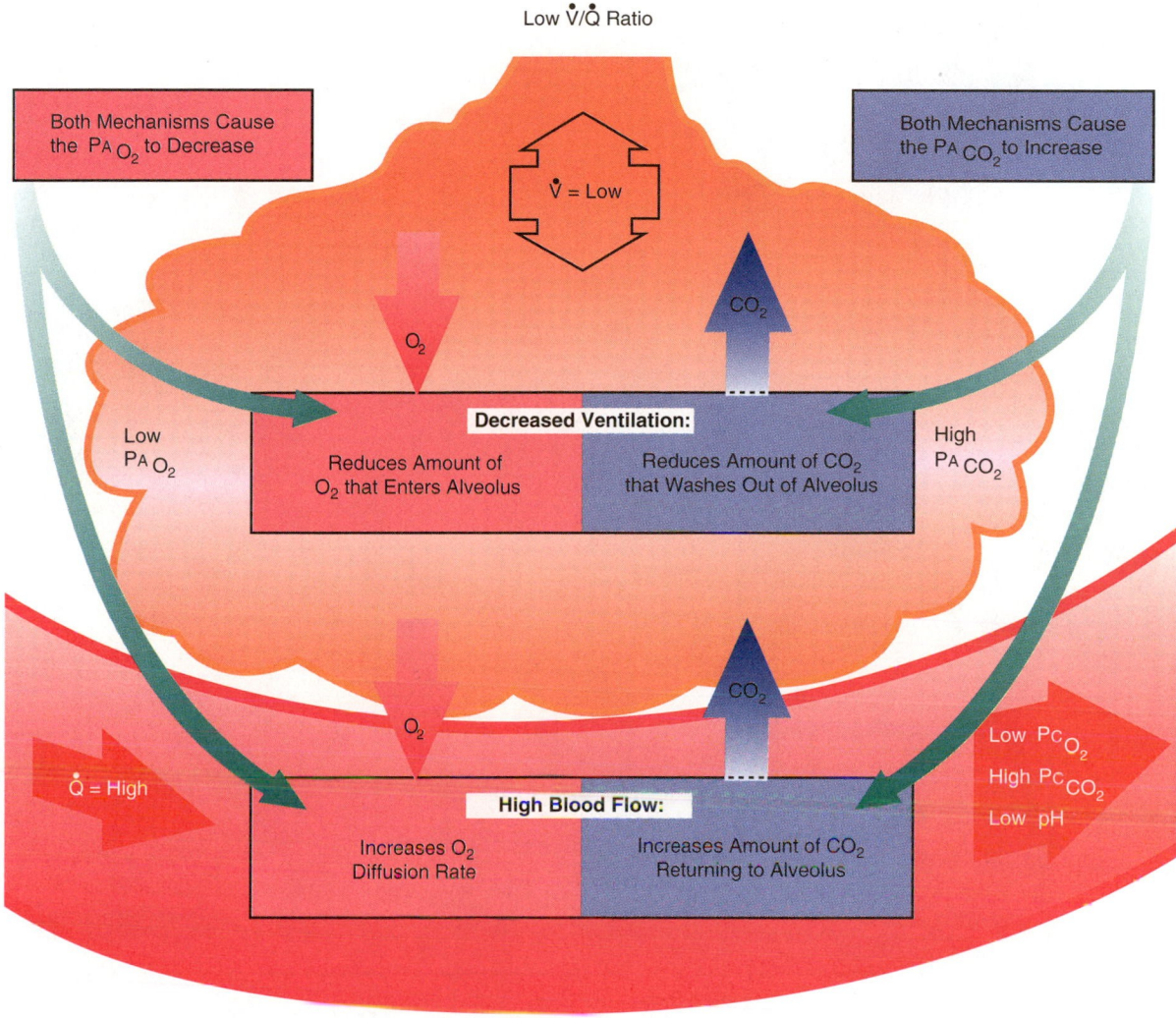

Figure 9–4. *When the $\dot{V}/\dot{Q}$ ratio is low, the alveolar oxygen pressure ($P_{A_{O_2}}$) decreases and the alveolar carbon dioxide pressure ($P_{A_{CO_2}}$) increases.*

olus (Figure 9–4). This $\dot{V}/\dot{Q}$ relationship is present in the lower segments of the upright lung (see Figure 9–2).

O_2–CO_2 Diagram

The effect of changing $\dot{V}/\dot{Q}$ ratios on the $P_{A_{O_2}}$ and $P_{A_{CO_2}}$ levels is summarized in the O_2–CO_2 diagram (Figure 9–5, page 270). The line in this diagram represents all the possible alveolar gas compositions as the $\dot{V}/\dot{Q}$ ratio decreases or increases. For example, the O_2–CO_2 diagram (nomogram) shows that in the upper lung regions,

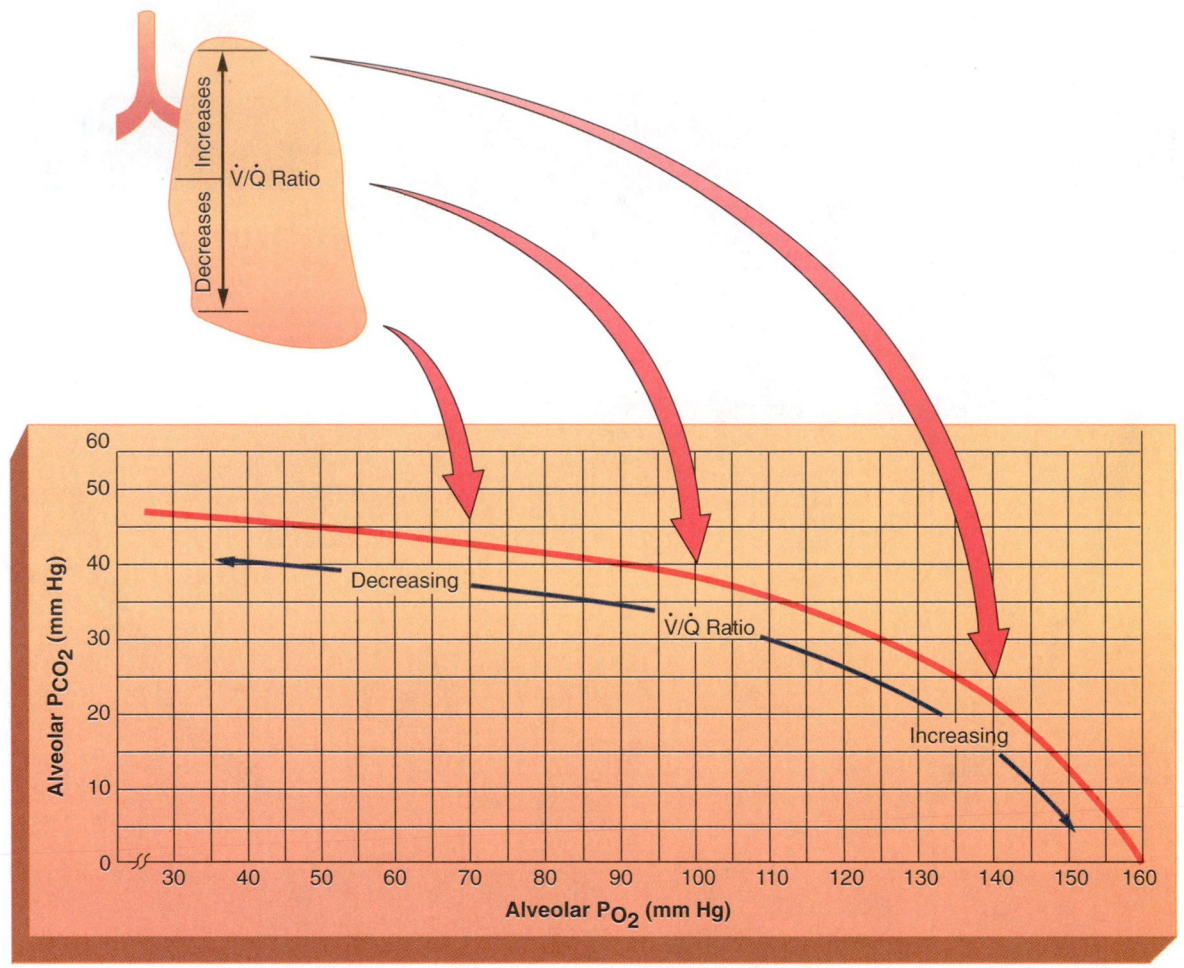

Figure 9–5. *The O$_2$–CO$_2$ diagram.*

the $\dot{V}/\dot{Q}$ ratio is high, the $P_{A_{O_2}}$ is up, and the $P_{A_{CO_2}}$ is down. In contrast, the diagram shows that in the lower lung regions, the $\dot{V}/\dot{Q}$ ratio is low, the $P_{A_{O_2}}$ is down, and the $P_{A_{CO_2}}$ is up.

HOW THE VENTILATION-PERFUSION RATIO AFFECTS THE END-CAPILLARY GASES

The oxygen and carbon dioxide pressures in the end-capillary blood ($P_{c_{O_2}}$ and $P_{c_{CO_2}}$) mirror the $P_{A_{O_2}}$ and $P_{A_{CO_2}}$ changes that occur in the lungs. Thus, as the $\dot{V}/\dot{Q}$ ratio progressively decreases from the top to the bottom of the upright lung, causing the $P_{A_{O_2}}$ to decrease and the $P_{A_{CO_2}}$ to increase, the $P_{c_{O_2}}$ and $P_{c_{CO_2}}$ also decrease and increase, respectively (see Figures 9–3 and 9–4).

Downstream, in the pulmonary veins, the different Pc_{O_2} and Pc_{CO_2} levels mix together and, under normal circumstances, produce a P_{O_2} of 100 mm Hg and a P_{CO_2} of 40 mm Hg (Figure 9–6). Clinically, the result of the Pc_{O_2} and Pc_{CO_2} mixture that occurs in the pulmonary veins is reflected downstream in the Pa_{O_2} and Pa_{CO_2} of an arterial blood gas sample (see Table 7–1, page 205).

It should also be noted that as the PA_{CO_2} decreases from the bottom to the top of the lungs, the progressive reduction of the CO_2 level in the end-capillary blood causes the pH to become more alkaline. The overall pH mixture in the pulmonary

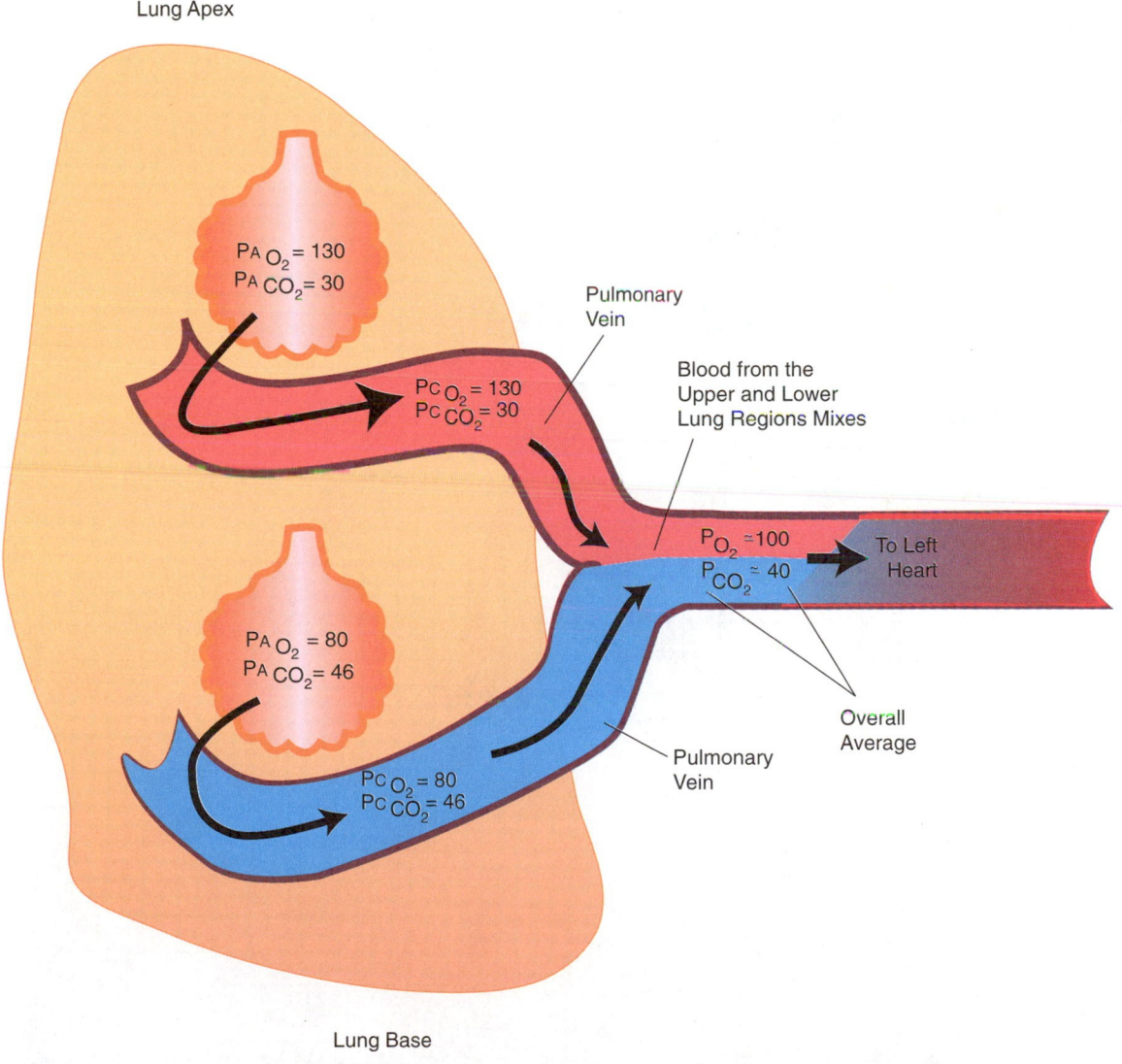

Figure 9–6. *The mixing of pulmonary capillary blood gases (Pc_{O_2} and Pc_{CO_2}) from the upper and lower lung regions.*

veins and, subsequently, in the arterial blood is normally about 7.35 to 7.45 (see Figure 7–1, page 206).

Figure 9–7 summarizes the important effects of changing $\dot{V}/\dot{Q}$ ratios.

RESPIRATORY QUOTIENT

Gas exchange between the systemic capillaries and the cells is called internal respiration. Under normal circumstances, about 250 ml of oxygen are consumed by the tissues during one minute. In exchange, the cells produce about 200 ml of car-

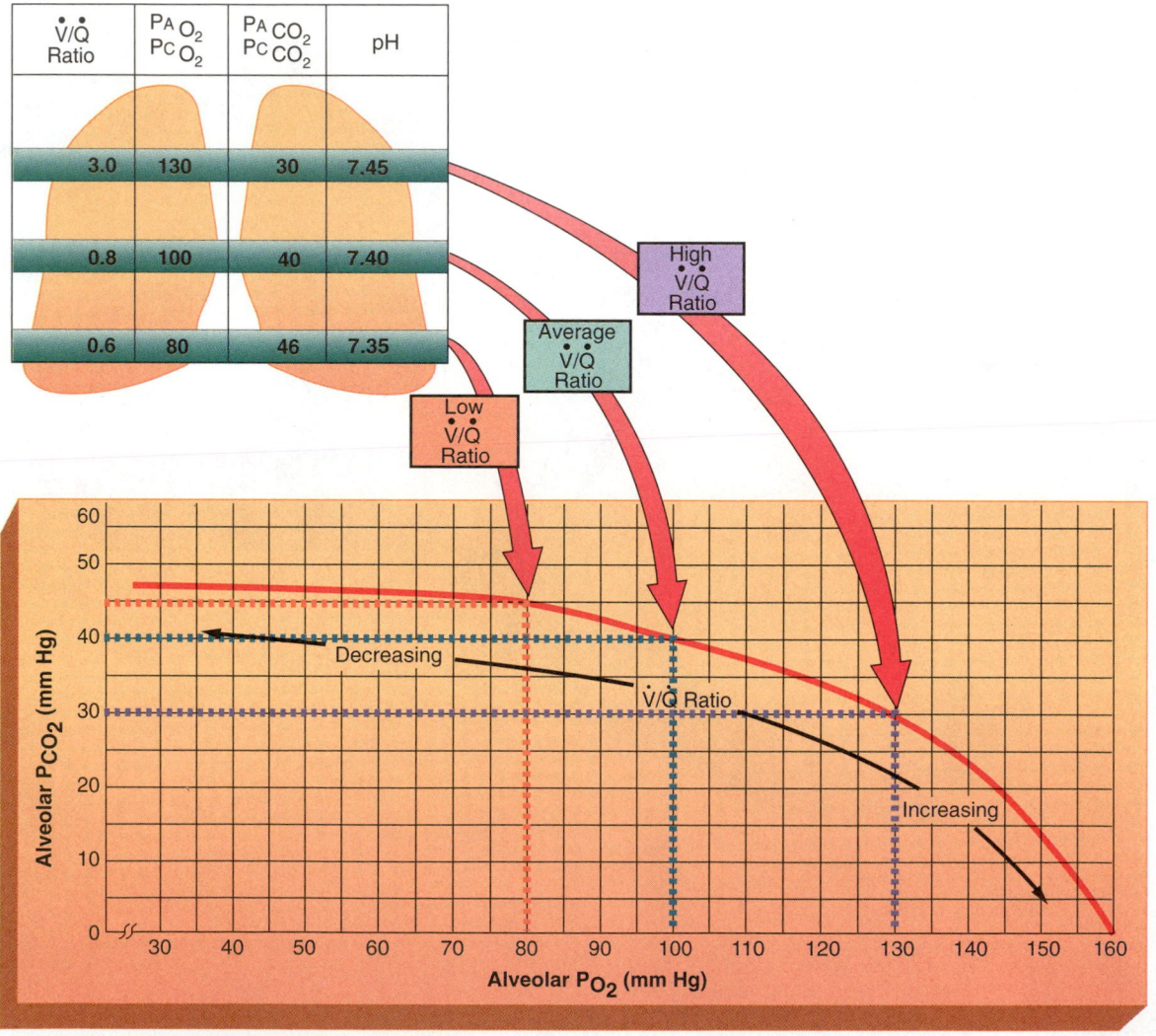

Figure 9–7. *How changes in the $\dot{V}/\dot{Q}$ ratio affect the $P_{A_{O_2}}$ and Pc_{O_2}, the $P_{A_{CO_2}}$ and Pc_{CO_2}, and the pH of the pulmonary blood.*

bon dioxide. Clinically, the ratio between the volume of oxygen consumed ($\dot{V}_{O_2}$) and the volume of carbon dioxide produced ($\dot{V}_{CO_2}$) is called the **respiratory quotient** (RQ) and is expressed as follows:

$$RQ = \frac{\dot{V}_{CO_2}}{\dot{V}_{O_2}}$$

$$= \frac{200 \text{ ml } CO_2/\text{min}}{250 \text{ ml } O_2/\text{min}}$$

$$= 0.8$$

RESPIRATORY EXCHANGE RATIO

Gas exchange between the pulmonary capillaries and the alveoli is called **external respiration**, since this gas exchange is between the body and the external environment. The quantity of oxygen and carbon dioxide exchanged during a period of one minute is called the **respiratory exchange ratio** (RR). Under normal conditions, the RR equals the RQ.

HOW RESPIRATORY DISORDERS AFFECT THE $\dot{V}/\dot{Q}$ RATIO

In respiratory disorders, the $\dot{V}/\dot{Q}$ ratio is always altered. For example, in disorders that diminish pulmonary perfusion, the affected lung area receives little or no blood flow in relation to ventilation. This condition causes the $\dot{V}/\dot{Q}$ ratio to increase. As a result, a larger portion of the alveolar ventilation will not be physiologically effective and is said to be **wasted** or **deadspace ventilation**. When the $\dot{V}/\dot{Q}$ ratio increases, the $P_{A_{O_2}}$ increases and the $P_{A_{CO_2}}$ decreases. Pulmonary disorders that increase the $\dot{V}/\dot{Q}$ ratio include the following:

- Pulmonary emboli
- Partial or complete obstruction in the pulmonary artery or some of the arterioles (e.g., atherosclerosis, collagen disease)
- Extrinsic pressure on the pulmonary vessels (e.g., pneumothorax, hydrothorax, tumors)
- Destruction of the pulmonary vessels (e.g., emphysema)
- Decreased cardiac output

In disorders that diminish pulmonary ventilation, the affected lung area receives little or no ventilation in relation to blood flow. This condition causes the $\dot{V}/\dot{Q}$ ratio to decrease. As a result, a larger portion of the pulmonary blood flow will not be physiologically effective in terms of gas exchange, and is said to be **shunted blood**. When the $\dot{V}/\dot{Q}$ ratio decreases, the $P_{A_{O_2}}$ decreases and the $P_{A_{CO_2}}$ increases. Pulmonary disorders that decrease the $\dot{V}/\dot{Q}$ ratio include the following:

- Obstructive lung disorders (e.g., emphysema, bronchitis, asthma)
- Restrictive lung disorders (e.g., pneumonia, silicosis, pulmonary fibrosis)
- Hypoventilation from any cause

Figure 9–8 summarizes the O_2–CO_2 effects of changing $\dot{V}/\dot{Q}$ ratios in response to respiratory disorders.

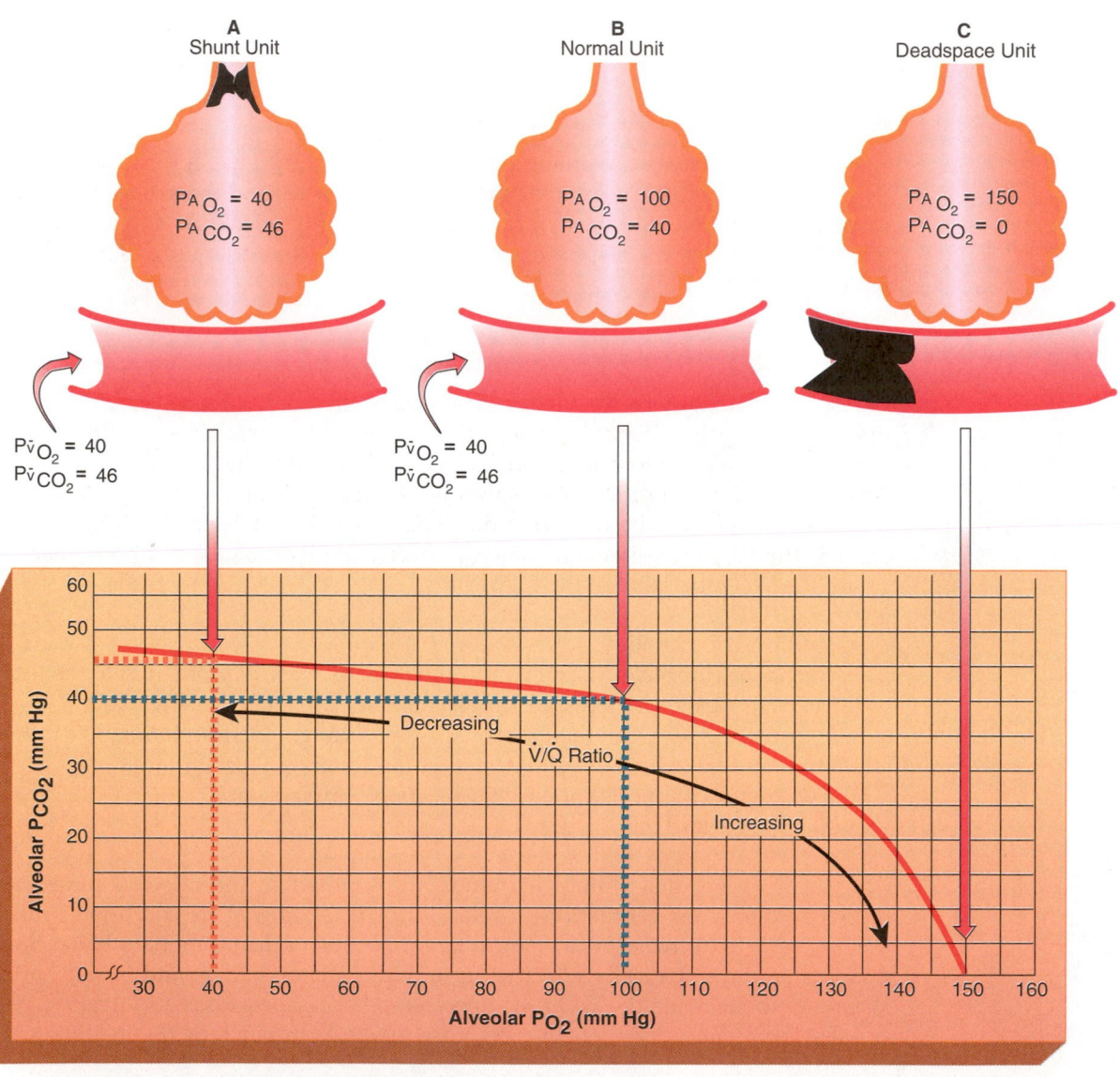

Figure 9–8. *Alveolar O_2 and CO_2 pressure changes that occur as a result of $\dot{V}/\dot{Q}$ ratio changes caused by respiratory disorders. A) shunt unit; B) normal unit; C) deadspace unit.*

CLINICAL APPLICATION

This 4-year-old boy presented in the emergency room in severe respiratory distress. An hour earlier, the patient's mother had brought home some groceries in a large box. After removing the groceries, she noticed a silver quarter in the bottom of the box. She removed the quarter and placed it on the kitchen counter. She then gave the box to her 4-year-old son to play with. Thinking he was occupied for a while, she went downstairs to the basement with her 10-year-old son to put a load of laundry in the washing machine. Moments later, they heard the youngest child cry.

Thinking that it was not anything serious, the mother asked the 10-year-old boy to go get his brother. Seconds later, the older boy called to his mother that his brother looked blue and that he had vomited. The mother quickly went up the stairs to the kitchen. She found her 4-year-old choking and expectorating frothy white sputum from his mouth. Immediately, she knew what had happened. The quarter was gone. Her 4-year-old had put the quarter in his mouth and aspirated it.

Having been trained in cardiopulmonary resuscitation (CPR), she initated the American Heart Association's Conscious-Obstructive CPR procedure. Her son's response, however, was not favorable. In fact, his choking appeared, and sounded, worse. Frothy white secretions continued to flow out of the patient's mouth, and a loud, brassy-like sound could be heard each time the patient inhaled. His inspiratory efforts were clearly labored. Alarmed, the mother immediately drove her son to the emergency room a few miles away. The 10-year-old tried to comfort his brother as they drove to the hospital.

In the emergency room, the patient was conscious, crying, and in obvious respiratory distress. His skin was cyanotic and pale. He appeared very fatigued. Inspiratory stridor could be heard without the aid of a stethoscope. He was sitting up on the side of the gurney, with his legs hanging over the edge, using his accessory muscles of inspiration. His vital signs were: blood pressure—89/50, heart rate—105 beats/min, and respiratory rate—6 breaths/min and labored. His breath sounds were very diminished. A portable chest x-ray film showed the quarter was lodged about 2 cm above the vocal cords (see below). The patient's oxygen saturation measured by pulse oximetry (Sp_{O_2}) was 87 percent. The patient was immediately transferred to surgery and placed under general anethesia. The quarter was removed moments later without difficulty.

DISCUSSION

This case illustrates a decreased ventilation-perfusion ratio caused by an upper airway obstruction (see below). Although an arterial blood gas sample was not drawn in this case, one can easily predict what the values would have been by considering the following factors: As a result of the upper airway obstruction, the patient had a low ventilation-perfusion ratio in both lungs. In addition, in the emergency room the patient was

(continues)

becoming fatigued (his respiratory rate was 6 breaths per minute). This further caused the patient's ventilation-perfusion ratio to fall.

Thus, as the patient's ventilation-perfusion ratio progressively decreased, his $P_{A_{O_2}}$ decreased while, at the same time, his $P_{A_{CO_2}}$ increased. This condition, in turn, caused the end-capillary oxygen pressure (Pc_{O_2}) and carbon dioxide pressure (Pc_{CO_2}) to decrease and increase, respectively. In addition, as the Pc_{CO_2} decreased, the pulmonary capillary blood pH also decreased (see Figure 9–4 and Figure 9–7). If these arterial blood gas trends had continued, the patient would have died. Fortunately, when the quarter was successfully removed, the patient's ventilation-perfusion ratio quickly returned (increased) to normal. Today, the mother has the quarter on a charm bracelet.

CLINICAL APPLICATION

This 34-year-old construction worker fell from a second-story platform and was impaled by a steel enforcement rod that was protruding vertically about three feet from a cement structure. The steel rod entered the side of the patient's lower right abdomen and exited from the left side of the abdomen, about two cm below the twelfth rib (see x-ray below). Although the steel rod pierced the side of the descending aorta, no other major organs were seriously damaged.

The patient was still conscious when workers cut through the steel rod to free him from the cement structure. While he was being cut free, an emergency medical team inserted an intravenous (IV) infusion line, placed a non-rebreathing mask over his face, and worked to stop the bleeding as best they could. When the patient was finally cut free, he was immediately transported to the trauma center. It was later estimated that the patient had lost about half of his blood volume at the accident site.

A full trauma team was in the emergency room when the patient arrived. The patient was unconscious and very cyanotic. Even though he still had spontaneous breaths, he had an oral airway in place and was being manually ventilated with an inspired oxygen concentration ($F_{I_{O_2}}$) of 1.0. His blood pressure was 65/40 and his heart rate was 120 beats per minute. The respiratory therapist intubated the patient and continued to manually ventilate the patient with an $F_{I_{O_2}}$ of 1.0.

Almost simultaneously a portable x-ray film was taken STAT to aid the trauma surgeons in the removal of the steel rod. A blood specimen was obtained for the following laboratory assays: glucose, BUN (blood urea nitrogen), creatinine, electrolytes, CBC (complete blood count), and a type and screen and blood gas analysis. The emergency room physician called the laboratory to alert lab staff that 10 units of uncrossmatched O negative blood would be needed STAT, and to stay 5 units ahead at all times. The patient was rushed to surgery. The surgical team learned during the operation that the patient's hematocrit was 15.3 percent and his hemoglobin level was 5.1 g%.

FOUR HOURS LATER

The patient was in stable condition in the surgical intensive care unit (ICU). The steel rod had been successfully removed and his aorta was repaired. Although he was still listed in critical condition, his prognosis was described as good to excellent. At this time, however, the patient was still unconscious because of the drugs administered during surgery. He was on mechanical ventilation with the following settings: tidal volume 900 ml, respiratory rate 12 breaths/min, $F_{I_{O_2}}$ 0.4, and continuous positive airway pressure (CPAP) 5 cm H_2O.

His blood pressure was 126/79 and his heart rate was 78 beats per minute. His arterial blood gas values were: pH 7.44, Pa_{CO_2} 36 mm Hg, HCO_3^- 24 mmol/L, and Pa_{O_2} 136 mm Hg. His oxygen saturation measured by a pulse oximeter

(Sp_{O_2}) was 98 percent. His hematocrit was 44 percent and his hemoglobin level was 14.6 g%. The patient's recovery went very well. Two days later he was conscious and no longer on the ventilator. He was discharged six days later.

DISCUSSION

This case illustrates an increased ventilation-perfusion ratio caused by an excessive amount of blood lost as a result of trauma (the penetrating steel rod). As the patient continued to lose blood, the blood flow through both of his lungs progressively decreased. As a result of this pathologic process, his alveolar ventilation progressively became greater than his pulmonary blood flow. Thus, the patient's alveolar ventilation was becoming more and more "ineffective" physiologically. In other words, more and more of the patient's alveolar ventilation was becoming **wasted** or **deadspace ventilation** (see Figure 2–28, page 88). The paradox of this condition is that even though the patient's PA_{O_2} and Pa_{O_2} increased in response to an increased ventilation-perfusion ratio, the actual amount of oxygen being transported decreased because of the reduced blood flow (see Table 7–10, page 226). Fortunately, this pathologic process was reversed in surgery.

REVIEW QUESTIONS

1. Overall, the normal $\dot{V}/\dot{Q}$ ratio is about
   a. 0.2
   b. 0.4
   c. 0.6
   d. 0.8
   e. 1.0
2. In the healthy individual in the upright position, the
   I. $\dot{V}/\dot{Q}$ ratio is highest in the lower lung regions
   II. PA_{O_2} is lowest in the upper lung regions
   III. $\dot{V}/\dot{Q}$ ratio is lowest in the upper lung regions
   IV. PA_{CO_2} is highest in the lower lung regions
   a. I only

    b. II only

    c. IV only

    d. I and IV only

    e. II and IV only

3. When the $\dot{V}/\dot{Q}$ ratio decreases, the

    I. $P_{A_{O_2}}$ falls

    II. Pc_{CO_2} increases

    III. $P_{A_{CO_2}}$ rises

    IV. Pc_{O_2} decreases

    a. I only

    b. III only

    c. I and II only

    d. II, III, and IV only

    e. I, II, III, and IV

4. When alveolar ventilation is 7 L/min and the pulmonary blood flow is 9.5 L/min, the $\dot{V}/\dot{Q}$ ratio is about

    a. 0.4

    b. 0.5

    c. 0.6

    d. 0.7

    e. 0.8

5. If a patient's tissue cells consume 275 ml of O_2 per minute and produce 195 ml of CO_2 per minute, what is the RQ?

    a. 0.65

    b. 0.7

    c. 0.8

    d. 0.96

    e. 1.25

10

CONTROL OF VENTILATION

OBJECTIVES

By the end of this chapter, the student should be able to:

1. Describe the function of the following *respiratory neurons* of the *medulla oblongata:*
   —The dorsal respiratory group
   —The ventral respiratory group
2. Describe the influence of the following *pontine respiratory centers* on the respiratory neurons of the medulla oblongata:
   —Apneustic center
   —Pneumotaxic center
3. List conditions that can depress the respiratory neurons.
4. Describe how the following regulate the respiratory neurons:

   —Central chemoreceptors
   —Peripheral chemoreceptors
   —Reflexes that influence ventilation
   • Hering-Breuer inflation reflex
   • Deflation reflex
   • Irritant reflex
   • Juxtapulmonary-capillary receptor reflex
   • Reflexes from the aortic and carotid sinus baroreceptors
   • Other stimuli that affect ventilation
5. Complete the review questions at the end of this chapter.

The intrinsic rhythmicity of respiration is primarily controlled by specific neural areas located in the reticular substance of the medulla and pons of the brain. These neural areas possess monitoring, stimulating, and inhibiting properties that continually adjust the ventilatory pattern to meet specific metabolic needs. Also received and coordinated in these respiratory neural areas are the voluntary signals transmitted by the cerebral cortex during a variety of ventilatory maneuvers such as talking, singing, sniffing, coughing, or blowing into a woodwind instrument.

To fully understand this subject, a basic knowledge of (1) the function of the major respiratory components of the medulla, (2) the influence of the pontine respiratory centers on the respiratory components of the medulla, (3) the major monitoring systems that influence the respiratory components of the medulla, and (4) the reflexes that influence ventilation is necessary.

THE RESPIRATORY COMPONENTS OF THE MEDULLA

Although knowledge concerning this subject is incomplete, it is now believed that two groups of respiratory neurons in the medulla oblongata are responsible for co-ordinating the intrinsic rhythmicity of respiration: these are (1) the dorsal respiratory group (DRG), and (2) the ventral respiratory group (VRG) (Figure 10–1).

DORSAL RESPIRATORY GROUP

The dorsal respiratory group (DRG) consists chiefly of inspiratory neurons. The DRG neurons are believed to be responsible for the basic rhythm of ventilation (see Figure 10–1). They (1) receive numerous signals from the body regarding the respiratory needs; (2) evaluate and prioritize the various signals; and, depending on the respiratory needs, (3) emit neural impulses every few seconds to the muscles of inspiration, primarily the diaphragm. The signals released by the DRG continue for about 1 to 2 seconds and then cease abruptly, causing the muscles of inspiration to

Figure 10–1. *Schematic illustration of the respiratory components of the lower brainstem (pons and medulla). PNC = pneumotaxic center; APC = apneustic center; DRG = dorsal respiratory group; VRG = ventral respiratory group; CC = central chemoreceptors.*

relax. During exhalation, which lasts for about 2 to 3 seconds, the natural elastic recoil forces of the lungs cause the lungs to deflate.

VENTRAL RESPIRATORY GROUP

The ventral respiratory group (VRG) contains both **inspiratory** and **expiratory neurons**. During normal quiet breathing, the VRG is almost entirely dormant, since the lungs passively return to their original size by virtue of their own elastic recoil forces. During heavy exercise or stress, however, the expiratory neurons of the VRG actively send impulses to the muscles of exhalation (e.g., abdominal muscles) and the accessory muscles of inspiration (e.g., sternocleidomastoid) innervated by the vagus nerve (see Figure 10–1).

THE INFLUENCE OF THE PONTINE RESPIRATORY CENTERS ON THE RESPIRATORY COMPONENTS OF THE MEDULLA

The pontine respiratory centers consist of the **apneustic center** and the **pneumotaxic center**. Although these centers are known to exist and can be made to operate under experimental conditions, their functional significance in man is still not fully understood. It appears that these centers function to some degree to modify and fine-tune the rhythmicity of respirations.

Apneustic Center

The apneustic center is located in the middle and lower pons (see Figure 10–1). If unrestrained, the apneustic center continually sends neural impulses to the DRG and VRG in the medulla. This action causes a prolonged, gasping type of inspiratory maneuver called **apneustic breathing**. Under normal conditions, however, the apneustic center receives numerous signals that suppress its function, thus permitting expiration to occur. Such signals include the strong inhibitory impulses transmitted by the pneumotaxic center and the Hering-Breuer inflation reflex.

Pneumotaxic Center

The pneumotaxic center is located in the reticular substance of the upper one-third of the pons (see Figure 10–1). By varying the neural impulses that suppress the apneustic center, the pneumotaxic area enhances the rhythmicity of the breathing pattern. Neural impulses from the pneumotaxic center simultaneously cause (1) the depth of breathing to decrease and (2) the rate of breathing to increase, by almost an equal amount. Because these two respiratory maneuvers (rapid and shallow breaths) offset each other, the total change in minute ventilation is unremarkable.

Some investigators believe the pneumotaxic center is closely related to the so-called **panting center** in animals such as dogs. For example, when the dog becomes overheated, the panting center causes the dog to breathe with rapid, shallow breaths that evaporate large amounts of water from the dog's upper airways, thus cooling the animal. In man, the pneumotaxic center appears to have an effect similar to the Hering-Breuer inflation reflex.*

---

*The Hering-Breuer inflation reflex is described in further detail later in this chapter, page 288.

FAILURE OF THE RESPIRATORY COMPONENTS OF THE MEDULLA

There are several clinical conditions that can depress the function of the respiratory components of the medulla. Such conditions include (1) reduced blood flow through the medulla as a result of excess pressure caused by a cerebral edema or some other intracerebral abnormality, (2) acute poliomyelitis, and (3) ingestion of drugs that depress the central nervous system.

MONITORING SYSTEMS THAT INFLUENCE THE RESPIRATORY COMPONENTS OF THE MEDULLA

From moment to moment, the respiratory components of the medulla (DRG and VRG) activate specific ventilatory patterns based upon information received from several different monitoring systems throughout the body. The major known monitoring systems are the (1) central chemoreceptors and (2) peripheral chemoreceptors. Certain neural impulses transmitted to the respiratory neurons during exercise and certain reflexes also influence ventilation.

CENTRAL CHEMORECEPTORS

The most powerful stimulus known to influence the respiratory components (DRG and VRG) of the medulla is an excess concentration of hydrogen ions [H^+] in the cerebrospinal fluid (CSF). The central chemoreceptors, which are located bilaterally and ventrally in the substance of the medulla, are responsible for monitoring the H^+ ion concentration of the CSF. In fact, a portion of the central chemoreceptors is actually in direct contact with the CSF. It is believed that the central chemoreceptors transmit signals to the respiratory components of the medulla by the following mechanism:

1. As the CO_2 level increases in the arterial blood (e.g., during hypoventilation), the CO_2 molecules diffuse across a semipermeable membrane, called the blood–brain barrier, which separates the blood from the CSF. The blood–brain barrier is very permeable to CO_2 molecules but relatively impermeable to H^+ and HCO_3^- ions.
2. As CO_2 moves into the CSF, it forms carbonic acid by means of the following reaction:

$$CO_2 + H_2O \rightleftharpoons H_2CO_3 \rightleftharpoons H+ + HCO_3^-$$

3. Because the CSF lacks hemoglobin and carbonic anhydrase and has a relatively low bicarbonate and protein level, the overall buffering system in the CSF is very slow. Because of the inefficient CSF buffering system, the H^+ generated from the above reaction rapidly increases and therefore significantly reduces the pH level in the CSF.

4. The liberated H^+ ions cause the central chemoreceptors to transmit signals to the respiratory component in the medulla, which, in turn, increases the alveolar ventilation.

5. The increased ventilation reduces the Pa_{CO_2} and, subsequently, the P_{CO_2} in the CSF. As the P_{CO_2} in the CSF decreases, the H^+ ion concentration of the CSF also falls. This action decreases the stimulation of the central chemoreceptors. Thus, the neural signals to the respiratory components in the medulla also diminish; this, in turn, causes alveolar ventilation to decrease.

6. In view of the above sequences, it should be understood that the central chemoreceptors regulate ventilation through the indirect effects of CO_2 on the pH level of the CSF (Figure 10–2).

Peripheral Chemoreceptors

The peripheral chemoreceptors are special oxygen-sensitive cells that react to reductions of oxygen levels in the arterial blood. They are located high in the neck at the bifurcation of the internal and external carotid arteries and on the aortic arch (Figure 10–3, page 284). They are close to, but distinct from, the *baroreceptors*, pressoreceptors (see Figure 5–10, page 165). The peripheral chemoreceptors are also called the *carotid and aortic bodies*.

The carotid and aortic bodies are composed of epithelial-like cells and neuron terminals in intimate contact with the arterial blood. When activated by a low Pa_{O_2},

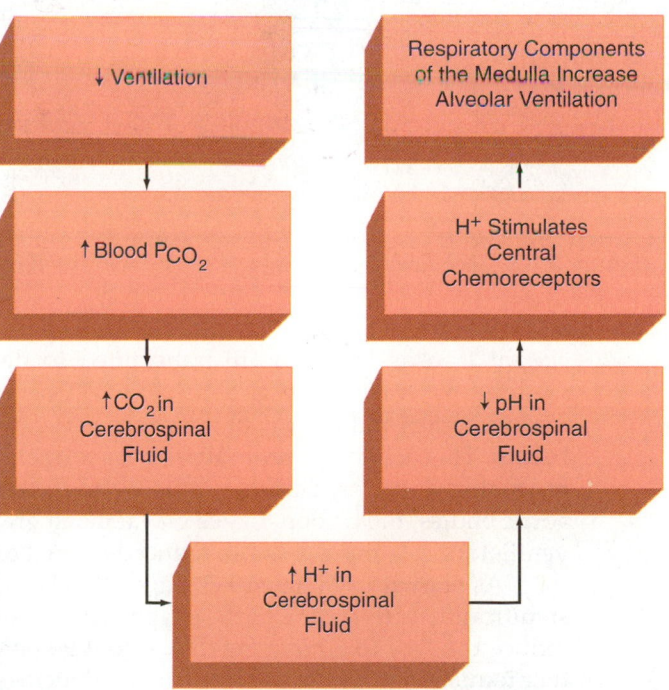

Figure 10–2. *How an increased carbon dioxide level increases alveolar ventilation.*

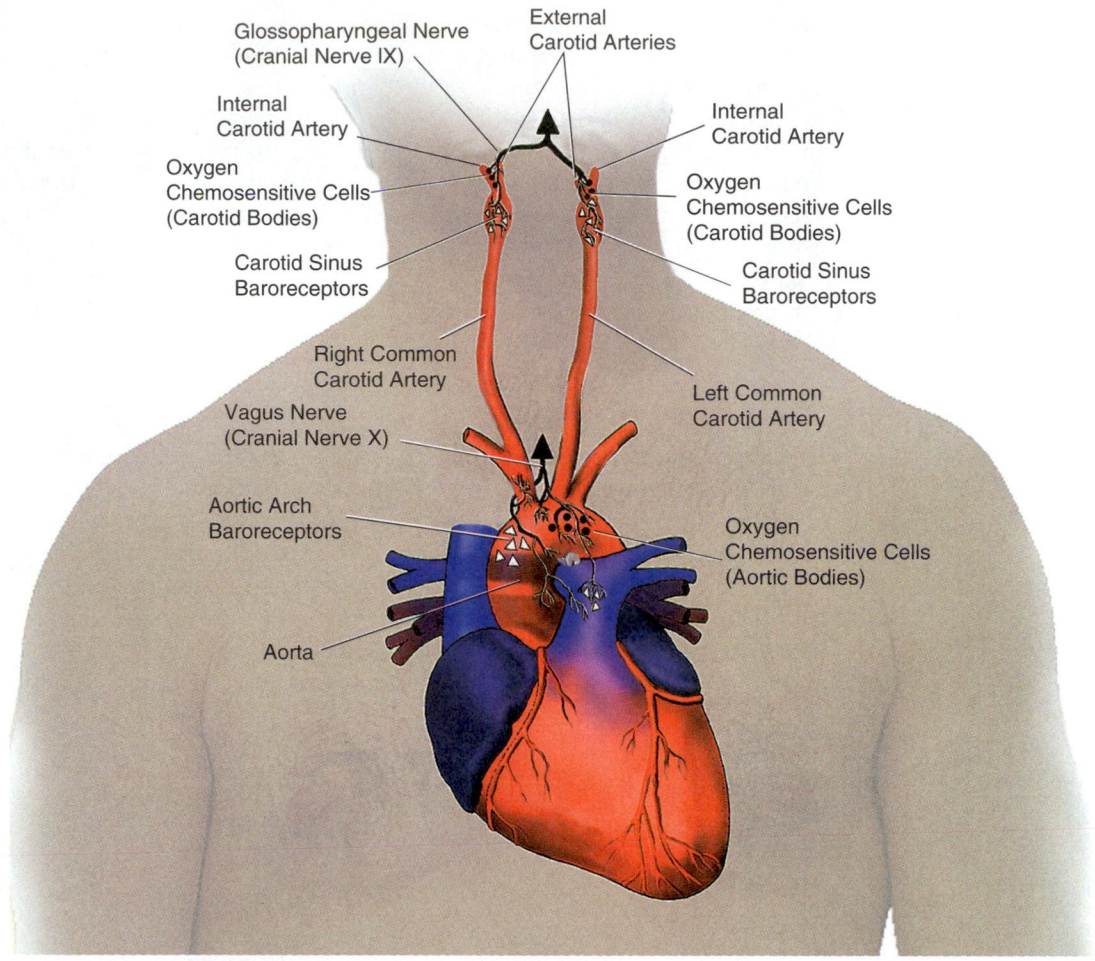

Glossopharyngeal Nerve
(Cranial Nerve IX)

External
Carotid Arteries

Internal
Carotid Artery

Internal
Carotid Artery

Oxygen
Chemosensitive Cells
(Carotid Bodies)

Oxygen
Chemosensitive Cells
(Carotid Bodies)

Carotid Sinus
Baroreceptors

Carotid Sinus
Baroreceptors

Right Common
Carotid Artery

Left Common
Carotid Artery

Vagus Nerve
(Cranial Nerve X)

Aortic Arch
Baroreceptors

Oxygen
Chemosensitive Cells
(Aortic Bodies)

Aorta

Figure 10–3. *Location of the carotid and aortic bodies (the peripheral chemoreceptors).*

afferent (sensory) signals are transmitted to the respiratory components in the medulla by way of the glossopharyngeal nerve (ninth cranial nerve) from the carotid bodies and by way of the vagus nerve (tenth cranial nerve) from the aortic bodies. This action, in turn, causes *efferent* (motor) signals to be transmitted to the respiratory muscles, causing ventilation to increase (Figure 10–4). Compared to the aortic bodies, the carotid bodies play a much greater role in initiating an increased ventilatory rate in response to reduced arterial oxygen levels.

As shown in Figure 10–5, page 286, the peripheral chemoreceptors are not significantly activated until the oxygen content of the inspired air is low enough to reduce the Pa_{O_2} to 60 mm Hg (Sa_{O_2} about 90 percent). Beyond this point, any further reduction in the Pa_{O_2} causes a marked increase in ventilation. *Suppression* of the peripheral chemoreceptors is seen, however, when the Pa_{O_2} falls below 30 mm Hg.

In the patient with a low Pa_{O_2} and a chronically high Pa_{CO_2} level (e.g., the end-stages of emphysema), the peripheral chemoreceptors may be totally re-

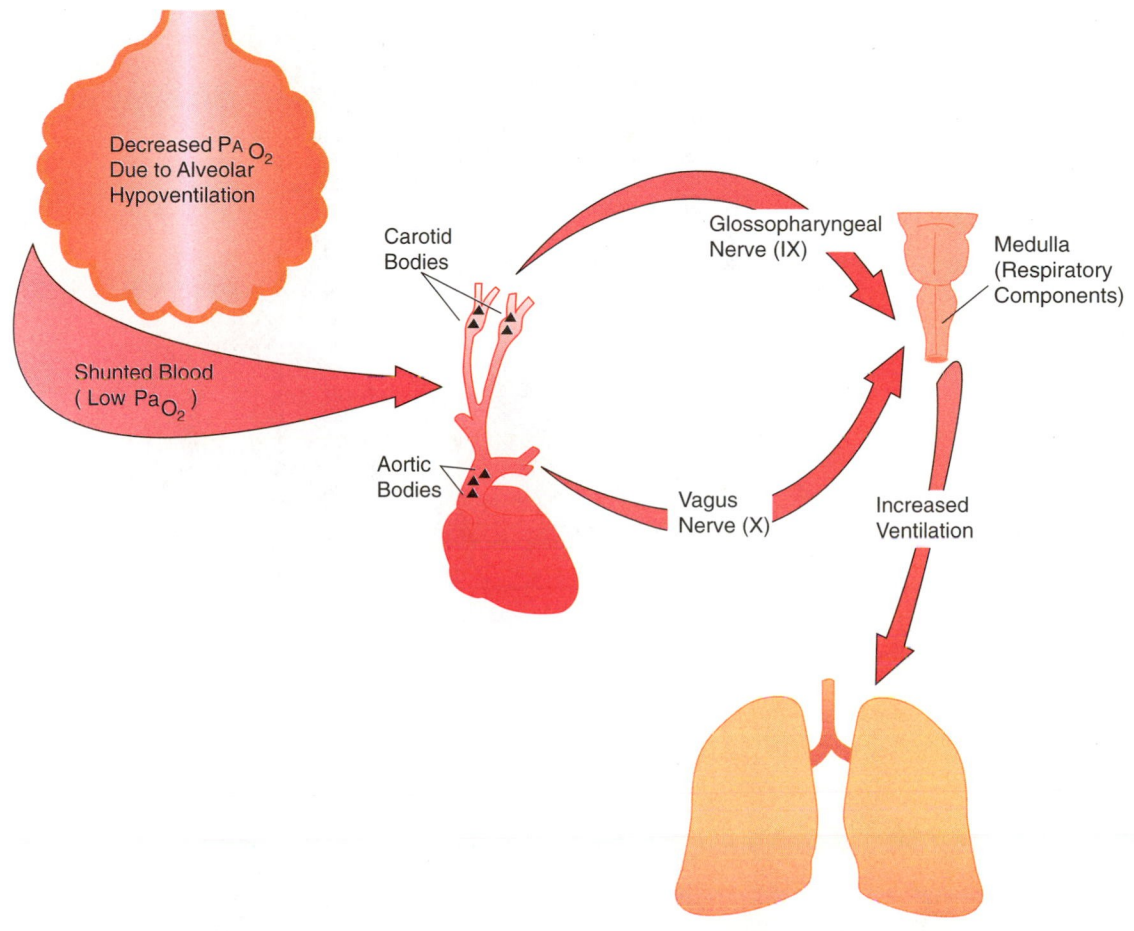

Figure 10–4. *Schematic illustration showing how a low Pa*$_{O_2}$ *stimulates the respiratory components of the medulla to increase alveolar ventilation.*

sponsible for the control of ventilation. This is because a chronically high CO_2 concentration in the CSF inactivates the H^+ sensitivity of the central chemoreceptor—that is, HCO_3^- moves into the CSF via the active transport mechanism and combines with H^+, thus returning the pH to normal. A compensatory response to a chronically high CO_2 concentration, however, is the enhancement of the sensitivity of the peripheral chemoreceptors at higher CO_2 levels (Figure 10–6, page 286).

Finally, it is important to understand that the peripheral chemoreceptors are specifically sensitive to the P_{O_2} of the blood and relatively insensitive to the oxygen content of the blood. The precise mechanism for this exclusive P_{O_2} sensitivity is not fully understood. It is known, however, that the blood flow through the peripheral chemoreceptors is very high in relation to metabolism. Thus, the overall extraction of oxygen is relatively low, and therefore the difference between the oxygen content in the arterial blood and the venous blood [$C(a - v)_{O_2}$] is small.

Figure 10–5. *The effect of low Pa_{O_2} levels on ventilation.*

Figure 10–6. *The effect of Pa_{O_2} on ventilation at three different Pa_{CO_2} values. Note that as the Pa_{CO_2} value increases, the sensitivity of the peripheral chemoreceptors increases.*

Clinically, this exclusive Pa_{O_2} sensitivity can be misleading. There are certain conditions in which the Pa_{O_2} is normal (and therefore the peripheral chemoreceptors are not stimulated), yet the oxygen content of the blood is dangerously low. Such conditions include chronic anemia, carbon monoxide poisoning, and methemoglobinemia.

Other Factors That Stimulate the Peripheral Chemoreceptors. Although the peripheral chemoreceptors are primarily stimulated by a reduced Pa_{O_2} level, they are also activated by a decreased pH (increased H^+ level). This is an important feature of the peripheral chemoreceptors, since there are many situations in which a change in arterial H^+ ion levels can occur by means other than a primary change in the P_{CO_2}. In fact, because the H^+ ions do not readily move across the blood–brain barrier, the peripheral chemoreceptors play a major role in initiating ventilation whenever the H^+ ion concentration increases for reasons other than an increased Pa_{CO_2}. For example, the accumulation of lactic acids or ketone acids in the blood stimulates hyperventilation almost entirely through the peripheral chemoreceptors (Figure 10–7).

The peripheral chemoreceptors are also stimulated by (1) hypoperfusion (e.g., stagnant hypoxia), (2) increased temperature, (3) nicotine, and (4) the direct effect of Pa_{CO_2}. The response of the peripheral chemoreceptors to Pa_{CO_2} stimulation, however,

Figure 10–7. *The accumulation of lactic acids leads to an increased alveolar ventilation primarily through the stimulation of the peripheral chemoreceptors.*

is minor and not nearly so great as the response generated by the central chemoreceptors. The peripheral chemoreceptors do respond faster than the central chemoreceptors to an increased Pa_{CO_2}. This occurs because the peripheral chemoreceptors are stimulated directly by the CO_2 molecule, whereas the central chemoreceptors are stimulated by the H^+ generated by the CO_2 hydration reaction in the CSF—a reaction that occurs slowly in the absence of carbonic anhydrase (see Figure 10–2).

Other Responses Activated by the Peripheral Chemoreceptors. In addition to the increased ventilation activated by the peripheral chemoreceptors, other responses can occur as a result of peripheral chemoreceptor stimulation, including the following:

- Peripheral vasoconstriction
- Increased pulmonary vascular resistance
- Systemic arterial hypertension
- Tachycardia
- Increase in left ventricular performance

REFLEXES THAT INFLUENCE VENTILATION

A number of reflexes are known to influence the rate of ventilation.

HERING-BREUER INFLATION REFLEX

The Hering-Breuer inflation reflex is generated by stretch receptors located in the walls of the bronchi and bronchioles that become excited when the lungs overinflate. Signals from these receptors travel through the vagus nerve to the respiratory components in the medulla, causing inspiration to cease. In essence, the lungs themselves provide a feedback mechanism to terminate inspiration. Instead of a reflex to control ventilation, the Hering-Breuer reflex appears to be a protective mechanism that prevents pulmonary damage caused by excessive lung inflation. The significance of the Hering-Breuer reflex in the adult at normal tidal volumes is controversial; it appears to have more significance in the control of ventilation in the newborn.

DEFLATION REFLEX

When the lungs are compressed or deflated, an increased rate of breathing results. The precise mechanism responsible for this reflex is not known. Some workers believe that the increased rate of breathing may be due to the reduced stimulation of receptors serving the Hering-Breuer inflation reflex rather than to the stimulation of specific deflation receptors. Others, however, think that the deflation reflex is not due to the absence of receptor stimulation of the Hering-Breuer reflex, since the reflex is still seen when the temperature of the bronchi and bronchioles is less than 8°C. The Hering-Breuer reflex is not seen when the bronchi and bronchioles are below this temperature.

IRRITANT REFLEX

When the lungs are exposed to noxious gases, the irritant receptors may also be stimulated. The irritant receptors are subepithelial mechanoreceptors located in the trachea, bronchi, and bronchioles. When the receptors are activated, a reflex response causes the ventilatory rate to increase. Stimulation of the irritant receptors may also produce a reflex cough and bronchoconstriction.

JUXTAPULMONARY-CAPILLARY RECEPTORS

Juxtapulmonary-capillary receptors, or *J receptors*, are located in the interstitial tissues between the pulmonary capillaries and the alveoli. It is believed that the J receptors are activated by the following:

- Pulmonary capillary congestion
- Capillary hypertension
- Edema of the alveolar walls
- Humoral agents (serotonin)
- Lung deflation
- Emboli

When the J receptors are stimulated, a reflex response triggers rapid, shallow breathing.

REFLEXES FROM THE AORTIC AND CAROTID SINUS BARORECEPTORS

The normal function of the aortic and carotid sinus baroreceptors, located near the aortic and carotid peripheral chemoreceptors (see Figure 5–10, page 165), is to initiate reflexes that cause (1) a decreased heart and ventilatory rate in response to an elevated systemic blood pressure and (2) an increased heart and ventilatory rate in response to a reduced systemic blood pressure.

OTHER STIMULI THAT AFFECT VENTILATION

Many stimuli can influence ventilation, including the following:

1. A sudden cold stimulus, such as plunging into very cold water, may cause respiration to temporarily cease.
2. A sudden pain may cause a temporary cessation of breathing. Prolonged pain, however, activates the general adaptation syndrome and increases the breathing rate.
3. Irritation of the pharynx or larynx by touch or chemicals can trigger an immediate cessation of breathing, followed by an episode of coughing.
4. The stretching of the anal sphincter triggers an increased respiratory rate. Clinically, this technique is sometimes used to activate respirations during emergencies—for example, during periods of apnea in newborn infants.
5. Light pressure applied to the thorax may increase ventilation. The significance of this chest wall reflex in humans is unknown.

CLINICAL APPLICATION 1

This 44-year-old female was found unconscious on her living room floor by her husband when he returned home from work. He immediately carried her to his car and drove her to the hospital. As he was driving, he called the hospital emergency room on his cellular telephone to alert the medical staff. He estimated that his time of arrival would be in about 15 minutes. While on the phone, he also reported that his wife had a long history of diabetes. He stated that his wife had passed out three times before, over the past two years, as a result of not taking her insulin as prescribed. The husband had no idea how long his wife had been unconscious before he found her.

Upon arrival, the patient was still unconscious and breathing very deeply and rapidly. The emergency room nurse placed an oxygen mask on the patient's face and started an intravenous (IV) infusion. A laboratory phlebotomist drew some blood, and the respiratory therapist obtained an arterial blood gas sample from the patient's radial artery. The patient's vital signs were: blood pressure—135/85, heart rate—97 beats/min, respiratory rate—22 breaths/min, and temperature 37° C. The patient's respiratory pattern was charted by the respiratory therapist as Kussmaul breathing (see page 97). The patient's arterial blood gas values were: pH 7.23, Pa_{CO_2} 24 mm Hg, HCO_3^- 19 mmol/L, and Pa_{O_2} 405 mm Hg. The respiratory therapist discontinued the patient's oxygen therapy. The second set of arterial blood gas values on room air were: pH 7.23, Pa_{CO_2} 24 mm Hg, HCO_3^- 19 mmol/L, and Pa_{O_2} 119 mm Hg.

The laboratory report showed that the patient had a glucose level of 837 mg/dl (normal is 70–150). The report also showed that her serum acetone level was 1 : 64 (normal is 0). The attending physician started to administer the patient insulin. Two hours later the patient was conscious and talking with her husband. Her vital signs were: blood pressure—122/68, heart rate—75 beats/min, respiratory rate—12 breaths/min, and normal temperature—37° C. Her arterial blood gas values on room air at this time were: pH 7.41, Pa_{CO_2} 39, HCO_3^- 24 mmol/L, and Pa_{O_2} 95 mm Hg. Her glucose level was 95 mg/dl and her acetone level was zero. The patient was discharged the next day.

DISCUSSION

This case illustrates how clinical factors other than an increased P_{CO_2} or decreased P_{O_2} can stimulate ventilation. Because the patient had not taken her insulin as prescribed, ketone acids (H^+) started to accumulate in her blood. As the ketone acid level increased, her pH decreased. As this pathologic process developed, the excessive ketone acids (H^+) stimulated the patient's peripheral chemoreceptors. Since the H^+ ion does not readily move across the blood–brain barrier, the peripheral chemoreceptors played a major role in causing the patient's ventilation to increase (see Figure 10–7).

In addition, it should be noted that as the patient's ventilation increased, her Pa_{CO_2} decreased (to 24 mm Hg in the emergency room). The reduction in the patient's Pa_{CO_2} was a compensatory mechanism—i.e., the decreased Pa_{CO_2} worked to offset the patient's acidic pH caused by the increased ketone acids. In other words, if the patient's Pa_{CO_2} had been closer to her normal level (around 40 mm Hg) in the emergency room, her pH would have been lower than 7.23.

It should also be noted that an increased respiratory rate does not necessarily mean that the patient is in need of oxygen therapy. In this case, however, oxygen in the emergency room was appropriate (because of the patient's rapid breathing) until the cause of the rapid breathing was determined. When the results of the first arterial blood gas analysis were available (the Pa_{O_2} was 405 mm Hg), the discontinuation of the oxygen therapy was the appropriate response.

C L I N I C A L   A P P L I C A T I O N 2

To facilitate the understanding of how the peripheral and central chemoreceptors control the ventilatory pattern, consider the following chain of events that develops when an individual who normally resides at sea level ascends to a high altitude (say, to the Colorado mountains to ski) for a period of two weeks.

CHANGES AT HIGH ALTITUDES
Stimulation of the Peripheral Chemoreceptors

1. As the individual ascends the mountain, the barometric pressure, and therefore the P_{O_2}, of the atmosphere progressively decrease. (Remember, however, that the oxygen percentage is still 21 percent).
2. As the atmospheric P_{O_2} decreases, the individual's arterial oxygen pressure (Pa_{O_2}) also decreases.
3. As the individual continues to ascend the mountain, the Pa_{O_2} eventually falls low enough (to about 60 mm Hg) to stimulate the medulla to increase ventilation.
4. The increased ventilation initiated by the peripheral chemoreceptors causes a secondary decrease in the Pa_{CO_2}. In other words, the individual hyperventilates in response to the reduced Pa_{O_2} level.
5. Because the peripheral chemoreceptors do not acclimate to a decreased oxygen concentration, hyperventilation will continue for the entire time the individual remains at the high altitude.

Readjustment of the Central Chemoreceptors

In response to the hyperventilation that occurs while the individual is at the high altitude, the central chemoreceptors readjust to the lower CO_2 level because of the following chain of events:

1. As the individual hyperventilates to offset the low atmospheric P_{O_2}, the individual's Pa_{CO_2} level decreases.

2. In response to the decreased Pa_{CO_2}, the CO_2 molecules in the CSF move into the blood until equilibrium occurs.
3. This reaction causes the pH of the CSF to increase.
4. Over the next 48 hours, however, HCO_3^- will also leave the CSF (via the active transport mechanism) to correct the pH back to normal. In short, the individual's CSF readjusts to the low CO_2 level.

CHANGES AFTER LEAVING A HIGH ALTITUDE
Stimulation of the Central Chemoreceptors

Interestingly, even after the individual returns to a lower altitude, hyperventilation continues for a few days. The reason for this is as follows:

1. As the individual moves down the mountain, the barometric pressure steadily increases, and therefore the atmospheric P_{O_2} increases.
2. As the atmospheric P_{O_2} increases, the individual's Pa_{O_2} also increases and eventually ceases to stimulate the peripheral chemoreceptors.
3. As the stimulation of the peripheral chemoreceptors decreases, the individual's ventilatory rate decreases.
4. As the ventilatory rate declines, however, the individual's Pa_{CO_2} progressively increases.
5. As the Pa_{CO_2} increases, CO_2 molecules move across the blood–brain barrier into the CSF.
6. As CO_2 moves into the CSF, H^+ ions are formed, causing the pH of the CSF to decrease.
7. The H^+ ions liberated in the above reaction stimulate the central chemoreceptors to increase the individual's ventilatory rate.
8. Eventually, HCO_3^- ions move across the blood–brain barrier into the CSF to correct the pH back to normal. When this occurs, the individual's ventilatory pattern will be as it was before the trip to the mountains.

REVIEW QUESTIONS

1. The respiratory components of the medulla consist of which of the following?
   I. Dorsal respiratory group
   II. Apneustic center
   III. Ventral respiratory group
   IV. Pneumotaxic center
      a. I only
      b. II only
      c. I and III only
      d. II and IV only
      e. I, II, III, and IV

2. Which of the following has the most powerful effect on the respiratory components of the medulla?
   a. Decreased O_2
   b. Increased H^+
   c. Decreased CO_2
   d. Increased pH
   e. Decreased HCO_3^-

3. Which of the following may cause a temporary cessation in breathing?
   I. Sudden pain
   II. Pharynx or larynx irritation
   III. Sudden cold
   IV. Inhalation of noxious gases
      a. I only
      b. II only
      c. IV only
      d. III and IV only
      e. I, II, and III only

4. Which of the following will readily diffuse across the blood–brain barrier?
   I. CO_2
   II. H^+
   III. HCO_3^-
   IV. H_2CO_3
      a. I only
      b. II only
      c. III only
      d. II and IV only
      e. II, III, and IV only

5. When the systemic blood pressure increases, the aortic and carotid sinus baroreceptors initiate reflexes that cause a/an:
   I. increased heart rate
   II. decreased ventilatory rate
   III. increased ventilatory rate

IV. decreased heart rate
   a. I only
   b. II only
   c. III only
   d. II and IV only
   e. I and III only

6. The peripheral chemoreceptors are significantly activated when the P_{O_2} decreases to about
   a. 80 mm Hg
   b. 75 mm Hg
   c. 70 mm Hg
   d. 65 mm Hg
   e. 60 mm Hg

7. Stimulation of the peripheral chemoreceptors can cause which of the following?
   I. Tachycardia
   II. Decreased left ventricular performance
   III. Increased pulmonary vascular resistance
   IV. Systemic arterial hypertension
      a. I only
      b. II only
      c. IV only
      d. I, III, and IV only
      e. I, II, III, and IV

8. Suppression of the peripheral chemoreceptors begins when the P_{O_2} falls below
   a. 50 mm Hg
   b. 40 mm Hg
   c. 30 mm Hg
   d. 20 mm Hg
   e. 10 mm Hg

9. In addition to a low P_{O_2}, the peripheral chemoreceptors are also sensitive to a/an:
   I. decreased H^+
   II. increased P_{CO_2}
   III. decreased pH
   IV. increased temperature
      a. I only
      b. II only
      c. III only
      d. I, II, and III only
      e. II, III, and IV only

10. Which of the following protects the lungs from excessive inflation?
   a. Juxtapulmonary-capillary receptors
   b. Hering-Breuer inflation reflex
   c. Deflation reflex
   d. Irritant reflex
   e. Reflexes from the aortic and carotid sinus baroreceptors

11

CARDIOPULMONARY PHYSIOLOGY OF THE FETUS AND THE NEWBORN

OBJECTIVES

By the end of this chapter, the student should be able to:

1. Describe the developmental events that occur during the following periods of fetal life:
   —Embryonic period
   —Pseudoglandular period
   —Canalicular period
   —Terminal sac period
2. Describe how the following components relate to the placenta:
   —Umbilical arteries
   —Cotyledons
   —Fetal vessels
   —Chorionic villi
   —Intervillous space
   —Spiral arterioles
   —Umbilical vein
3. List the three major reasons why oxygen transfers from maternal to fetal blood.
4. List the factors believed to cause the wide variance between the maternal and fetal P_{O_2} and P_{CO_2}.
5. Describe how the following structures relate to the fetal circulation:
   —Umbilical vein
   —Liver
   —Ductus venosus
   —Inferior vena cava
   —Right atrium
   —Superior vena cava
   —Foramen ovale
   —Pulmonary veins
   —Left ventricle
   —Right ventricle
   —Ductus arteriosus
   —Common iliac arteries
   —External and internal iliacs
6. Describe what happens to the following special structures of fetal circulation after birth:
   —Placenta
   —Umbilical arteries
   —Umbilical vein
   —Ductus venosus
   —Foramen ovale
   —Ductus arteriosus
7. Describe how the fetal lung fluid is removed from the lungs at birth.
8. List the number of alveoli at birth and at 12 years of age.

(continues)

9. Describe the pressure-volume changes of the lungs of the newborn during the first two weeks of life.
10. Identify the average newborn values for the following:
    —Compliance
    —Airway resistance
11. Describe how the following circulatory changes develop at birth:
    —Decrease in pulmonary vascular resistance
    —Closure of the foramen ovale
    —Constriction of the ductus arteriosus
12. Describe the role of the following in the control of ventilation of the newborn:
    —Peripheral chemoreceptors
    —Central chemoreceptors
    —Infant reflexes
      • Trigeminal reflex
      • Irritant reflex
      • Head paradoxical reflex
13. List the following normal clinical parameters of the newborn:
    —Lung volumes and capacities
    —Respiratory rate
    —Heart rate
    —Blood pressure
14. Complete the review questions at the end of this chapter.

FETAL LUNG DEVELOPMENT

During fetal life, the development of the lungs is arbitrarily divided into four periods: **embryonic, pseudoglandular, canalicular,** and **terminal sac.**

EMBRYONIC PERIOD

This period encompasses the developmental events that occur during the first 5 weeks after fertilization. The lungs first appear as a small bud arising from the esophagus on the 24th day of embryonic life (Figure 11–1). On about the 28th day of gestation, it branches into the right and left lung buds. Between the 30th and 32nd day, primitive lobar bronchi begin to appear—two on the left lung bud and three on the right lung bud. By the end of the 5th week, cartilage can be seen in the trachea, and the main stem bronchi are surrounded by primitive cellular mesoderm, which gradually differentiates into bronchial smooth muscle, connective tissue, and cartilaginous plates, as the lungs develop.

PSEUDOGLANDULAR PERIOD

This period includes the developmental processes that occur between the 5th and the 16th week of gestation. By the 6th week, all the segments are present and the subsegmental bronchi are also well represented. The subsegmental bronchi con-

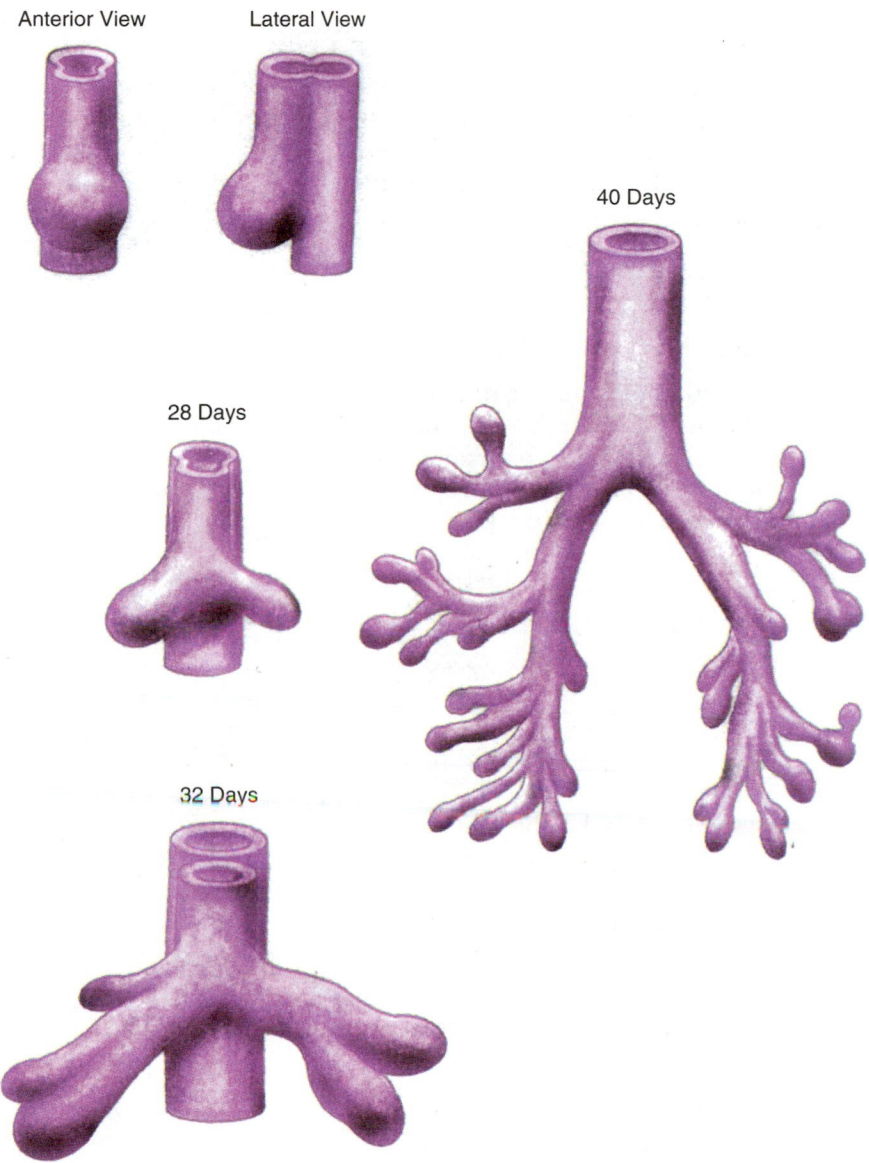

Figure 11–1. *Schematic representation of the developmental events that occur in the human lung during the embryonic and pseudoglandular periods (see text for explanation).*

tinue to undergo further branching throughout this developmental stage, and by the 16th week all the subsegmental bronchi are present.

By the 10th week, ciliated columnar epithelial cells, a deeper basal layer of irregular cells, and a primitive basement membrane appear in the conducting airways. Goblet cells also begin to appear at this time in the trachea and large bronchi. Between the 10th and 14th weeks, there is a sudden burst of bronchial branching. It is estimated that as many as 75 percent of the conducting airways develop at this time.

At 11 weeks of gestation, cartilage begins to appear in the lobar bronchi. Cartilaginous airways continue to form until about 24 weeks gestation. By the 12th week, the bronchial mucous glands start to appear. Immature smooth muscle cells are also noted at this time in the pulmonary arteries. As the tracheobronchial tree develops, new bronchial glands form until 25 to 26 weeks gestation. At birth, the concentration of bronchial glands is about 17 glands per square millimeter (mm^2). In the adult, the concentration drops to about 1 gland/mm^2, as a result of bronchial elongation and widening. By the 16th week, there are about 20 generations of bronchial airways.

CANALICULAR PERIOD

This period includes the developmental events between the 17th and 24th week of gestation. During this time, the terminal bronchioles continue to proliferate and primitive respiratory bronchioles begin to appear. The lung mass becomes highly vascularized and the lung lobes are clearly recognizable. At about the 20th week of gestation, the lymphatic vessels begin to appear.

TERMINAL SAC PERIOD

This period begins at the 24th week of gestation and continues until term (between the 38th and 41st week of gestation). The structures that appeared in the canalicular period continue to proliferate and the entire acinus (respiratory bronchioles, alveolar ducts, alveolar sacs, and alveoli) develops. The type I and type II alveolar cells can be identified at this time, and pulmonary surfactant begins to appear. Although pulmonary capillaries begin to appear at the 24th week, the air–blood interface between the alveoli and the pulmonary capillaries is poorly defined. By the 28th week, the air–blood interface and the quantity of pulmonary surfactant are usually sufficient to support life. By the 34th week, the respiratory acini are well developed. The smooth muscle fibers in the conducting airways begin to appear during the last few weeks of gestation. These muscles continue to mature after birth.

PLACENTA

Following conception, the fertilized egg moves down the **uterine tube** (Fallopian tube) and implants into the wall of the uterus. The placenta develops at the point of implantation. Throughout fetal life, the placenta transfers maternal oxygen and nutrients to the fetus and transfers waste products out of the fetal circulation. When fully developed, the placenta appears as a reddish brown disk about 20 cm long and 2.5 cm thick. Anatomically, the placenta consists of about 15 to 20 segments called **cotyledons** (Figure 11–2). Each cotyledon is composed of **fetal vessels, chorionic villi,** and **intervillous spaces** (Figure 11–3, page 300). Functionally, the cotyledons provide an interface between the maternal and fetal circulation.

Deoxygenated blood is carried from the fetus to the placenta by way of two **umbilical arteries**, which are wrapped around the **umbilical vein** (see Figure

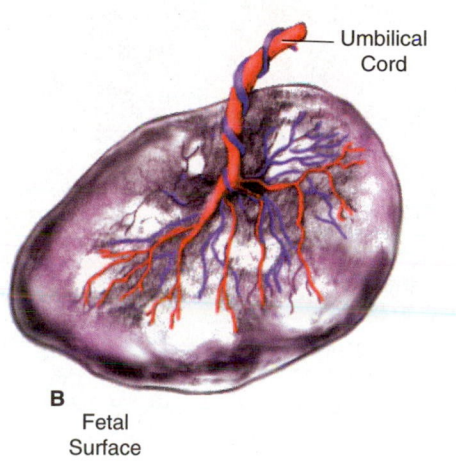

Figure 11–2. *The placenta. A) maternal surface; B) fetal surface.*

11–3). Normally, the P_{O_2} in the umbilical arteries is about 20 mm Hg and the P_{CO_2} is about 55 mm Hg. Once in the placenta, the umbilical arteries branch and supply each cotyledon. As the umbilical arteries enter the cotyledon, they again branch into the fetal vessels, which then loop around the internal portion of the fingerlike projections of the chorionic villi. Externally, the chorionic villi are surrounded by the intervillous space (see Figure 11–3).

Maternal blood from the uterine arteries enters the intervillous space through the **spiral arterioles**. The spiral arterioles continuously spurt jets of oxygenated blood and nutrients around the chorionic villi. Although the maternal blood P_{O_2} is usually normal during the last trimester of pregnancy (80 to 100 mm Hg), the P_{CO_2} is frequently lower than expected (about 33 mm Hg). This decreased maternal P_{CO_2} is caused by the alveolar hyperventilation that develops as the growing infant restricts the mother's diaphragmatic excursion.

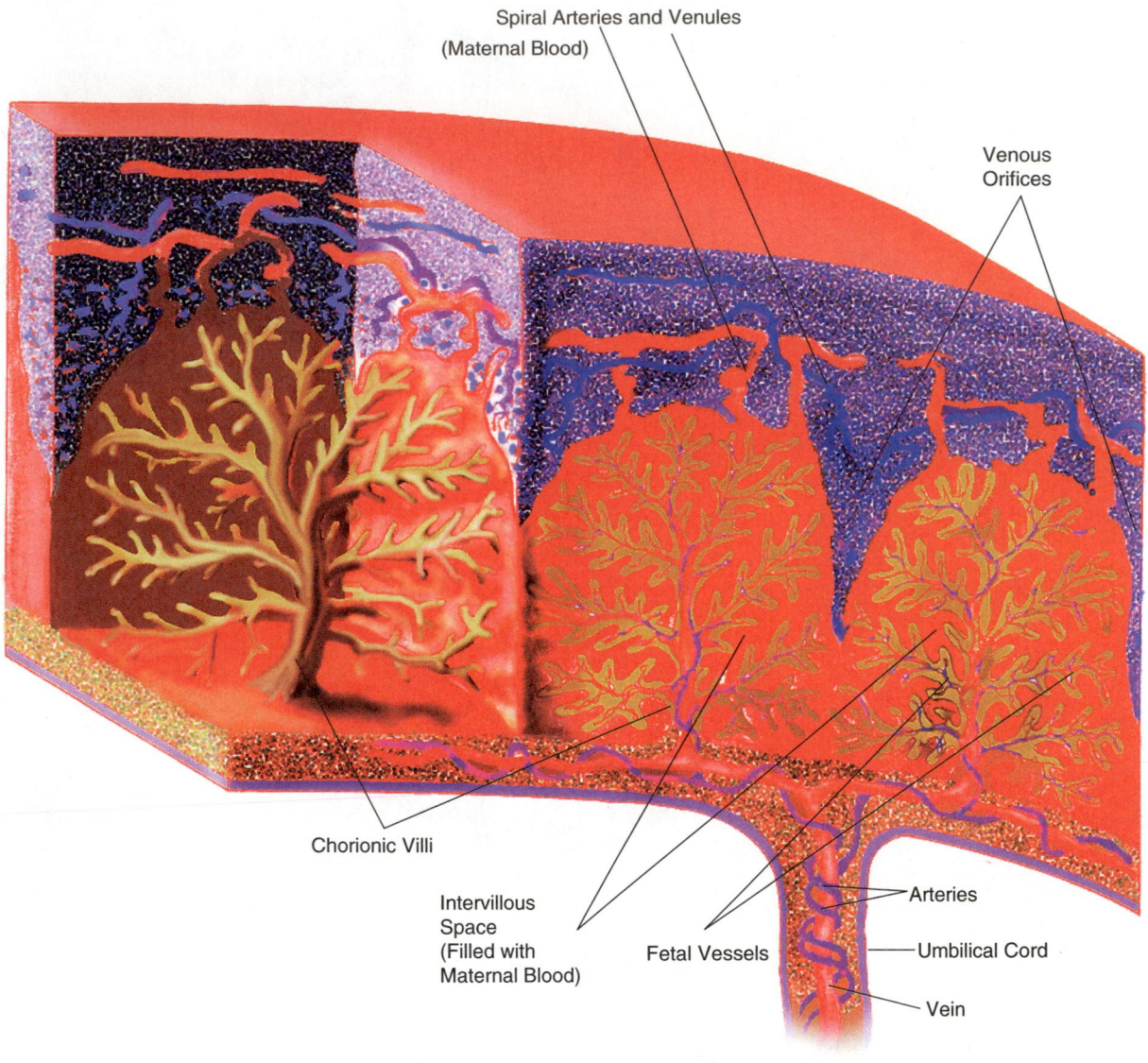

Figure 11–3. *Anatomic structure of the cotyledon of the placenta.*

Once in the intervillous space, oxygen and nutrients in the maternal blood move through the tissues of the chorionic villi and enter the fetal blood. Oxygen transfers from the maternal to fetal blood because of the (1) maternal–fetal P_{O_2} gradient, (2) higher hemoglobin concentration in the fetal blood as compared to maternal blood, and (3) greater affinity of fetal hemoglobin (Hb F) for oxygen as compared to adult hemoglobin (Hb A). While the maternal oxygen and nutrients are moving into the fetal blood, carbon dioxide (P_{CO_2} of about 55 mm Hg) and other waste products are moving out of the fetal blood and enter the maternal blood. The blood-to-blood barrier (chorionic villi) is about 3.5 microns (μ) thick.

Oxygenated fetal blood (actually a P_{O_2} of about 30 mm Hg and a P_{CO_2} of about 40 mm Hg) flows out of the chorionic villi via the fetal vessels and returns to the fetus by way of the umbilical vein (see Figure 11–3). The wide variance between the maternal and fetal P_{O_2} and P_{CO_2} is thought to be due to the following factors:

- The placenta itself is an actively metabolizing organ
- The permeability of the placenta varies from region to region with respect to respiratory gases
- There are fetal and maternal vascular shunts

The fetal waste products in the maternal blood move out of the intervillous space by virtue of the arteriovenous pressure gradient. The pressure in the spiral arteries is about 75 mm Hg and the pressure of the **venous orifices**, which are found adjacent to the spiral arteries, is about 8 mm Hg.

FETAL CIRCULATION

The **umbilical vein** carries oxygenated blood and nutrients from the placenta to the fetus (Figure 11–4, page 302). The umbilical vein enters the navel of the fetus and ascends anteriorly to the liver. About one-half of the blood enters the liver, and the rest flows through the **ductus venosus** and enters the **inferior vena cava**. This results in oxygenated fetal blood mixing with deoxygenated blood from the lower parts of the fetal body. The newly mixed fetal blood then travels up the inferior vena cava and enters the **right atrium**, where it again mingles with deoxygenated blood from the **superior vena cava**.

Once in the right atrium, most of the blood flows directly into the left atrium through the **foramen ovale**. While in the left atrium, the fetal blood again mingles with a small amount of deoxygenated blood from the pulmonary veins. The blood then enters the left ventricle and is pumped primarily to the heart and brain.

The rest of the blood in the right atrium moves into the right ventricle and is pumped into the pulmonary artery. Once in the pulmonary artery, most of the blood bypasses the lungs and flows directly into the aorta through the **ductus arteriosus**. A small amount of blood (about 15 percent) flows through the lungs and returns to the left atrium via the pulmonary veins. The Pa_{O_2} in the descending aorta is about 20 mm Hg. Downstream, the **common iliac arteries** branch into the **external** and **internal iliacs**. The blood in the internal iliac branch passes into the umbilical arteries and again flows back to the placenta to pick up oxygen and to drop off waste products.

After birth—and once the lungs and the renal, digestive, and liver functions are established—the special structures of the fetal circulation are no longer required. These special structures go through the following changes:

- The placenta is passed by the mother
- The umbilical arteries atrophy and become the lateral umbilical ligaments

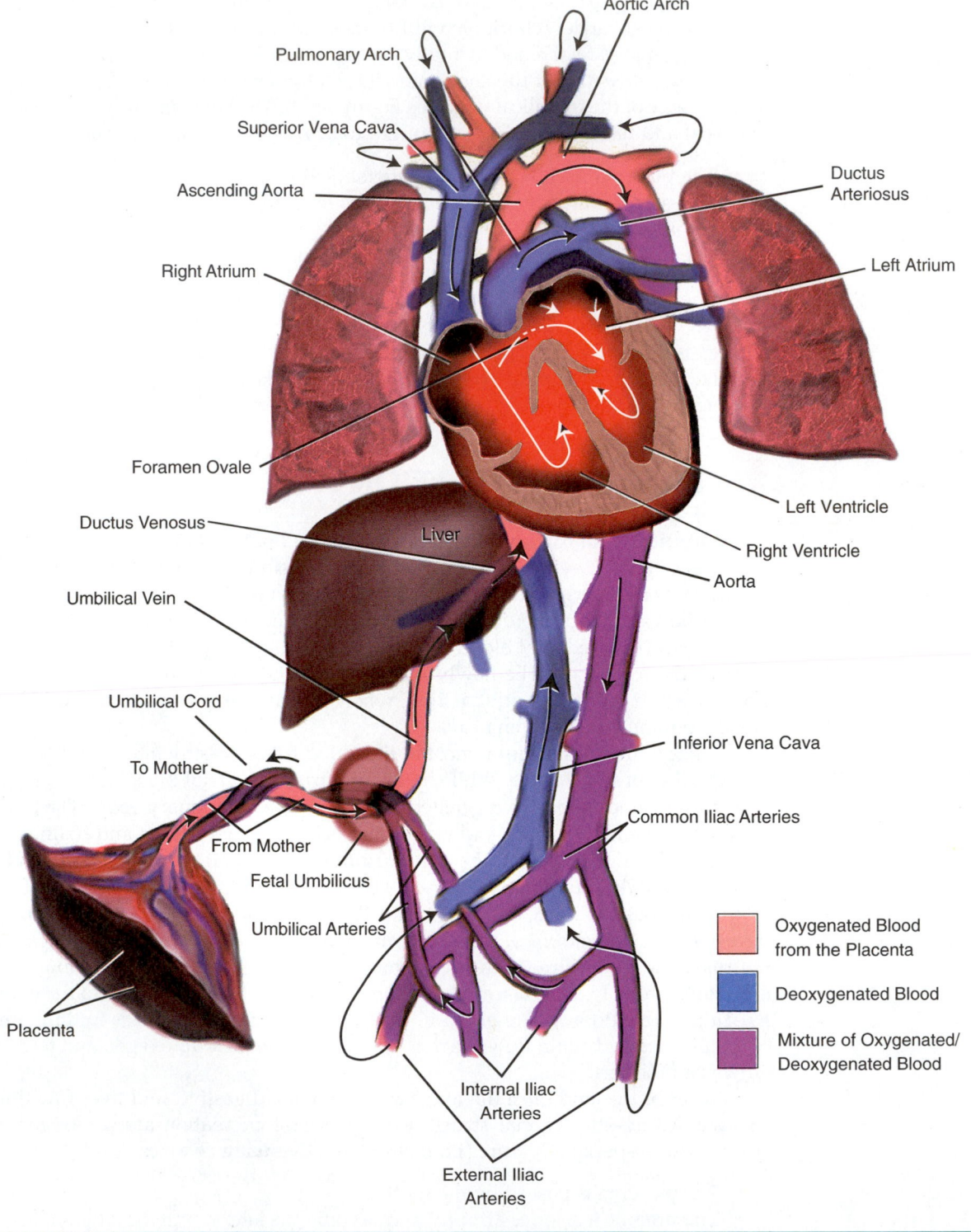

Figure 11–4. *Fetal circulation.*

- The umbilical vein becomes the round ligament (*ligamentum teres*) of the liver
- The ductus venosus becomes the *ligamentum venosum*, which is a fibrous cord in the liver
- The flap on the foramen ovale usually closes and becomes a depression in the interatrial septum called the *fossa ovalis*
- The ductus arteriosus atrophies and becomes the *ligamentum arteriosum*

FETAL LUNG FLUIDS

It is estimated that, at birth, the lungs are partially inflated with liquid approximately equal to the newborn's functional residual capacity. It was once thought that this liquid originated from the aspiration of amniotic fluid, since the fetus normally demonstrates periods of rapid and irregular breathing during the last trimester of gestation. It is now known, however, that this is not the case. The fluid apparently originates from the alveolar cells during fetal development. At birth the fluid is removed from the lungs during the first 24 hours of life primarily by the following mechanisms:

- About one-third of the fluid is squeezed out of the lungs as the infant passes through the birth canal
- About one-third of the fluid is absorbed by the pulmonary capillaries
- About one-third of the fluid is removed by the lymphatic system

NUMBER OF ALVEOLI AT BIRTH

About 24 million primitive alveoli are present at birth. This number, however, represents only about 10 percent of the adult gas exchange units. The number of alveoli continue to increase until about 12 years of age. Thus, it is important to note that respiratory problems during childhood can have a dramatic effect on the anatomy and physiology of the mature pulmonary system.

BIRTH

Moments after birth, an intriguing and dramatic sequence of anatomic and physiologic events occurs. The function of the placenta is suddenly terminated, the lungs rapidly establish themselves as the organ of gas exchange, and all the features of adult circulation are set in place.

FIRST BREATH

At birth, the infant is bombarded by a variety of external sensory stimuli (e.g., thermal, tactile, and visual). At the same time, the placenta ceases to function, causing the fetal blood P_{O_2} to decrease, the P_{CO_2} to increase, and the pH to decrease. Although the exact mechanism is unknown, the sensitivity of both the central and the peripheral chemoreceptors of the newborn increases dramatically at birth. In response to all these stimuli, the infant *inhales*.

To initiate the first breath, however, the infant must generate a remarkable negative intrapleural pressure to overcome the viscous fluid in the lungs. It is estimated that the intrapleural pressure has to decrease to about -40 cm H_2O before any air enters the lungs. Intrapleural pressures as low as -100 cm H_2O have been reported. About 40 ml of air enter the lungs during the first breath. On exhalation, the infant expels about one-half of the volume obtained on the first breath, thus establishing the first portion of the residual volume. Figure 11–5 illustrates the typical pressure-volume changes of the lungs that occur in the newborn during the first 2 weeks of life. The average *lung compliance* of the newborn is about .005 L/cm H_2O (5 ml/cm H_2O); the *airway resistance* is about 30 cm H_2O/L/sec.

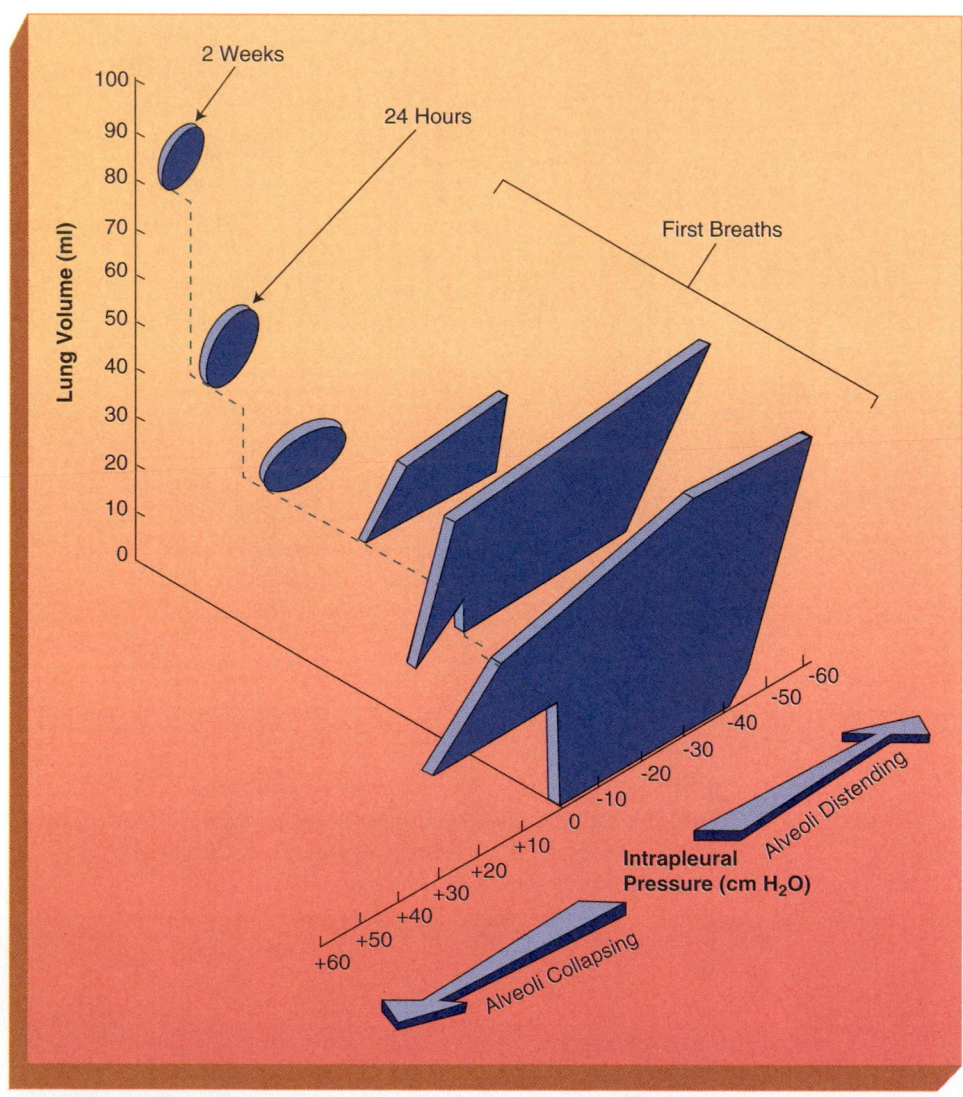

Figure 11–5. *The pressure-volume changes of the newborn lungs during the first two weeks of life.*

CIRCULATORY CHANGES AT BIRTH

As the infant inhales for the first time, the pulmonary vascular resistance falls dramatically. Two major mechanisms account for the decreased pulmonary vascular resistance: (1) the sudden increase in the alveolar P_{O_2}, which offsets the hypoxic vasoconstriction, and (2) the mechanical increase in lung volume, which widens the caliber of the extra-alveolar vessels.

As the pulmonary vascular resistance decreases, a greater amount of blood flows through the lungs, and therefore more blood returns to the left atrium. This causes the pressure in the left atrium to increase and the flap of the foramen ovale to close functionally. The closure of the foramen ovale is further aided by the fall in pressure that occurs in the right atrium as the umbilical flow ceases. A few minutes later, the smooth muscles of the ductus arteriosus constrict in response to the increased P_{O_2}.

Clinically, however, the newborn's P_{O_2} must increase to more than 45 to 50 mm Hg in order for the ductus arteriosus to close. If this P_{O_2} level is not reached, the ductus arteriosus will remain open, and the pulmonary vascular resistance will remain elevated, producing the syndrome known as **persistent pulmonary hypertension of the neonate (PPHN)** (previously known as persistent fetal circulation). Furthermore, should the fetal P_{O_2} increase sufficiently to close the ductus arteriosus but then fall within the first 24 to 48 hours after birth, the ductus arteriosus will reopen.

It is believed that other substances released at birth (such as bradykinin, serotonin, and prostaglandin inhibitors) contribute to the constriction of the ductus arteriosus.

CONTROL OF VENTILATION IN THE NEWBORN

Within moments after birth, the newborn infant initiates the first breath. Although they are inhibited during fetal life, the peripheral and central chemoreceptors play a major role in activating the first breath. It is not precisely understood why these chemoreceptors are dormant during fetal life but are suddenly activated at birth.

PERIPHERAL CHEMORECEPTORS

The exact role of the peripheral chemoreceptors in the newborn is not clearly defined. It is known, however, that in both the preterm and term infant, hypoxia elicits a transient rise in ventilation, followed by a marked fall. The magnitude of the increase is similar whether the infant is in the rapid eye-movement (REM) state, quiet sleep state, or awake state. However, the late fall is less marked or is absent when the infant is in the quiet sleep state. One to two weeks after birth, the infant demonstrates the adult response of sustained hyperventilation. The response to hypoxia is greater and more sustained in the term infant that in the preterm infant. While it is known that the peripheral chemoreceptors of the adult are responsive to CO_2, little information is available about the peripheral chemoreceptors' sensitivity to changes in CO_2 and pH during the newborn period.

CENTRAL CHEMORECEPTORS

The central chemoreceptors of the newborn respond to the elevated CO_2 levels in a manner similar to that of the adult. The response to an increased CO_2 level is primarily an increased tidal volume, with little change in inspiratory time or ventilatory rate. The response of the central chemoreceptors may be more marked with increasing gestational age, although not all researchers agree.

INFANT REFLEXES

Trigeminal Reflex

Stimulation of the newborn's trigeminal nerve (i.e., the face and nasal and nasopharyngeal mucosa) causes a decrease in the infant's respiration and heart rate. In fact, it has been reported that even gentle stimulation of the malar region in both the preterm and term infant may cause significant respiratory slowing. Thus, the various procedures (such as nasopharyngeal suctioning) may be hazardous to the newborn. Clinically, facial cooling has been used as a means of terminating paroxysms of supraventricular tachycardia in the newborn.

Irritant Reflex

Epithelial irritant receptors, located throughout the airways, respond to direct tactile stimulation, lung deflation, and irritant gases. This response is mediated by myelinated vagal fibers. Based upon gestational age, these receptors elicit different responses. In preterm infants of less than 35 weeks gestation, tracheal stimulation (e.g., endotracheal suctioning or intubation) is commonly followed by respiratory slowing or apnea. In the term infant, however, stimulation causes marked hyperventilation. The inhibitory response seen in the preterm infant may be due to vagal nerve immaturity (i.e., the vagal nerves are not adequately myelinated). Unmyelinated neurons are unable to transmit high-frequency discharges.

Head Paradoxical Reflex

The head paradoxical reflex is a deep inspiration that is elicited by lung inflation. In other words, the infant inhales and then tops the inspiration with a deep breath before exhalation occurs. This reflex is seen in the term infant and is thought to be mediated by the irritant receptors. The head parodoxical reflex may play a role in sighing, which is frequently seen in the newborn. This reflex is thought to be valuable in maintaining lung compliance by offsetting alveolar collapse.

NORMAL CLINICAL PARAMETERS IN THE NEWBORN

Table 11–1 lists the average pulmonary function findings of the newborn. The normal vital signs of the newborn are listed in Table 11–2. Figure 11–6 illustrates graphically the average pH, Pa_{CO_2}, HCO_3^-, and Pa_{O_2} values of the normal infant over a period of 72 hours after birth.

TABLE 11–1. **Approximate Lung Volumes and Capacities of the Newborn**

Tidal volume (V$_T$)	15 ml	Vital capacity (VC)	115 ml
Residual volume (RV)	40 ml	Functional residual capacity (FRC)	80 ml
Expiratory reserve volume (ERV)	40 ml	Inspiratory capacity (IC)	75 ml
Inspiratory reserve volume (IRV)	60 ml	Total lung capacity (TLC)	155 ml

TABLE 11–2. **Normal Vital Sign Ranges of the Newborn**

Respiratory rate (RR)	35–50/min
Heart rate (HR)	130–150/min
Blood pressure (BP)	60/40–70/45

Figure 11–6. *The average pH, Pa$_{CO_2}$, HCO$_3^-$, and Pa$_{O_2}$ values of the normal infant during the first 72 hours of life.*

CLINICAL APPLICATION

This patient was a 1620 g (3 lb, 9 oz) boy born 12 weeks early (at 28 weeks gestation). His Apgar scores at delivery were 4 and 5.* On observation the baby's skin was cyanotic and he was in obvious respiratory distress. He demonstrated nasal flaring and intercostal retractions. A grunt-like sound could be heard without the aid of a stethoscope during each exhalation. The baby was transferred to the neonatal intensive care unit (ICU) and placed on continuous positive airway pressure (CPAP) via nasal prongs at a pressure setting of 3 cm H_2O and an inspired oxygen concentration ($F_{I_{O_2}}$) of 0.4.

The baby's vital signs were: respiratory rate—64 breaths/min, blood pressure—48/22, and apical heart rate—175 beats/min. On auscultation bilateral crackles could be heard. A portable chest x-ray showed a "ground-glass" appearance and air bronchogram throughout both lung fields, consistent with Idiopathic (infant) Respiratory Distress Syndrome (IRDS). Umbilical arterial blood gas values were: pH 7.53, Pa_{CO_2} 28 mm Hg, HCO_3^- 21 mmol/L, and Pa_{O_2} 41 mm Hg. The neonatologist entered the following diagnosis in the infant's progress notes: "IRDS and PPHN" (persistent pulmonary hypertension of the neonate).

Over the next 72 hours the infant's clinical progress was stormy. Three hours after the baby was born, he was intubated and placed on a time-cycled, pressure-limited synchronized intermittent mandatory ventilation (SIMV) rate of 35 breaths per minute, inspiratory time 0.5 seconds, peak inspiratory pressure (PIP) of 22 cm H_2O, an $F_{I_{O_2}}$ of 0.8, and positive end-expiratory pressure (PEEP) of 7 cm H_2O. The baby received Exosurf® treatments (a synthetic pulmonary surfactant) through his endotracheal tube on day two. On day four, his clinical condition stabilized.

Although the baby was still intubated on day five, he no longer required SIMV. The ventilator was set on the CPAP mode at a pressure setting of 3 cm H_2O with an $F_{I_{O_2}}$ of 0.4. The baby's vital signs were: blood pressure—73/48, heart rate (apical) 122 beats/min, and respiratory rate—40 breaths/min. Normal vesicular breath sounds were heard over both lung fields. A chest x-ray showed substantial improvement throughout both lungs. The baby's umbilical arterial blood gas values were: pH 7.41, Pa_{CO_2} 38 mm Hg, HCO_3^- 24 mmol/L, and Pa_{O_2} 158 mm Hg. The $F_{I_{O_2}}$ was decreased to 0.3. The neonatologist wrote the following assessment in the patient's chart: "IRDS has significantly improved and PPHN no longer appears to be present." The baby progressively improved and was discharged three days later.

DISCUSSION

This case illustrates the possible adverse effects of a premature birth on the infant's (1) alveolar-capillary gas exchange units, and (2) pulmonary circulation. During fetal development, the alveolar-capillary system and the quantity of pulmonary surfactant are usually not sufficient to support life until the 28th week of gestation or beyond. In this case, the baby was born at the very beginning of this time period. Thus, because of the immaturity of the baby's alveolar-capillary system, the ability of the type II cells to produce pulmonary surfactant was inadequate (see Figure 1–21, page 29, and Figure 2–16, page 74).

As a result of the insufficient amount of pulmonary surfactant, the pathologic processes of a common newborn respiratory disease called Idiopathic Respiratory Distress Syndrome (IRDS) developed. The anatomic alterations of the lungs

---

*The Apgar score evaluates five factors: heart rate, respiratory effort, muscle tone, reflex irritability, and color. Each factor is rated either 0, 1, or 2. The scoring system provides a clinical picture of the infant's condition following delivery. An Apgar score is taken at 1 minute after delivery. A second Apgar score is taken at 5 minutes after delivery to assess the infant's ability to recover from the stress of birth and adapt to extrauterine life. The baby is usually considered to be out of danger when the score is greater than 7.

associated with IRDS include interstitial and intra-alveolar edema and hemorrhage, alveolar consolidation, intra-alveolar hyaline membrane formation, and atelectasis. All of these pathologic processes cause the alveolar-capillary membrane's thickness to increase. As this condition progressively worsened in this case, the diffusion of oxygen between the alveoli and pulmonary capillary blood decreased (see Figure 3–6, page 117), and the infant's lung compliance decreased (see Figure 2–6, page 64). Clinically, the decreased diffusion of oxygen was manifested by cyanosis, increased respiratory rate and heart rate, and decreased Pa_{O_2}. The decreased lung compliance was manifested

by nasal flaring, intercostal retractions, exhalation grunting, bilateral crackles, and a ground-glass appearance and air bronchogram on the chest x-ray.

Finally, because the baby's Pa_{O_2} was less than 45 mm Hg shortly after he was born, the ductus arteriosus remained open, or patent, producing the syndrome known as *persistent pulmonary hypertension of the neonate* (PPHN). As the infant's condition improved and his Pa_{O_2} increased, the ductus arteriosis closed and the signs and symptoms associated with PPHN disappeared. At the time of this writing, the baby was a perfectly normal 3-year-old boy who was attending half-day preschool sessions five days a week.

CLINICAL APPLICATION 2

While in her third trimester of pregnancy, this 28-year-old female experienced vaginal bleeding, abdominal pain, uterine tenderness, and uterine contractions. Concerned, she alerted her husband, who immediately drove her to the hospital. In the emergency room, the patient was provisionally diagnosed as having an *abruptio placentae* (premature partial or total separation of the placenta from the uterus). Because of the excessive hemorrhage, the medical staff felt that abruptio placentae was extensive and that both the mother and the fetus were in a life-threatening situation. The patient received medication—STAT—for shock treatment and blood replacement. She was then transferred to surgery and prepped for a cesarean section. Shortly after the delivery of the baby (and placenta), the bleeding stopped. The presence of a near-total abruptio placentae was confirmed during the surgery.

The initial assessment of the baby showed a premature female infant born 6 weeks early (at

34 weeks gestation). She weighed only 1610 g (3 lb, 7 oz). Her first Apgar score at delivery was 4. Her heart rate was less than 100 beats per minute, her respiratory rate was weak and irregular, her skin color was blue, she demonstrated no grimace reflex when suctioned, and her muscle tone showed only moderate flexion. The baby was manually ventilated aggressively with an inspired oxygen concentration (FI_{O_2}) of 1.0 and responded favorably within a few minutes. Her second Apgar score was 8. Her heart rate was greater than 100 beats per minute, she had a strong cry, her skin was pink, she demonstrated a grimace reflex when suctioned, and her muscle tone was improving.

The baby was transferred to the neonatal intensive care unit (ICU) for close observation. Two hours later the baby's vital signs were: respiratory rate—44 breaths/min, blood pressure—66/42, and apical heart rate—135 beats/min. On auscultation, normal vesicular breath sounds were heard bilaterally. A portable chest x-ray was normal. The

(continues)

baby's umbilical arterial blood gas values were: pH 7.33, Pa_{CO_2} 44 mm Hg, HCO_3^- 23 mmol/L, and Pa_{O_2} 52 mm Hg. Four days later, both the mother and the baby were discharged in good health.

DISCUSSION

This case illustrates the important function of the placenta as a lifeline between the mother and the baby during fetal life. In this case, because the placenta separated from the wall of the uterus, the maternal-placenta–fetal interface was seriously compromised. In short, the ability of the fetus to absorb oxygen, nutrients, and other substances and excrete carbon dioxide and other wastes was interrupted. Complete separation brings about immediate death of the fetus. Bleeding from the site of separation may cause abdominal pain, uterine tenderness, and uterine contraction. Bleeding may be concealed within the uterus or may be evident externally, sometimes as sudden massive hemorrhage (as was the occurrence in this case). In severe cases, shock and death can occur in minutes. Cesarean section must be performed immediately and rapidly. Fortunately, in this case the mother and the baby were treated in a timely manner.

REVIEW QUESTIONS

1. During the embryonic period, the lungs first appear at about the
   a. 10th day after fertilization
   b. 24th day after fertilization
   c. 6th week after fertilization
   d. 12th week after fertilization
   e. 16th week after fertilization
2. The lungs are usually sufficiently mature to support life by the
   a. 24th week of gestation
   b. 28th week of gestation
   c. 32nd week of gestation
   d. 36th week of gestation
   e. 40th week of gestation
3. At birth, the number of alveoli represent about how much of the total adult gas exchange units?
   a. 10%
   b. 20%
   c. 30%
   d. 40%
   e. 50%
4. The number of alveoli continues to increase until about
   a. 6 years of age
   b. 8 years of age
   c. 10 years of age
   d. 12 years of age
   e. 16 years of age

5. The average P_{O_2} in the umbilical arteries during fetal life is about
   a. 20 mm Hg
   b. 40 mm Hg
   c. 60 mm Hg
   d. 80 mm Hg
   e. 100 mm Hg

6. The average P_{O_2} in the umbilical vein during fetal life is about
   a. 10 mm Hg
   b. 20 mm Hg
   c. 30 mm Hg
   d. 40 mm Hg
   e. 50 mm Hg

7. The average P_{CO_2} in the umbilical arteries during fetal life is about
   a. 25 mm Hg
   b. 35 mm Hg
   c. 45 mm Hg
   d. 55 mm Hg
   e. 65 mm Hg

8. In the placenta, maternal blood is continuously pumped through the
   a. umbilical arteries
   b. chorionic villi
   c. fetal vessels
   d. umbilical vein
   e. intervillous space

9. In the fetal circulation, once blood enters the right atrium, most of the blood enters the left atrium by passing through the
   a. ductus arteriosus
   b. pulmonary veins
   c. ductus venosus
   d. pulmonary arteries
   e. foramen ovale

10. Shortly after birth the ductus arteriosus constricts in response to
    I. increased P_{O_2}
    II. decreased P_{CO_2}
    III. increased pH
    IV. prostaglandins
       a. I only
       b. II only
       c. III and IV only
       d. I and IV only
       e. II and IV only

CHAPTER TWELVE

RENAL FAILURE AND ITS EFFECTS ON THE CARDIOPULMONARY SYSTEM

O B J E C T I V E S

By the end of this chapter, the student should be able to:

1. Describe how the following relate to the kidneys:
   —Hilum
   —Ureters
   —Cortex
   —Medulla
   —Renal pelvis
   —Major calyces
   —Minor calyces
   —Renal papillae
   —Renal pyramid
   —Nephron

2. Describe how the following relate to the nephron:
   —Glomerulus
   —Bowman's capsule
   —Renal corpuscle
   —Proximal convoluted tubule
   —Descending limb of the loop of Henle
   —Ascending limb of the loop of Henle
   —Distal convoluted tubule
   —Collecting duct

3. Describe how the following blood vessels relate to the nephron:
   —Renal arteries
   —Interlobar arteries
   —Arcuate arteries
   —Interlobular arteries
   —Afferent arterioles
   —Efferent arterioles
   —Peritubular capillaries
   —Interlobular veins
   —Arcuate vein
   —Interlobar vein
   —Renal vein

4. Describe the role of the following in the formation of urine:
   —Glomerular filtration
   —Tubular reabsorption
   —Tubular secretion

5. Describe the role of the following in the control of urine concentration and volume:
   —Countercurrent mechanism
   —Selective permeability

(continues)

6. Describe the role of the kidneys in the regulation of the following:
   —Sodium
   —Potassium
   —Calcium, magnesium, and phosphate
   —Acid-base balance
7. Describe the role of the following in controlling the blood volume:
   —Capillary fluid shift system
   —The renal system
8. Identify common causes of renal disorders, including the following:
   —Congenital disorders
   —Infections
   —Obstructive disorders
   —Inflammation and immune responses
   —Neoplasms

9. Identify causes of the following types of renal disorders:
   —Prerenal conditions
   —Intrarenal conditions
   —Postrenal conditions
10. Describe how mechanical ventilation alters urinary output.
11. Describe cardiopulmonary problems that can develop with renal failure, including the following:
    —Hypertension and edema
    —Metabolic acidosis
    —Electrolyte abnormalities
      • Chloride
      • Potassium
    —Anemia
    —Bleeding
    —Cardiovascular problems
12. Complete the review questions at the end of this chapter.

The composition of blood is largely determined by what the kidneys retain and excrete. The kidneys filter dissolved particles from the blood and selectively reabsorb the substances that are needed to maintain the normal composition of body fluids. When the renal system fails, a variety of indirect cardiopulmonary problems develop, including hypertension, congestive heart failure, pulmonary edema, anemia, and changes in acid-base balance. Because of this fact, a basic understanding of the etiology, classification, and clinical manifestations associated with renal failure is essential in respiratory care.

THE KIDNEYS

The kidneys are two bean-shaped organs that are located against the posterior wall of the abdominal cavity, one on each side of the vertebral column (Figure 12–1). In the adult, each kidney is about 12 cm long, 6 cm wide, and 3 cm thick. Medially, in the central concave portion of each kidney there is a longitudinal fissure called the hilum. The renal artery, renal vein, and nerves enter and leave kidneys through the hilum. The ureters, which transport urine from the kidneys to the bladder, also exit the kidneys through the hilum.

   As shown in Figure 12–2 (page 316), the cortex, which is the outer one-third of the kidney, is a dark brownish red layer. The middle two-thirds of the kidney,

Inferior
Vena Cava

Aorta

Right
Adrenal Gland

Left
Adrenal Gland

Right
Renal Artery
and Vein

Left Renal
Artery and
Vein

Right Kidney

Left Kidney

Left Ureter

Right Ureter

Urinary
Bladder

Urethra

Figure 12–1. *The organs of the urinary system. Urine is formed by the kidneys and flows through the ureters to the bladder, where it is eliminated via the urethra.*

the medulla, can be seen as a light-colored layer. Within the kidney, the ureter expands to form a funnel-shaped structure called the renal pelvis. The renal pelvis subdivides into two or three tubes called major calyces (singular, calyx). These, in turn, divide into several smaller tubes called minor calyces. A series of small structures called renal papillae (or *papillary ducts*) extend from the calyx toward the cortex of the kidney to form a triangular-shaped structure called the renal pyramid. The peripheral portions of the papillary ducts serve as collecting ducts for the waste products selectively filtered and excreted by the nephrons.

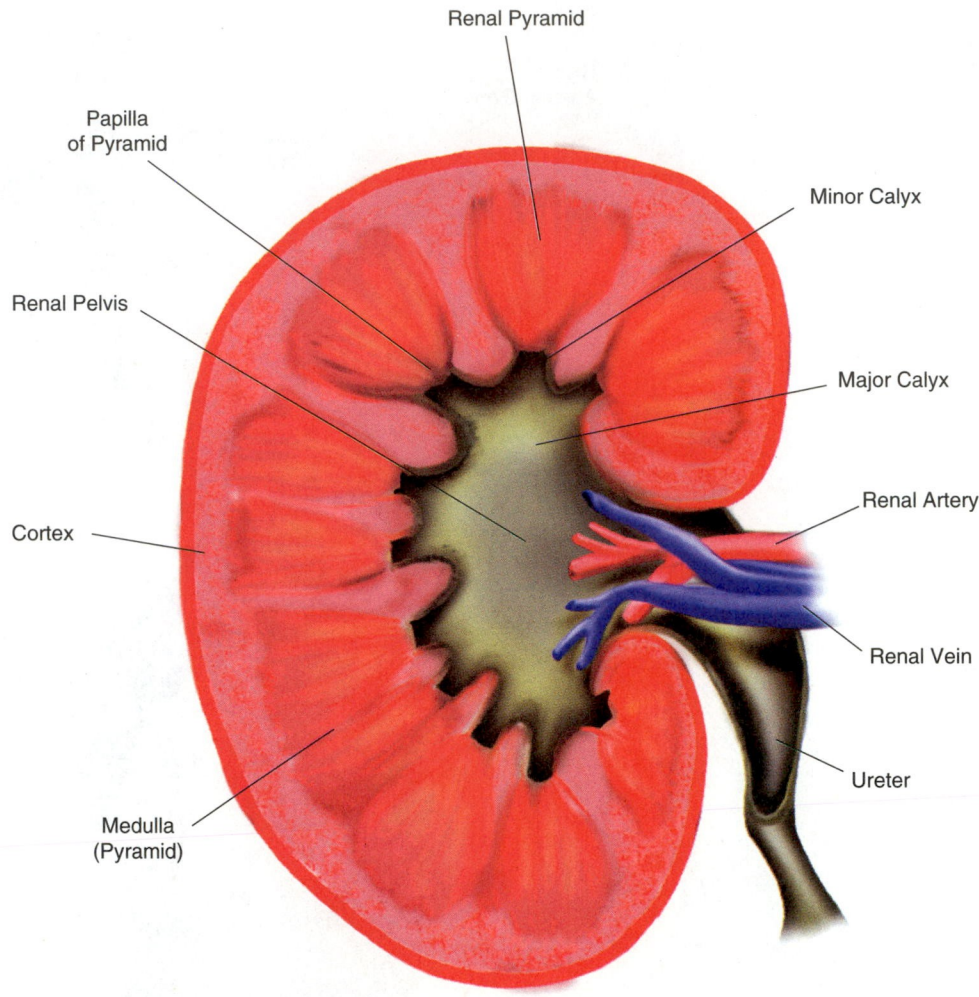

Figure 12–2. *Cross-section of the kidney.*

THE NEPHRON

The nephrons are the functional units of the kidneys (Figure 12–3). Each kidney contains about one million nephrons. Each nephron consists of a **glomerulus, proximal tubule, loop of Henle,** and **distal tubule**. The distal tubules empty into the collecting ducts. Although the collecting ducts are technically not part of the renal pyramid, they are considered a functional part of the nephron because of their role in urine concentration, ion salvaging, and acid-base balance.

The **glomerulus** consists of a network of interconnected capillaries encased in a thin-walled, saclike structure called **Bowman's capsule**. The glomerulus and Bowman's capsule constitute what is known as a **renal corpuscle**. Urine formation begins with the filtration of fluid and low-molecular-weight particles through the glomerular capillaries into Bowman's capsule. The substances that are filtered pass into the **proximal convoluted tubule**, which lies in the cortex.

Figure 12–3. *The nephron.*

The proximal tubule dips into the medulla to form the *descending* limb of the loop of Henle. The tubule then bends into a U-shaped structure to form the loop of Henle. As the tubule straightens, it ascends back toward the cortex as the *ascending* limb of the loop of Henle. The tubule again becomes convoluted as it enters the cortex. This portion of the nephron is called the **distal convoluted tubule** (see Figure 12–3). The distal convoluted tubule empties into the **collecting duct**. The collecting duct then passes through the renal pyramid to empty into the minor and major calyces, which in turn drain into the renal pelvis (see Figure 12–2). From the renal pelvis, the mixture of waste products (collectively referred to as urine) drains into the ureter, where it is carried by peristalsis to the urinary bladder. The urine is stored in the urinary bladder until it is discharged from the body through the urethra (see Figure 12–1).

BLOOD VESSELS OF THE KIDNEYS

As shown in Figure 12–4, the right and left renal arteries carry blood to the kidneys. Shortly after passing through the hilum of the kidney, the renal artery divides into several branches called the interlobar arteries. At the base of the renal pyramids, the interlobar arteries become the arcuate arteries. Divisions of the arcuate arteries form a series of interlobular arteries, which enter the cortex and branch into the afferent arterioles.

Figure 12–4. *Blood vessels of the kidney.*

The afferent arterioles deliver blood to the capillary cluster that forms the glomerulus. After passing through the glomerulus, the blood leaves by way of the efferent arterioles. The efferent arterioles then branch into a complex network of capillaries called the peritubular capillaries, which surround the various portions of the renal tubules of the nephron (see Figure 12–3).

The peritubular capillaries eventually reunite to form the interlobular veins, followed by the arcuate vein, the interlobar vein, and the renal vein. The renal vein eventually joins the inferior vena cava as it courses through the abdominal cavity.

URINE FORMATION

The formation of urine involves glomerular filtration, tubular reabsorption, and tubular secretion.

GLOMERULAR FILTRATION

Urine formation begins at the renal corpuscle. Water and dissolved substances such as electrolytes are forced out of the glomerular capillaries by means of the blood pressure (*hydrostatic pressure*). The filtration of substances through the capillary membrane of the glomerulus is similar to the filtration of other capillaries throughout the body. The permeability of the glomerular capillary, however, is much greater than that of the capillaries in other tissues. As the filtrate leaves the glomerular capillaries, it is received in Bowman's capsule.

The rate of filtration is directly proportional to the hydrostatic pressure of the blood. The hydrostatic pressure in the glomerular capillary is about 55 mm Hg. This pressure, however, is partially offset by the hydrostatic pressure in Bowman's capsule of about 15 mm Hg. The osmotic pressure of the plasma is another important factor that offsets glomerular filtration. In other words, in the capillaries the hydrostatic pressure acting to move water and dissolved particles outward is opposed by the inward osmotic pressure generated by the presence of protein in the plasma. Under normal conditions, the magnitude of the osmotic pressure is about 30 mm Hg. As shown in Table 12–1, the net filtration pressure, which is the algebraic sum of the three relevant forces, is about 10 mm Hg. The glomeruli filter

TABLE 12–1. **Forces of Glomerular Filtration**

FACTORS	FORCE
Enhances Filtration	
Glomerular capillary blood pressure	+55 mm Hg
Opposes Filtration	
Fluid pressure in Bowman's capsule	−15 mm Hg
Osmotic force (caused by the protein concentration difference)	−30 mm Hg
Net Filtration Pressure	+10 mm Hg

about 125 ml of fluid per minute (about 180 L/day). Of the 125 ml, however, only about 1 ml is excreted as urine. The average urine output is about 60 ml per hour, or 1440 ml per day.

TUBULAR REABSORPTION

As the glomerular filtrate passes through the (1) proximal convoluted tubule, (2) loop of Henle, and (3) distal convoluted tubule, water, sodium, glucose, and other substances leave the tubule and enter the blood in the peritubular capillaries. Some substances, such as glucose and amino acids, are completely reabsorbed. About 99 percent of the filtered water and sodium is reabsorbed. About 50 percent of urea is reabsorbed and the electrolyte reabsorption is generally a function of need.

Although tubular reabsorption occurs throughout the entire renal tubule system, the bulk of it occurs in the proximal convoluted portion. Certain sections of the tubule, however, reabsorb specific substances, using particular modes of transport. For example, the proximal tubule reabsorbs glucose by means of *active transport*, while water reabsorption occurs throughout the renal tubule by *osmosis*.

TUBULAR SECRETION

Tubular secretion is the mechanism by which various substances are transported from the plasma to the peritubular capillaries to the fluid of the renal tubule (the *opposite* direction of tubular reabsorption). In essence, this mechanism constitutes a second pathway through which fluid can gain entrance into the renal tubule (the first being *glomerular filtration*). The most important substances transported into the tubules by means of secretion are hydrogen (H^+) and potassium (K^+) ions. In fact, most of the hydrogen and potassium ions found in the urine enter the tubules by secretion. Thus, the mechanisms that control the rates of hydrogen and potassium tubular secretion regulate the level of these substances in the blood.

URINE CONCENTRATION AND VOLUME

The composition and volume of extracellular fluids are controlled by the kidney's ability to produce either a dilute or concentrated urine. The kidneys are able to do this by virtue of two mechanisms: the **countercurrent mechanism** and the **selective permeability of the collecting ducts**.

COUNTERCURRENT MECHANISM

The countercurrent mechanism controls water reabsorption in the distal tubules and collecting ducts. It accomplishes this function through the unique anatomic position of various nephrons. About one out of every five nephrons descends deep into the renal medulla. These nephrons are called **juxtamedullary nephrons**. The normal osmolality of the glomerular filtrate is approximately 300 mOsm/L.* The osmolality of the interstitial fluid increases from about 300 mOsm/L in the cortex

---

*Milliosmols (mOsm/L) = 1000 milliosmols equal 1 osmol, which is the unit in which osmotic pressure is expressed. We speak of osmols or milliosmols per liter.

to about 1200 mOsm/L as the juxtamedullary nephron descends into the renal medulla. This sets up a strong active transport of sodium out of the descending limb of Henle. The increased amount of sodium in the interstitial fluid, in turn, prevents water from returning to the peritubular capillaries surrounding the tubules.

SELECTIVE PERMEABILITY

As shown in Figure 12–5, the permeability of the collecting ducts is regulated by the antidiuretic hormone (ADH). ADH is produced in the hypothalamus and is

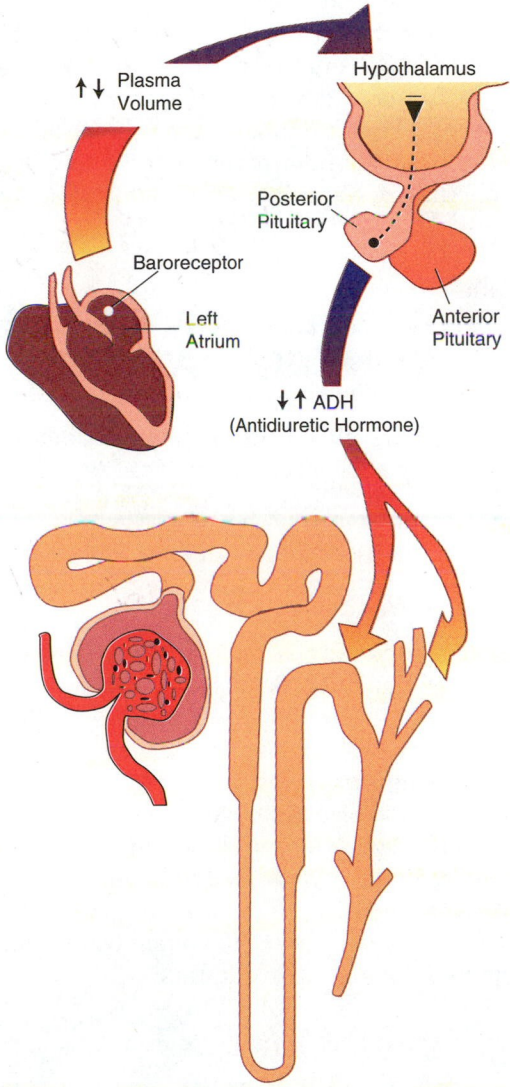

Figure 12–5.   *The pathway by which ADH is controlled. When the baroreceptors in the left atrium sense an increased pressure (increased plasma volume), they send neural impulses to the hypothalamus that cause the production of ADH to decrease. In contrast, a decreased pressure (decreased plasma volume) causes the production of ADH to increase.*

released by the pituitary gland. The hypothalamic cells manufacture ADH in response to input from numerous vascular baroreceptors, particularly a group found in the left atrium (see Figure 12–5). For example, when the atrial blood volume and, therefore, pressure increase, the baroreceptors are activated to transmit neural impulses to the hypothalamus, causing the production of ADH to be inhibited. This causes tubules to be impermeable to water and the urine to be greater in volume and more dilute.

In contrast, decreased atrial pressure (*dehydration*) decreases the neural impulses originating from the baroreceptors and causes the production of ADH to increase. The result is the rapid movement of water out of these portions of the tubules of the nephron and into the interstitium of the medullary area by osmosis. This causes the urine volume to decrease and its concentration to increase.

The specific gravity (*osmolality*) of urine varies with its concentration of solutes. The urine produced by the healthy kidney has a specific gravity of about 1.018 to 1.040 under normal conditions. During periods of diminished renal function, the urine specific gravity may fall to levels of 1.008 to 1.012.

REGULATION OF ELECTROLYTE CONCENTRATION

The kidneys play a major role in maintaining a normal cellular environment by regulating the concentration of various ions. Some of the more important ions regulated by the kidneys are sodium, potassium, calcium, magnesium, and phosphate.

SODIUM IONS

Sodium ions (Na^+) account for over 90 percent of the positively charged ions in the extracellular fluid. Because the sodium ions cause almost all of the osmotic pressure of the fluids, it follows that the sodium ion concentration directly affects the osmolality of the fluids. Thus, when the sodium concentration increases, there is a corresponding increase in the extracellular fluid osmolality. In contrast, the extracellular fluid osmolality decreases when there is a decreased sodium concentration.

The kidneys control the concentration of sodium primarily by regulating the amount of water in the body. When the sodium level becomes too high, the amount of water in the body increases by (1) secretion of antidiuretic hormone (ADH), which causes the kidney to retain water, and (2) stimulation of thirst, which causes the individual to drink liquids.

POTASSIUM IONS

A balanced potassium (K^+) level is essential for normal nerve and muscle function. Clinically, when the potassium level becomes too low, muscle weakness, diarrhea, metabolic alkalosis, and tachycardia develop. An excessively high potassium concentration causes muscle weakness, metabolic acidosis, and life-threatening arrhythmias. In response to a high K^+ level, the kidneys work to return the concentration to normal by means of two negative feedback control mechanisms: (1) the direct effect the excess potassium has on the epithelial cells of the renal tubules to cause an increased transport of potassium out of the peritubular capillaries and into the tubules of the nephrons, where it is subsequently passed in the urine, and (2) the stimulating effect the elevated potassium level has on the adrenal cortex, causing it to release increased quantities of *aldosterone*. Aldosterone stimulates the tubular epithelial cells to transport potassium ions into the nephron tubules and, hence, into the urine. The extracellular potassium concentration is normally 3.5 to 5 mEq/L.

CALCIUM, MAGNESIUM, AND PHOSPHATE IONS

The precise mechanisms by which calcium, magnesium, and phosphate concentrations are regulated by the kidneys are not well understood. It is known, however, that elevated levels of any one of these ions in the extracellular fluid cause the tubules to decrease reabsorption and to pass the substances into the urine. In contrast, when any one of these substances is low in concentration, the tubules rapidly reabsorb the substance until its concentration in the extracellular fluids returns to normal.

ROLE OF THE KIDNEYS IN ACID-BASE BALANCE

In addition to the natural acid-base buffers (see Chapter Eight) of the body fluids (e.g., HCO_3^-, phosphate, and protein buffers), and the respiratory system's ability to regulate the elimination of CO_2, the renal system also plays an important role in maintaining a normal acid-base balance by virtue of its ability to regulate the excretion of hydrogen ions and the reabsorption of bicarbonate ions.

All the renal tubules are capable of secreting hydrogen ions. The rate of secretion is directly proportional to the hydrogen ion concentration in the blood. Thus, when the extracellular fluids become too acidic, the kidneys excrete hydrogen ions into the urine. In contrast, when the extracellular fluids become too alkaline, the kidneys excrete basic substances (primarily sodium bicarbonate) into the urine.

This principle is illustrated in Figure 12–6, page 324, which shows that at point A, the extracellular fluid is 7.55. Because this is on the alkaline side, the pH of the urine is also alkaline (pH 7.5), since the kidneys excrete alkaline substances from the body fluids. In contrast, the extracellular pH at point B is 7.25 and the pH of the urine is very acidic (pH 5.25), because of excretion of large quantities of acidic substances (primarily hydrogen ions) from the body fluids. In both of these examples, the excretion of acidic or alkaline substances moves the pH toward normal.

BLOOD VOLUME

In the adult, the normal blood volume is about 5 liters, and it rarely increases or decreases more than a few hundred milliliters from that value. The capillary fluid shift system and the renal system are the two major mechanisms responsible for this constancy of the blood volume.

Figure 12–6. *The effect of extracellular fluid pH on the urine pH.*

Capillary Fluid Shift System

Under normal circumstances, the pressure in the capillaries of the systemic system is about 17 mm Hg. When the pressure rises above this value, fluid begins to leak into the tissue spaces, causing the blood volume to decrease toward normal. In contrast, when the blood volume falls, the capillary pressure decreases and fluid is then absorbed from the interstitial spaces, causing the blood volume to move back toward normal. This mechanism, however, has its limitations, since the tissue spaces cannot expand indefinitely when the blood volume becomes too high, nor can the tissue spaces supply an inexhaustible amount of fluid when the blood volume is low.

The Renal System

When the blood volume increases, the glomerular pressure in the kidney rises, causing the amount of the glomerular filtrate and the volume of the urine to increase. In addition, the pressure in the peritubular capillaries decreases fluid reabsorption from the tubules, which further increases the volume of urine.

An increased blood volume increases the glomerular pressure (normally 60 mm Hg) by means of two mechanisms: (1) the increased blood volume increases the blood flow through the afferent arterioles that lead into the kidneys and thus increases the intrarenal pressure, and (2) the increased blood volume stretches the atria of the heart, which contain stretch receptors called **volume receptors**. When the volume receptors in the atria are stretched, a neural reflex is initiated that causes the renal afferent arterioles to dilate. This causes the blood flow into the kidneys to increase and thus increases the amount of urine formed. Furthermore, when the volume receptors are stretched, the secretion of ADH by the posterior pituitary gland is inhibited, which in turn increases the urine output.

RENAL FAILURE

The renal system is subject to the same types of disorders as other body parts. The more common causes of renal failure are (1) congenital disorders, (2) infections, (3) obstructive disorders, (4) inflammation and immune responses, and (5) neoplasms.

COMMON CAUSES OF RENAL DISORDERS

Congenital Disorders

Approximately 10 percent of the infants born each year have a potentially life-threatening malformation of the renal system. Such abnormalities include unilateral renal agenesis, renal dysplasia, and polycystic disease of the kidney.

Infections

Urinary tract infections are the second most common type of bacterial infections (respiratory tract infections are the most common). Urinary tract infections are seen more often in women than men. Approximately 20 percent of all females will develop at least one urinary tract infection during their lifetime. These infections range from bacteriuria to severe kidney infections that cause irreversible damage to the kidneys.

Obstructive Disorders

Urinary obstruction can affect all age groups and can occur at any part of the urinary tract. About 90 percent of obstructions are located below the level of the glomerulus. Some factors that predispose individuals to urinary flow obstruction are listed in Table 12–2. Persons who have a urinary obstruction are prone to infections, a heightened susceptibility to calculus formation, and permanent kidney damage.

TABLE 12–2. **Factors that Obstruct Urinary Flow**

Calculi (bladder or kidney stones)
Normal pregnancy
Prostatic hypertrophy
Infection and inflammation causing scar tissue
Neurologic disorders (e.g., spinal cord injury and diabetic neuropathy)

Inflammation and Immune Responses

Kidney inflammation is caused by altered immune responses, drugs and related chemicals, and radiation. Inflammation can cause significant alterations in the glomerulus, tubules, and interstitium. The various forms of glomerulonephritis are believed to be caused by natural immune responses.

Neoplasms

Cancer of the kidneys accounts for 1 to 2 percent of all cancers. Although cancer of the kidneys is relatively rare in the adult, one form of cancer—Wilms' tumor—accounts for about 70 percent of all cancers of early childhood.

CLASSIFICATION OF RENAL DISORDERS

Renal disorders are commonly classified according to the anatomic portion of the renal system responsible for the renal decline. The major classifications are (1) prerenal, (2) renal, and (3) postrenal.

Prerenal Conditions

Prerenal conditions consist of abnormalities that impair blood flow to the kidneys. Prerenal problems are the most common and, generally, are reversible if identified and treated early. Table 12–3 lists some common prerenal causes of renal failure.

Normally, about 20 to 25 percent of the cardiac output is filtered by the kidneys. When the volume of blood falls (e.g., in cardiac failure or hemorrhage), the blood flow to the kidneys may decrease sharply. Thus, one of the early clinical manifestations of prerenal failure is a sharp reduction in urine output.

Renal Conditions

Renal abnormalities involve conditions that obstruct flow through the kidneys. Table 12–4 lists the five categories of renal abnormalities.

TABLE 12–3. Prerenal Abnormalities

Hypovolemia
  Decrease of gastrointestinal tract fluid
  Hemorrhage
  Fluid sequestration (e.g., burns)
Septicemia
Heart failure
Renal artery atherosclerosis

TABLE 12–4.   Renal Abnormalities

Renal ischemia
Injury to the glomerular membrane caused by nephrotoxic agents
   Aminoglycoside agents (e.g., gentamicin, kanamycin)
   Heavy metals (e.g., lead, mercury)
   Organic solvents (e.g., ethylene glycol)
   Radiopaque contrast media
   Sulfonamides
Acute tubular necrosis
Intratubular obstruction
   Uric acid cystals
   Hemolytic reactions (e.g., blood transfusion reactions)
Acute inflammatory conditions
   Acute pyelonephritis
   Necrotizing papillitis

Postrenal Conditions

An obstruction of the urinary tract at any point between the calyces and the urinary meatus is known as a postrenal obstruction. Table 12–5 lists some abnormalities included in the postrenal category.

MECHANICAL VENTILATION AS CAUSE OF RENAL FAILURE

It is well documented that mechanical ventilation can alter urinary output. *Positive pressure ventilation* decreases urinary output, whereas *negative pressure ventilation* increases urinary output. It is believed that this is due in part to the blood pressure changes that occur in response to mechanical ventilation. For example, in positive pressure ventilation, the venous return is often impeded, causing the blood volume and, therefore, the pressure in the atria to diminish. The reduced pressure stimulates the volume receptors in the atria to send more impulses to the pituitary gland. This causes more ADH to be released. As the concentration of ADH increases, the amount of urine formed by the kidneys decreases.

TABLE 12–5.   Postrenal Abnormalities

Ureteral obstruction (e.g., calculi, tumors)
Bladder outlet obstruction (e.g., prostatic hypertrophy)

CARDIOPULMONARY PROBLEMS CAUSED BY RENAL FAILURE

In chronic renal failure, a variety of cardiopulmonary problems can develop. In acute renal failure, the body's ability to eliminate nitrogenous wastes, water, and electrolytes is impaired. As the renal system declines further, the blood urea nitrogen (BUN), creatinine, potassium, and phosphate levels rapidly increase, and metabolic acidosis develops. Water retention gives rise to peripheral edema and pulmonary congestion. During the end stages, virtually every portion of the body is affected. In terms of specific cardiopulmonary problems, the following problems can be expected in patients with renal failure:

HYPERTENSION AND EDEMA

When the renal function is impaired, the kidneys lose their ability to excrete sodium. Consequently, the ingestion of excess sodium commonly leads to hypertension and edema.

METABOLIC ACIDOSIS

With the decline in renal function, the kidney's ability to secrete hydrogen ions (H^+) and to conserve bicarbonate (HCO_3^-) progressively decreases. Furthermore, during the more advanced stages of renal failure, hyperkalemia is a frequent finding. Thus, because of the increased H^+ and K^+ ion levels and the loss of HCO_3^-, *metabolic acidosis* is an almost inevitable clinical manifestation in severe renal failure.

RENAL ACID-BASE DISTURBANCES CAUSED BY ELECTROLYTE ABNORMALITIES

Chloride abnormalities can lead to acid-base disturbances through the renal system. For example, when the plasma chloride (Cl^-) level falls below normal, the amount of Cl^- available for glomerular filtration decreases. Under normal circumstances, when the positive sodium ion (Na^+) is reabsorbed by the tubules, the negative Cl^- ion must also be reabsorbed to maintain electrical neutrality. In the absence of adequate amounts of Cl^-, however, the electrical balance is maintained by the secretion of hydrogen ions (H^+). The loss of H^+ results in *hypochloremic alkalosis*. In contrast, when the plasma Cl^- level is higher than normal, the secretion of H^+ ions is reduced. This in turn causes a reduction in bicarbonate reabsorption and *hyperchloremic acidosis*.

Potassium abnormalities can also lead to acid-base disturbances through the renal system. For example, under normal conditions the potassium ion (K^+) behaves similarly to the H^+ ion in that it is secreted in the renal tubules in exchange for Na^+. In the absence of Na^+, neither K^+ nor H^+ can be secreted. When the K^+ level is higher than normal, however, the competition with H^+ for Na^+ exchange increases. When this happens, the amount of H^+ ions secreted is reduced, which in turn decreases the amount of bicarbonate reabsorption. The end-product of this process is *hyperkalemic acidosis.* When the K^+ level is lower than normal, the competition with H^+ for Na^+ exchange decreases. Consequently, the amount of H^+ secreted is increased, which in turn increases the amount of HCO_3^- reabsorption. The end-product of this process is *hypokalemic alkalosis.*

ANEMIA

The kidneys are a primary source of the hormone *erythropoietin,* which stimulates the bone marrow to produce red blood cells. When the renal system fails, the production of erythropoietin is often inadequate to stimulate the bone marrow to produce a sufficient amount of red blood cells. In addition, the toxic wastes that accumulate as a result of renal failure also suppress the ability of bone marrow to produce red blood cells. Both of these mechanisms contribute to the anemia seen in chronic renal failure.

BLEEDING

Approximately 20 percent of persons with chronic renal failure have a tendency to bleed as a result of platelet abnormalities. Clinically, this is manifested by epistaxis (nose bleed), gastrointestinal bleeding, and bruising of the skin and subcutaneous tissues.

CARDIOVASCULAR PROBLEMS

Hypertension is often an early sign of renal failure. In severe cases, the increased extracellular fluid volume, caused by sodium and water retention, gives rise to edema, congestive heart failure, and pulmonary edema. Pericarditis is also seen in about 50 percent of persons with chronic renal failure. This condition develops as a result of the pericardium being exposed to the metabolic end-products associated with renal decline.

CLINICAL APPLICATION

This 73-year-old female was admitted to the hospital for severe renal failure and left ventricular heart failure. An electrocardiogram (ECG) revealed a slow, irregular sinus rhythm with occasional premature ventricular contractions (PVCs). Her ankles, hands, and eyelids were swollen. Her skin was pale, damp, and cool. She had a spontaneous cough, productive of a small amount of white, frothy sputum. A chest x-ray showed white, fluffy patches that spread outward from the hilar areas to the peripheral borders of both lungs. Her left ventricle appeared moderately enlarged.

The patient's vital signs were: blood pressure—183/97, heart rate—101 beats/min, respiratory rate—18 breaths/min and deep, and temperature 98.8°F. The laboratory report showed that the patient's blood urea nitrogen (BUN), creatinine, potassium, and phosphate levels were all higher than normal. The patient had no urine output. On room air, her arterial blood gas values were: pH 7.29, Pa_{CO_2} 32 mm Hg, HCO_3 17 mmol/L,

(continues)

and Pa_{O_2} 64 mm Hg. The respiratory therapist started the patient on 4 L/min of oxygen via a nasal cannula and drew a second arterial blood gas sample twenty-five minutes later. The results showed a pH of 7.28, Pa_{CO_2} 30, HCO_3^- 16, and Pa_{O_2} 86 mm Hg. No remarkable change was seen in the patient's vital signs.

Although the patient received aggressive medical treatment to correct her cardiac and renal problems, her pulmonary congestion did not significantly improve until she started to produce urine, which was twenty hours after admission. On day four the patient's condition was upgraded. Her skin color was normal and her skin was warm and dry to the touch. She no longer had a productive cough. When the patient was asked to produce a strong cough, no sputum was produced.

Her peripheral edema was no longer present, and her vital signs were: blood pressure—132/84, heart rate—74 beats/min, and respiratory rate—10 breaths/min. Her laboratory report showed no remarkable problems, and her ECG was normal. A second chest x-ray showed normal lungs and normal heart size. On room air, her arterial blood gas values were: pH 7.39, Pa_{CO_2} 39 mm Hg, HCO_3^- 24 mmol/L, and Pa_{O_2} 93 mm Hg. On day five the patient was discharged.

DISCUSSION

This case illustrates the adverse effects of poor blood circulation on the function of both the kidneys and lungs. Essentially, all of the clinical manifestations in this case can be traced back to the patient's left ventricular failure (a prerenal abnormality). As pointed out in this chapter, prerenal problems are the most common and generally are reversible if identified and treated early. One of the early clinical manifestations of prerenal failure is a sharp reduction in urine output. On admission, the patient had no urine output. With the decline in renal function, the kidneys' ability to secrete hydrogen ions (H^+) and to conserve bicarbonate (HCO_3^-) progressively decreases. Furthermore, during the more advanced stages of renal failure, hyperkalemia (increased K^+) is a frequent finding. Thus, because of the increased H^+ and K^+ ion levels and the loss of HCO_3^-, *metabolic acidosis* is an inevitable clinical manifestation in severe renal failure.

Because of the left ventricular failure, fluid progressively accumulated in the patient's lungs and extremities. The fluid accumulation, in turn, increased the density of the alveolar-capillary membranes, causing the white fluffy patches on the patient's chest x-ray. In addition, as the fluid accumulation in her lungs worsened, the oxygen diffusion across the alveolar-capillary membrane decreased (see Figure 3–6, page 117). This pathologic process was verified by the Pa_{O_2} of 64 mm Hg on admission. Moreover, because the blood flow through the pulmonary system was impeded (because of the left ventricular failure), blood accumulated throughout the patient's extremities, thus causing swelling in the patient's ankles, hands, and eyelids. Fortunately, the patient was treated aggressively and in a timely manner to reverse all of these potentially fatal pathologic processes.

CLINICAL APPLICATION

This 42-year-old male firefighter was found unconscious in a smoke-filled room on the fourth floor of a burning office building. He had second- and third-degree burns over portions of his left shoulder, left arm, and left hand, and over the anterior portion of his chest and abdominal region. His pulse was rapid and his respiration was slow and gasping. The patient was quickly carried out of the burning building and placed in a waiting ambulance. It was later estimated that the patient had been unconscious in the smoke-filled room for more than ten minutes. En route to the hospital the patient was manually ventilated with 100 percent oxygen. An intravenous infusion was started and Ringer's lactate solution was administered. The patient's clothing was cut away and the burn wounds were covered to prevent shock, fluid loss, and heat loss.

When the patient arrived in the emergency room, his skin that was not burned appeared cherry red. His vital signs were: blood pressure—96/55 and heart rate—124 beats/min. He was still being manually ventilated with 100 percent oxygen. Bilateral bronchospasm and crackles were heard when his lungs were auscultated. The patient was intubated. Black, frothy secretions were suctioned from the patient's lungs. A chest x-ray showed white fluffy densities throughout both lung fields. His arterial blood gas values were: pH 7.52, Pa_{CO_2} 28 mm Hg, HCO_3^- 22 mmol/L, Pa_{O_2} 47 mm Hg. His *carboxyhemoglobin* (CO_{Hb}) level was 47 percent. The emergency room physician felt the patient was hypovolemic and going into shock.

The patient was transferred to the intensive care unit (ICU) and placed on a mechanical ventilator. The patient's progress was stormy during the first 24 hours. The respiratory-care team had to make several aggressive ventilator adjustments. The patient's hemodynamic profile was classified as critical (see Hemodynamic Profile No. 1). His cardiopulmonary status, however, was finally stabilized on the second day. At this time, the patient's ventilator settings were a ventilatory rate of 12 breaths/min, an inspired oxygen concentration ($F_{I_{O_2}}$) of 1.0, and a positive end-expiratory pressure (PEEP) of +15 cm H_2O. His arterial blood gas values were: pH 7.38, Pa_{CO_2} 37 mm Hg, HCO_3^- 24 mmol/L, Pa_{O_2} 78 mm Hg, and Sa_{O_2} 93 percent.

Two days later, the patient's cardiopulmonary status was upgraded to fair. His ventilator settings at this time were a mechanical ventilator rate of 6 breaths/min, and $F_{I_{O_2}}$ 0.5, and a PEEP of +8 cm H_2O. The patient's arterial blood gas

HEMODYNAMIC PROFILE

Parameter*	Profile No. 1	Profile No. 2
BP	63/39	125/83
CVP	12	3
RAP	13	3
$\overline{PA}$	25	14
CO	2.7	5.8
URINE ml/hr	0	54

*BP = blood pressure; CVP = central venous pressure; RAP = right atrial pressure; $\overline{PA}$ = mean pulmonary artery pressure; CO = cardiac output.

values were: pH 7.41, Pa_{CO_2} 38 mm Hg, HCO_3^- 24 mmol/L, Pa_{O_2} 84 mm Hg, and Sa_{O_2} 93 percent. His carboxyhemoglobin (CO_{Hb}) level was 11 percent. His hemodynamic status had significantly improved and he was producing urine (see Profile No. 2). The patient progressively improved and was discharged two weeks later.

DISCUSSION

Similar to Case 1, this case illustrates a prerenal abnormality. The patient's burns caused fluid sequestration, which in turn lead to *hypovolemia* (see Table 12–3). As a result of the hypovolemia, the blood flow though the patient's kidneys decreased. Again, one of the early clinical manifestations of prerenal failure is a sharp reduction in urine output. Note the low cardiac output and no urine output charted in Hemodynamic Profile No. 1. Fortunately, the patient responded favorably to the therapy and his hemodynamic status and urine output returned to normal (see Hemodynamic Profile No. 2).

It should also be noted that the patient's pulmonary status, unrelated to the poor kidney function, was very serious on admission. The patient's pathologic lung changes in the distal airways and alveoli were most likely caused by the irritant and toxic gases, and suspended soot particles associated with incomplete combustion and smoke. Many of the substances found

(*continues*)

in smoke are extremely caustic to the tracheo-bronchial tree and poisonous to the body. The injuries that develop from smoke inhalation include inflammation of the tracheobronchial tree, bronchospasm, excessive bronchial secretions and mucus plugging, decreased mucosal ciliary transport mechanism, atelectasis, alveolar edema, and frothy secretions. Evidence of this condition was documented by the white, fluffy densities throughout both lung fields and the low Pa_{O_2} of 47 mm Hg at admission. Finally, the patient's carbon monoxide level (his CO_{Hb} was 47 percent) was dangerously high in the emergency room. Though the patient initially responded slowly to respiratory care, the above pathologic processes were ultimately reversed and the cardiopulmonary status was perfectly normal at the time of discharge.

REVIEW QUESTIONS

1. The outer one-third of the kidney is called the
   a. renal pelvis
   b. medulla
   c. minor calyces
   d. renal pyramid
   e. cortex
2. Glomerular filtration is directly proportional to
   a. blood cell size
   b. hydrostatic pressure
   c. osmotic pressure
   d. protein size
   e. the patient's fluid intake
3. Tubular reabsorption occurs primarily in the
   a. renal corpuscle
   b. proximal convoluted tubule
   c. loop of Henle
   d. distal convoluted tubule
   e. collecting duct
4. The major substance(s) transported by means of tubular secretion is/are:
   I. H^+
   II. Cl^-
   III. K^+
   IV. HCO_3^-
   V. Na^+
      a. I only
      b. IV only
      c. V only
      d. I and III only
      e. IV and V only

5. The urine produced by the healthy kidney has a specific gravity of about
   a. 1.000–1.001
   b. 1.006–1.020
   c. 1.018–1.040
   d. 1.060–1.080
   e. 1.080–1.100
6. Which of the following can be classified as a prerenal condition?
   I. Heart failure
   II. Intratubular obstruction
   III. Bladder outlet obstruction
   IV. Hypovolemia
       a. I only
       b. II only
       c. IV only
       d. II and III only
       e. I and IV only
7. Which of the following is the functional unit(s) of the kidneys?
   a. Cortex
   b. Collecting ducts
   c. Major calyces
   d. Peritubular capillaries
   e. Nephrons
8. Which of the following empties urine into the bladder?
   a. Collecting ducts
   b. Ureters
   c. Distal convoluted tubules
   d. Urethra
   e. Major calyces
9. Normally, the net glomerular filtration pressure is about
   a. 5 mm Hg
   b. 10 mm Hg
   c. 15 mm Hg
   d. 20 mm Hg
   e. 25 mm Hg
10. Which of the following is/are part of the nephron?
    I. Proximal convoluted tubules
    II. Loop of Henle
    III. Glomerulus
    IV. Distal convoluted tubules
        a. II only
        b. III only
        c. II, III, and IV only
        d. I, II, and III only
        e. I, II, III, and IV

CHAPTER THIRTEEN

AGING AND ITS EFFECTS ON THE CARDIOPULMONARY SYSTEM

OBJECTIVES

By the end of this chapter, the student should be able to:

1. Describe the effects of aging on the following components of the *respiratory system:*
   —Static mechanical properties
   - Elastic recoil of the lungs
   - Lung compliance
   - Thoracic compliance
   —Lung volumes and capacities
   —Dynamic maneuvers of ventilation
   —Pulmonary diffusing capacity
   —Alveolar deadspace ventilation
   —Pulmonary gas exchange
   —Arterial blood gases
   —Arterial-venous oxygen content difference
   —Hemoglobin concentration
   —Control of ventilation
   —Exercise tolerance
   —Pulmonary diseases in the aged
2. Describe the effects of aging on the following components of the *cardiovascular system:*
   —Structure of the heart
   —Work of the heart
   —Heart rate
   —Stroke volume
   —Cardiac output
   —Peripheral vascular resistance
   —Blood pressure
3. Complete the review questions at the end of this chapter.

The aging process is normal, progressive, and physiologically irreversible. Aging occurs in spite of optimal nutrition, genetic background, environmental surroundings, and activity patterns. The biological aging process, however, may demonstrate altered rates of progression in response to an individual's genetic background and day-to-day living habits.

Assuming that the death rate remains the same in the United States, the number of people 74 to 85 years of age will double (to 10.6 million) by the year 2000. The number of people older than 85 will increase by more than 80 percent (to 3.8 million). Between the years 2010 and 2030, those born 1946 to 1964 during the post–World War II baby boom (the biggest baby boom in history) will be turning

65. During this period, it is estimated that the number of people over 65 years of age will increase from the present 25 million to some 50 million. By the year 2020, the 75-and-over population, who have specific activity limitations due to chronic ailments, will increase 2.5 times (to 10.7 million). Figure 13–1 illustrates the actual and projected population of persons 55 years and older for four different age groups between the years of 1900 and 2040.

It is also projected that the number of short-stay hospital days of persons 65 years and older will increase from the 105,358 in 1980 to over 286,000 by the year 2050 (Figure 13–2). Because the mortality and morbidity rates rise sharply after age

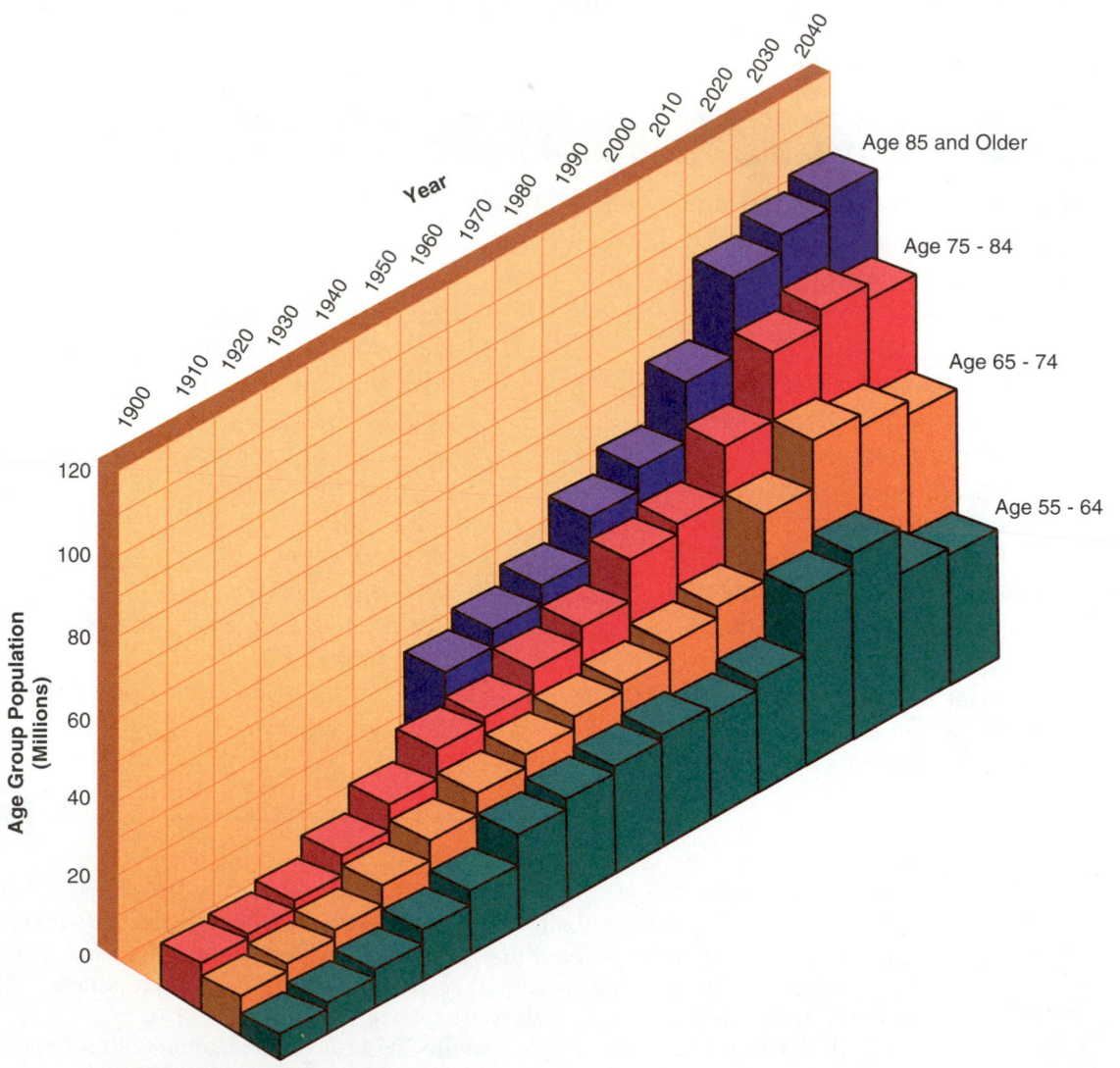

Figure 13–1. *The actual and projected population of persons 55 years and older for four different age groups between the years 1900 and 2040.*

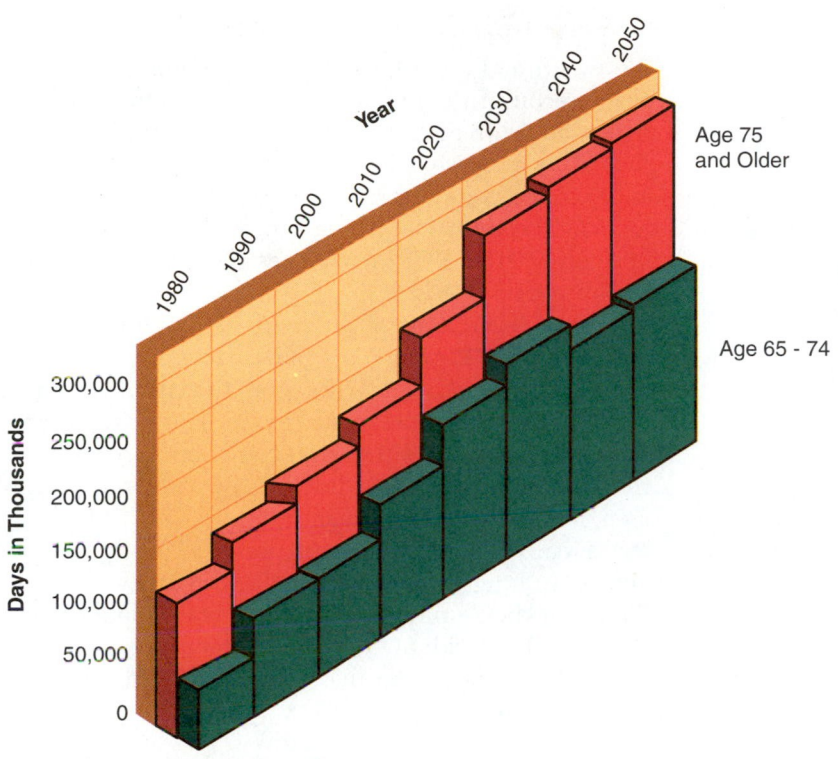

Figure 13–2. *The actual and projected short-stay hospital days of persons 65 years and older between the years 1980 and 2050.*

65, the large size of this population will undoubtedly pose a tremendous challenge to the health care industry. A basic understanding of how the aging process influences the cardiopulmonary system is critical for the respiratory care practitioner.

THE INFLUENCE OF AGING ON THE RESPIRATORY SYSTEM

The growth and development of the lungs is essentially complete by about 20 years of age. Most of the pulmonary function indices reach their maximum levels between 20 and 25 years of age and then progressively decline. The precise influence of aging on the respiratory system is difficult to determine, since changes associated with time are often indistinguishable from those of disease. For example, factors such as chronic exposure to environmental pollutants, repeated pulmonary infections, smoking, and some working conditions can cause alterations in the respiratory system that are not easily differentiated from changes due to aging alone. In spite of these difficulties, the conclusions reached here appear to be well founded.

STATIC MECHANICAL PROPERTIES

The **functional residual capacity** is the volume remaining in the lungs when the elastic recoil of the lungs exactly balances the natural tendency of the chest wall to expand. With aging, the elastic recoil of the lungs decreases, causing lung compliance to increase. This is illustrated graphically as a shift to the left (steeper slope) of the volume-pressure curve (Figure 13–3). The decrease in lung elasticity develops because the alveoli progressively deteriorate and enlarge after age 30. Structurally, the alveolar changes resemble the air sac changes associated with emphysema.

Even though the potential for greater lung expansion exists as an individual becomes older, it cannot be realized because of the structural limitations that develop in the chest wall. With aging the costal cartilages of the thoracic wall progressively calcify, causing the ribs to slant downward, and this structural change causes the thorax to become less compliant. Because of these anatomic changes, the transpulmonary pressure difference, which is responsible for holding the airways open, is diminished with age.

Finally, the reduction in chest wall compliance is slightly greater than the increase in lung compliance, resulting in an overall moderate decline in total compliance of the respiratory system. It is estimated that the work expenditure of a 60-year-old individual to overcome static mechanical forces during normal breathing is 20 percent greater than that of a 20-year-old person. The decreased compli-

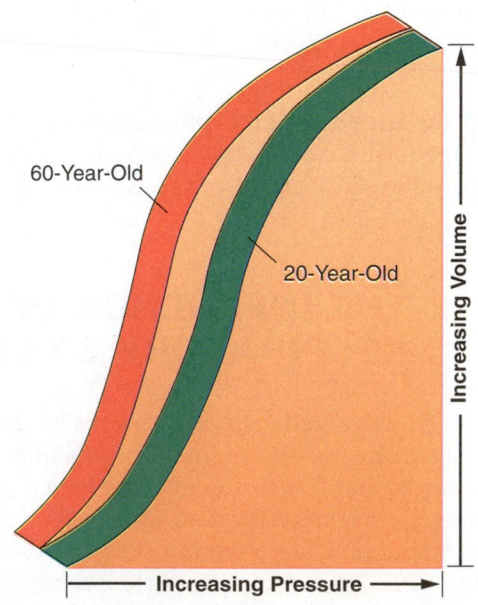

Figure 13–3. *Comparison of the pressure-volume curve of a 60-year-old person with that of a 20-year-old individual. With aging, the curve shifts to the left.*

ance of the respiratory system associated with age is offset by increased respiratory frequency rather than by increased tidal volume during exertion.

LUNG VOLUMES AND CAPACITIES

Figure 13–4 shows the changes that occur in the lung volumes and capacities with aging. Although studies are in conflict, it is generally agreed that the total lung capacity (TLC) essentially remains the same throughout life. Should the TLC decrease, however, it is probably due to the decreased height that typically occurs with age.

It is well documented that the residual volume (RV) increases with age. This is primarily due to age-related alveolar enlargement and to small airway closure. As the RV increases, the RV/TLC ratio also increases. The RV/TLC ratio increases from approximately 20 percent at age 20 to about 35 percent at age 60. This increase occurs predominantly after the age of 40. As the RV increases, moreover, the expiratory reserve volume (ERV) decreases. Most studies show that the functional residual capacity (FRC) increases with age, but not as much as the RV and the RV/TLC. Since the FRC typically increases with age, the inspiratory capacity (IC) decreases.

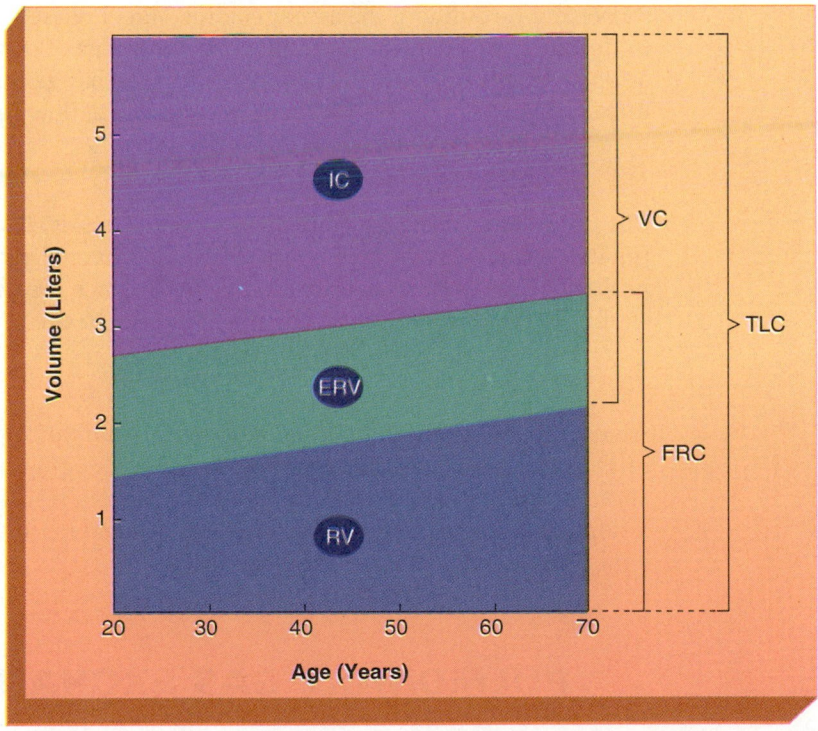

Figure 13–4. *Schematic representation of the changes that occur in lung volumes and capacities with aging. Abbreviations are explained in text.*

Because the vital capacity (VC) is equal to the TLC minus the RV, the VC inevitably decreases as the RV increases. It is estimated that in the male, the VC decreases about 25 ml/year. In the female, the VC decreases about 20 ml/year. In general, the VC decreases about 40 to 50 percent by age 70.

DYNAMIC MANEUVERS OF VENTILATION

Because of the loss of lung elasticity associated with aging, there inevitably is a marked effect on the dynamics of ventilation. In fact, one of the most prominent physiologic changes associated with age is the reduced efficiency in forced air expulsion. This normal deterioration is reflected by a progressive decrease in the following dynamic lung functions:

- Forced vital capacity (FVC)
- Peak expiratory flow rate (PEFR)
- Forced expiratory flow$_{25-75\%}$ (FEF$_{25-75\%}$)
- Forced expiratory volume in 1 second (FEV$_1$)
- Forced expiratory volume in 1 second/forced vital capacity ratio (FEV$_1$/FVC ratio)
- Maximum voluntary ventilation (MVV)

It is estimated that these dynamic lung functions decrease approximately 20 to 30 percent throughout the average adult's life. Precisely what causes the flow rates to decline is still controversial. Since, however, gas flow is dependent upon (1) the applied pressure and (2) the airway resistance, changes in either or both of these factors could be responsible for the reduction of gas flow rates seen in the elderly.

PULMONARY DIFFUSING CAPACITY

The pulmonary diffusing capacity (D$_{L_{CO}}$) progressively decreases with age. It is estimated that the D$_{L_{CO}}$ falls about 20 percent over the course of adult life. This is probably the result of decreased alveolar surface area and decreased pulmonary capillary blood flow, both of which are known to occur with aging.

ALVEOLAR DEADSPACE VENTILATION

Alveolar deadspace ventilation increases with advancing age. This is probably due to the decreased cardiac index associated with aging and to the structural alterations of the pulmonary capillaries that occur as a result of the normal alveolar deterioration. It is estimated that the alveolar deadspace ventilation increases about 1 ml per year throughout adult life.

 # PULMONARY GAS EXCHANGE

The alveolar-arterial oxygen tension difference P$_{(A-a)O_2}$ progressively increases with age. Although controversial, factors that may increase the P$_{(A-a)O_2}$ include the physiologic shunt, the mismatching of ventilation and perfusion, and a decreased diffusing capacity.

ARTERIAL BLOOD GASES

The Pa_{O_2} progressively decreases with age. Because lung degeneration and relative hypoxemia are a normal part of aging, an acceptable Pa_{O_2} range for individuals between 60 and 90 years of age can be calculated by subtracting 1 mm Hg from the minimal 80 mm Hg level for every year over 60 (see Table 7–1, page 205). Thus, a Pa_{O_2} of 65 mm Hg should be acceptable for a 75-year-old individual.

The Pa_{CO_2} remains constant throughout life. A possible explanation for this is the greater diffusion ability of carbon dioxide through the alveolar-capillary barrier. Because the Pa_{CO_2} remains the same in the healthy adult with age, the pH and HCO_3^- levels also remain constant.

ARTERIAL-VENOUS OXYGEN CONTENT DIFFERENCE

The maximum arterial-venous oxygen content difference $C(a - v)_{O_2}$ tends to decrease with age. Contributory factors include (1) decline in physical fitness, (2) less efficient peripheral blood distribution, and (3) reduction in tissue enzyme activity.

HEMOGLOBIN CONCENTRATION

Anemia is a common finding among the elderly. Several factors predispose the aged to anemia. Red bone marrow has a tendency to be replaced by fatty marrow, especially in the long bones. Gastrointestinal atrophy, which is commonly associated with advancing age, may slow the absorption of iron or vitamin B_{12}. Gastrointestinal bleeding is also more prevalent in the elderly. Perhaps the most important reasons for anemia in the aged are sociologic rather than medical—for example, insufficient income to purchase food or decreased interest in cooking and eating adequate meals.

CONTROL OF VENTILATION

The ventilatory response to both hypoxia and hypercapnia diminishes with age. This is probably due to a reduced sensitivity of the peripheral and central chemoreceptors. The incidence of snoring and obstructive sleep apnea also increases with aging.

EXERCISE TOLERANCE

In healthy individuals of any age, the respiratory function does not limit exercise tolerance. The oxygen transport system is more critically dependent on the cardiovascular system than on respiratory function. The maximal oxygen uptake ($\dot{V}_{O_2max}$), which is the parameter most commonly used to evaluate an individual's aerobic exercise tolerance, peaks at age 20 and progressively and linearly decreases with age. Although there is considerable variation among individuals, it is estimated that from 20 to 60 years of age, a person's maximal oxygen uptake decreases by approximately 35 percent. Evidence indicates, however, that regular physical conditioning throughout life increases oxygen uptake and therefore enhances the capacity for exertion during work and recreation.

PULMONARY DISEASES IN THE AGED

Although the occurrence of pulmonary diseases increases with age, it is difficult to determine the precise relationship aging has to pulmonary disease. This is because aging is also associated with the presence of chronic diseases (e.g., lung cancer, bronchitis, and emphysema). It is known, however, that the incidence of serious infectious pulmonary diseases is significantly greater in the elderly. While the incidence has decreased dramatically in recent years, the mortality from pneumonia is still a major cause of death in the elderly. Evidence suggests that this is partly due to the impaired defense mechanisms in the aged.

THE INFLUENCE OF AGING ON THE CARDIOVASCULAR SYSTEM

A variety of adverse changes develops in the cardiovascular system with age. In fact, the major causes of death in the aging population are diseases of the cardiovascular system. The major changes in the cardiovascular system that develop as a function of age are as follows.

STRUCTURE OF THE HEART

Between 30 and 80 years of age, the thickness of the left ventricular wall increases by about 25 percent. Cardiac hypertrophy, however, is not considered a primary change associated with aging. In the ventricles, the muscle fiber size progressively increases. Fibrosis develops in the lining of the chambers and fatty infiltration occurs in the wall of the chambers. The amount of connective tissue increases, causing the heart to become less elastic. Thus, the compliance of the heart is reduced and the heart functions less efficiently as a pump. The heart valves thicken from calcification and fibrosis. This structural change causes the valves to be more rigid and less effective. As the valves become more rigid and distorted, the blood flow may be impeded and systolic murmurs may develop.

WORK OF THE HEART

The work of the heart, which is defined as stroke volume times mean systolic blood pressure, decreases approximately 1 percent per year (Figure 13–5).

HEART RATE

Although the effect of age on the resting heart rate is controversial, it is known that the increase in heart rate in response to stress is less in the elderly. The maximum heart rate can be estimated by the following formula:

maximum heart rate = 220 − age

Thus, the maximum heart rate for a 60-year-old is about 160 (220 − 60 = 160). (Recent research has shown that some older subjects can achieve higher heart rates than those predicted by this method.) The reasons for the decreased maximum

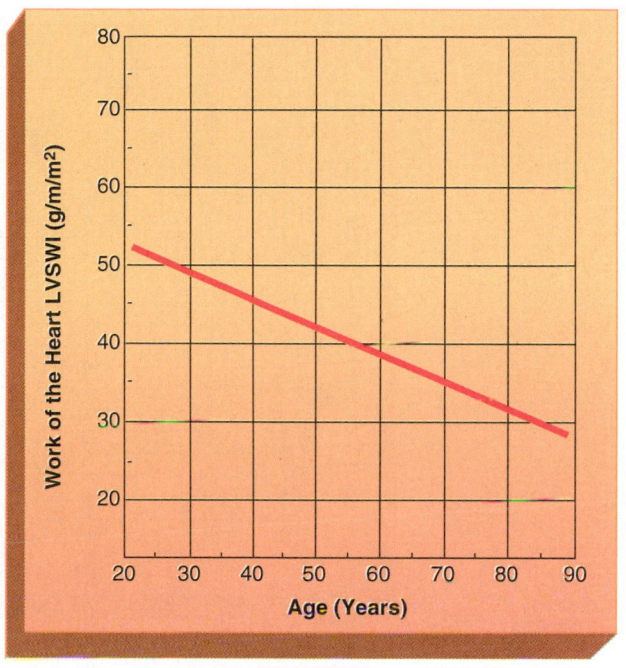

Figure 13–5. *Schematic representation of the effects of aging on the work of the heart.*

heart rate are unclear (Figure 13–6, page 344). It may be due to the diminished myocardial oxygen supply associated with advanced age. Another possibility is the decreased compliance of the heart in the aged. The increase in heart rate in response to stress may be impaired because of increased connective tissue in the sinoatrial and atrioventricular nodes and in the bundle branches. The number of catecholamine receptors on the muscle fibers may also be reduced.

With aging, moreover, it not only takes more time for the heart to accelerate, but it also takes more time to return to normal after a stressful event. Because of this, the expected increase in pulse rate in response to certain clinical situations (e.g., anxiety, pain, hemorrhage, and infectious processes) is often not as evident in the elderly.

STROKE VOLUME

The stroke volume diminishes with age. The precise reason for the reduction in the stroke volume is unknown. It is suggested, however, that the decline in stroke volume may be a reflection of poor myocardial perfusion, decreased cardiac compliance, and poor contractility. As the stroke volume declines, the *stroke volume index* (stroke volume divided by body surface area) also decreases.

CARDIAC OUTPUT

As the stroke volume diminishes, the cardiac output inevitably declines. After the age of 20, the cardiac output decreases in a linear fashion about 1 percent per year

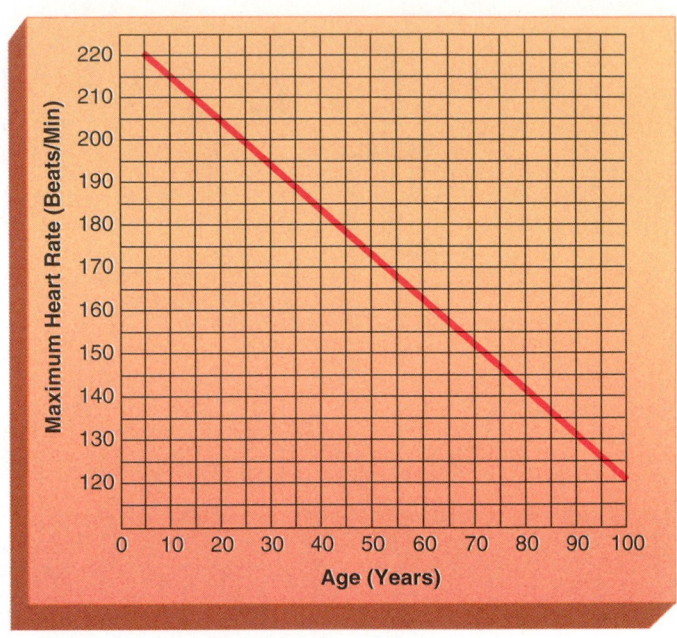

Figure 13–6. *Schematic representation of the effects of aging on the maximum heart rate.*

(Figure 13–7). Between the ages of 30 and 80, the cardiac output decreases about 40 percent in both men and women. As the cardiac output declines, the *cardiac index* (cardiac output divided by body surface area) also decreases.

PERIPHERAL VASCULAR RESISTANCE

It is well documented that the elasticity of the major blood vessels decreases with advancing age. Both the arteries and veins undergo age-related changes. The intima thickens and the media becomes more fibrotic (see Figure 1–24, page 33). Collagen and extracellular materials accumulate in both the intima and media. As the peripheral vascular system stiffens, its ability to accept the cardiac stroke volume declines. This age-related development increases the *resting pulse pressure* and the *systolic blood pressure*. It is estimated that the *total* peripheral resistance increases about 1 percent per year (Figure 13–8).

As the peripheral resistance increases, the perfusion of the body organs decreases. This progressive decline in organ perfusion partly explains the many organ debilities seen in the elderly. As the vascular system stiffens with age, its tolerance to change diminishes. For example, a sudden move from the horizontal to the vertical position may cause a marked drop in systemic blood pressure, causing dizziness, confusion, weakness, and fainting. Arterial stiffening also makes the baroreceptors, located in the carotid sinuses and aortic arch, sluggish and less able to moderate blood pressure changes.

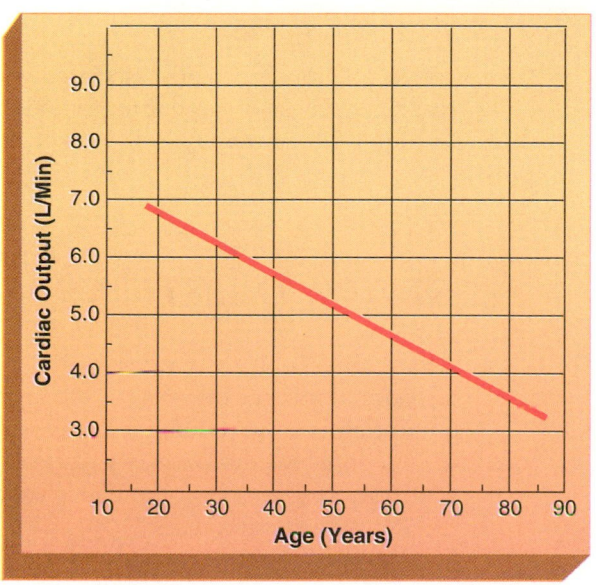

Figure 13–7. *Schematic representation of the effects of aging on the cardiac output.*

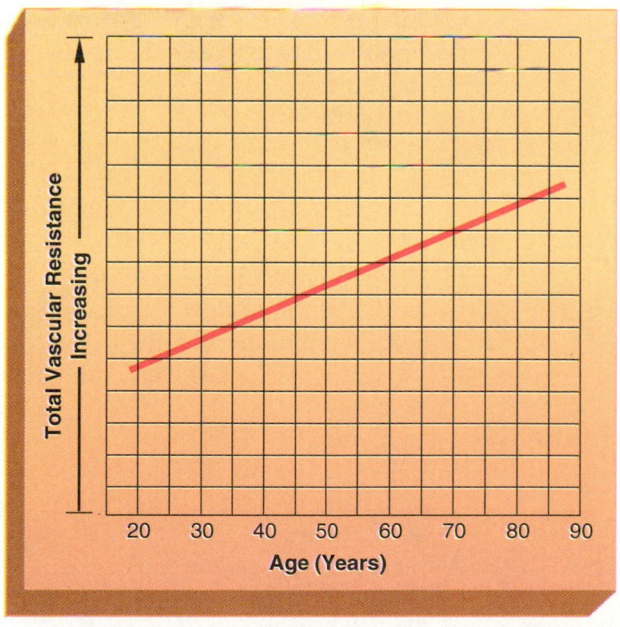

Figure 13–8. *Schematic representation of the effects of aging on the total vascular resistance.*

BLOOD PRESSURE

As described previously, factors associated with aging that increase blood pressure are increasing stiffness of large arteries and increasing total peripheral resistance. Other factors, such as obesity, salt intake, and stress, can also elevate the blood pressure.

REVIEW QUESTIONS

1. As an individual grows older, the
   a. residual volume decreases
   b. expiratory reserve volume increases
   c. functional residual capacity decreases
   d. inspiratory reserve volume increases
   e. vital capacity decreases
2. Most of the lung function indices reach their maximum levels between
   a. 1–5 years of age
   b. 5–10 years of age
   c. 10–15 years of age
   d. 15–20 years of age
   e. 20–25 years of age
3. With advancing age, the
   I. lung compliance decreases
   II. chest wall compliance increases
   III. lung compliance increases
   IV. chest wall compliance decreases
      a. I only
      b. II only
      c. III only
      d. I and II only
      e. III and IV only
4. As an individual grows older, the
   I. forced vital capacity increases
   II. peak expiratory flow rate decreases
   III. forced expiratory volume in 1 second increases
   IV. maximum voluntary ventilation increases
      a. I only
      b. II only
      c. II and IV only
      d. III and IV only
      e. II, III, and IV only
5. With advancing age, the
   I. Pa_{CO_2} increases
   II. Pa_{O_2} decreases
   III. $P_{(A-a)O_2}$ decreases

   IV. $C(a - v)_{O_2}$ decreases
- a. I only
- b. II only
- c. III only
- d. II and IV only
- e. III and IV only

6. The maximum heart rate of a 45-year-old person is
- a. 155 beats/min
- b. 165 beats/min
- c. 175 beats/min
- d. 185 beats/min
- e. 195 beats/min

7. Over the course of life, the diffusion capacity decreases by about
- a. 5%
- b. 10%
- c. 15%
- d. 20%
- e. 25%

8. Between 30 and 80 years of age, the cardiac output decreases by about
- a. 10%
- b. 20%
- c. 30%
- d. 40%
- e. 50%

9. With advancing age, the
   I. blood pressure increases
   II. stroke volume decreases
   III. cardiac output increases
   IV. heart work decreases
- a. I only
- b. II only
- c. III and IV only
- d. II and III only
- e. I, II, and IV only

10. Between 20 and 60 years of age, the RV/TLC ratio
- a. increases from 20% to 25%
- b. increases from 20% to 30%
- c. increases from 20% to 35%
- d. increases from 20% to 40%
- e. remains the same

CHAPTER FOURTEEN

EXERCISE AND ITS EFFECTS ON THE CARDIOPULMONARY SYSTEM

OBJECTIVES

By the end of this chapter, the student should be able to:

1. Describe the effects of exercise on the following components of the cardiopulmonary system:
   —Ventilation
   —Oxygen consumption
   —Arterial blood gases
   —Oxygen diffusion capacity
   —Alveolar-arterial oxygen tension difference
   —Circulation
   • Sympathetic discharge
   • Increased cardiac output
   • Increased arterial blood pressure
   • Pulmonary vascular pressures
   • Opening of muscle capillaries

2. Describe the interrelationships between muscle work, oxygen consumption, and cardiac output.
3. Describe the influence of training on the heart and on cardiac output.
4. Differentiate between stroke volume and heart rate in increasing the cardiac output.
5. Describe how body temperature and cutaneous blood flow relate to a number of symptoms collectively referred to as heat stroke.
6. List the benefits of cardiovascular rehabilitation.
7. Complete the review questions at the end of this chapter.

During heavy exercise, components of the cardiopulmonary system may be stressed close to their limit. Alveolar ventilation may increase as much as 20-fold, oxygen diffusion capacity as much as 3-fold, cardic output as much as 6-fold, muscle blood flow as much as 25-fold, oxygen consumption as much as 20-fold, and heat production as much as 20-fold.

Muscle training can increase muscle size and strength 30 to 60 percent. The efficiency of intracellular metabolism may increase by 30 to 50 percent. The size of the heart chambers and the heart mass of well-trained athletes, such as marathon runners, may be increased by 40 percent. When the level of exercise is greater, however, than the ability of the cardiopulmonary system to provide a sufficient supply of oxygen to the muscles, anaerobic metabolism ensues. The point at which anaerobic metabolism develops is called the **anaerobic threshold**.

VENTILATION

CONTROL OF VENTILATION

The precise mechanism responsible for increased alveolar ventilation during exercise is not well understood. Exercise causes the body to consume a large amount of oxygen and, simultaneously, to produce a large amount of carbon dioxide. However, alveolar ventilation increases so much that the concentration of these gases in the body does not change significantly. In addition, no oxygen or carbon dioxide chemoreceptors have been identified on the venous side of circulation, or in the lungs, that could account for the increased alveolar ventilation during exercise. Thus it is unlikely that the increased ventilation seen in exercise is caused by either of these gases.

It has been suggested that the increased ventilation is caused by neural impulses sent to the medulla by way of the following pathways (Figure 14–1):

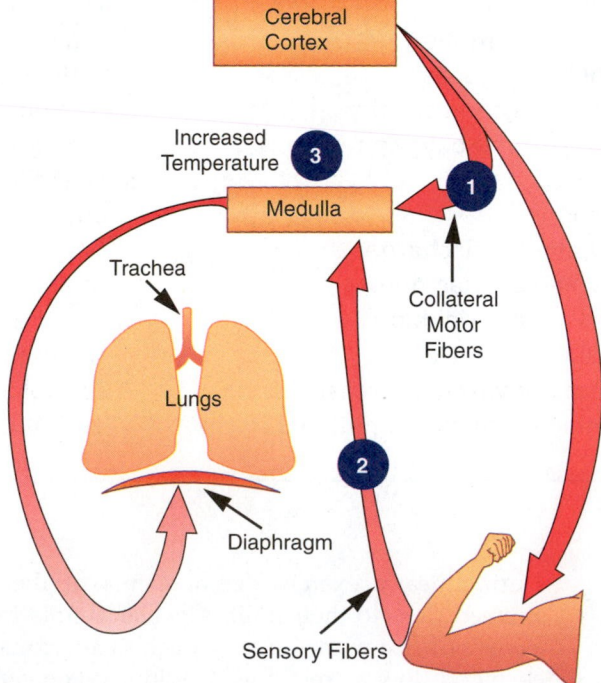

Figure 14–1. *Mechanisms by which exercise stimulates ventilation. (1) Collateral fibers from the motor neurons go to the medulla; (2) sensory signals from the exercising limbs are sent to the medulla; (3) the increase in body temperature during exercise may also increase ventilation.*

1. The cerebral cortex sending neural signals to the exercising muscles may also send collateral signals to the medulla to increase the rate and depth of breathing.
2. Proprioceptors in the moving muscles, tendons, and joints transmit sensory signals via the spinal cord to the respiratory centers of the medulla.
3. The increase in body temperature during exercise may also contribute to increased ventilation.

ALVEOLAR VENTILATION

During normal quiet breathing, an adult exchanges about 6 liters of air per minute. During strenuous exercise, this can increase to 120 liters per minute, a 20-fold increase. Depending on the intensity and duration of the exercise, alveolar ventilation must increase to (1) supply sufficient oxygen to the blood, and (2) eliminate the excess carbon dioxide produced by the skeletal muscles. The increased alveolar ventilation is produced mainly by an increased depth of ventilation (increased tidal volume) rather than by an increased rate of ventilation. During very heavy exercise, however, both an increased depth and frequency of ventilation is seen. The tidal volume is usually about 50 percent of the vital capacity, and the respiratory rate is usually between 40 and 50 breaths per minute.

There are three distinct consecutive breathing patterns seen during mild and moderate exercise. The **first stage** is characterized by an increase in alveolar ventilation, within seconds after the onset of exercise. The **second stage** is typified by a slow, gradual further increase in alveolar ventilation developing over approximately the first 3 minutes of exercise. Alveolar ventilation during this period increases almost linearly with the amount of work performed. During the **third stage**, alveolar ventilation stabilizes. When an individual stops exercising, alveolar ventilation decreases abruptly (Figure 14–2).

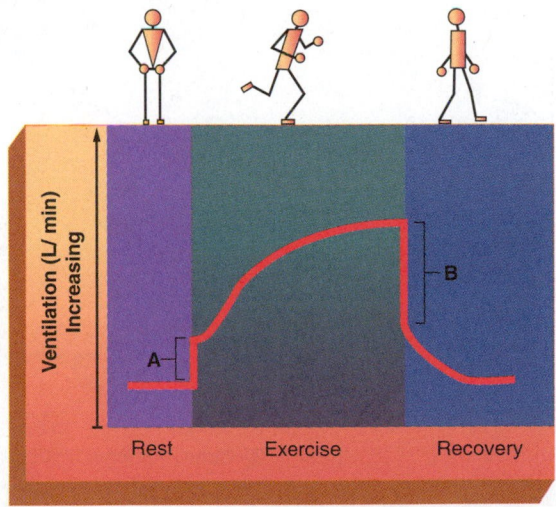

Figure 14–2. *The relationship of exercise and ventilation. Note the abrupt increase in ventilation at the outset of exercise (A) and the even larger, abrupt decrease in ventilation at the end of exercise (B).*

During very heavy exercise, the steady-state third stage may not be seen. In fact, when approximately 60 to 70 percent of the maximal exercise level is reached during the linear second stage, alveolar ventilation increases proportionately more than the oxygen uptake. The additional stimulation is thought to be caused primarily by the accumulation of lactic acids in the blood after the anaerobic threshold has been reached. It is suggested that the H^+ ions generated by the lactic acids stimulate the carotid chemoreceptors, which, in turn, send neural impulses to the medulla to increase alveolar ventilation (see Figure 10–3, page 284).

The maximum alveolar ventilation generated during heavy exercise under normal conditions is only about 50 to 65 percent of the maximum voluntary ventilation (also called maximum breathing capacity). This provides the athlete with an important reserve of alveolar ventilation, which may be required in such conditions as short bursts of increased exercise, exercise at high altitudes, or exercise during very hot and humid conditions. Because there is normally a large alveolar ventilatory reserve during exercise, it is not the limiting factor in the delivery of oxygen to the muscles during maximal muscular aerobic metabolism. As discussed later, the inability of the heart to pump sufficient blood to the working muscles is the major limiting factor.

OXYGEN CONSUMPTION

At rest, normal oxygen consumption ($\dot{V}_{O_2}$) is about 250 ml per minute. The skeletal muscles account for approximately 35 to 40 percent of the total $\dot{V}_{O_2}$. During ex-

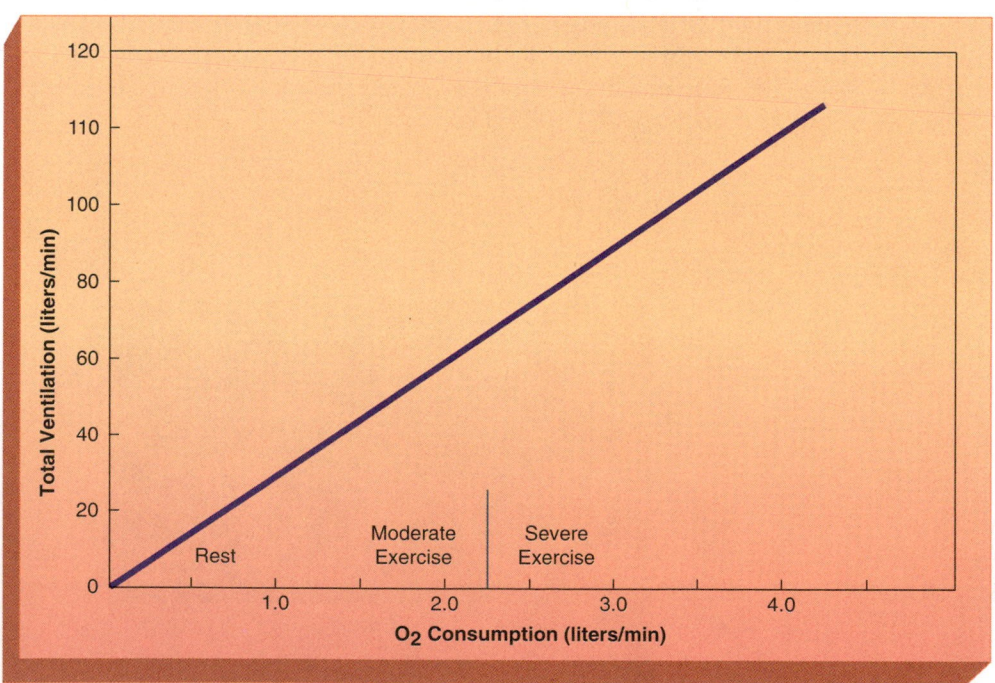

Figure 14–3. *There is a linear relationship between oxygen consumption ($\dot{V}_{O_2}$) and alveolar ventilation as the intensity of exercise increases.*

ercise, the skeletal muscles may account for more than 95 percent of the $\dot{V}_{O_2}$. During heavy exercise, the $\dot{V}_{O_2}$ of an untrained person may be more than 3500 ml of O_2 per minute. The $\dot{V}_{O_2}$ of a well-trained athlete while running a marathon may be over 5000 ml O_2 per minute. Figure 14–3 shows the linear relationship between $\dot{V}_{O_2}$ and alveolar ventilation as the intensity of exercises increases.

ARTERIAL BLOOD GASES DURING EXERCISE

No significant Pa_{O_2}, Pa_{CO_2}, or pH changes are seen between rest and approximately 60 to 70 percent of maximal $\dot{V}_{O_2}$. During very heavy exercise, however, when lactic acidosis is present, both the pH and Pa_{CO_2} decline. Although controversial, it is believed that arterial acidosis stimulates the carotid chemoreceptors, causing increased alveolar ventilation and promoting respiratory acid-base compensation. The Pa_{O_2} remains constant during mild, moderate, and heavy exercise (Figure 14–4).

OXYGEN DIFFUSION CAPACITY

The oxygen diffusion capacity increases linearly in response to the increased oxygen consumption ($\dot{V}_{O_2}$), during exercise (Figure 14–5, page 354). The oxygen diffusion capacity may increase as much as 3-fold during the state of maximum exercise. It has been shown that the increased oxygen diffusion capacity results from

Figure 14–4. *The effect of oxygen consumption on Pa_{O_2} and Pa_{CO_2} as the intensity of exercise increases.*

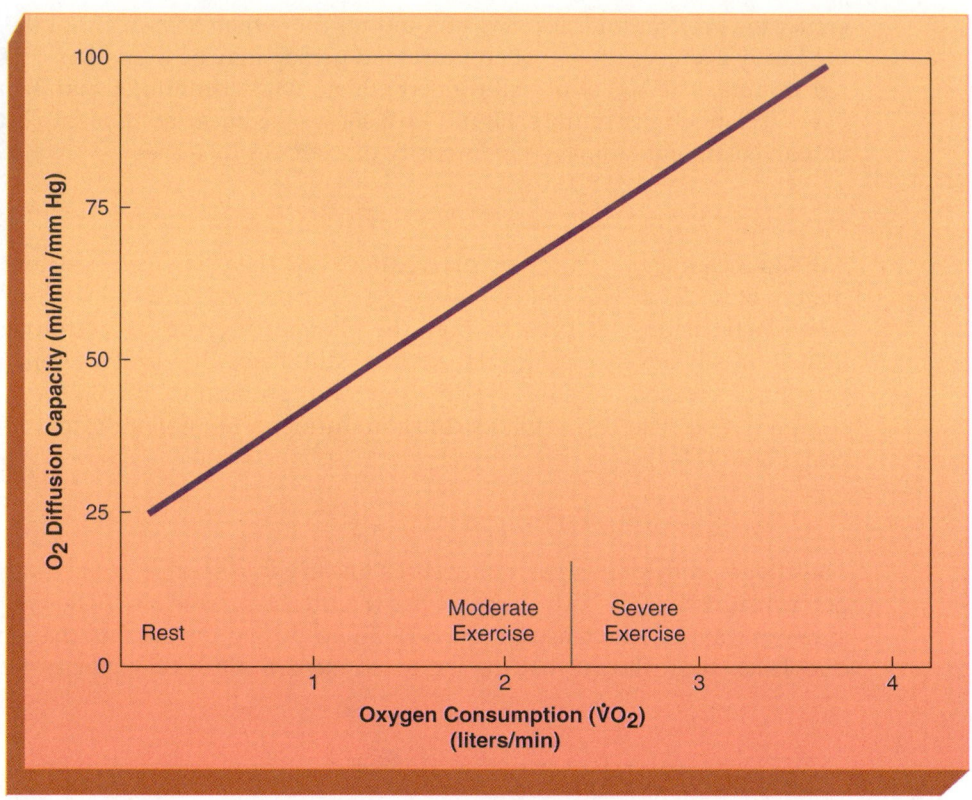

Figure 14–5. *Oxygen diffusion capacity increases linearly in response to increased oxygen consumption, as the intensity of exercise increases.*

the increased cardiac output during exercise. The increased cardiac output causes the intravascular pressure in the pulmonary artery and left atrium to increase, which in turn serves to (1) distend the pulmonary capillaries that are not fully dilated, and (2) open, or recruit, closed pulmonary capillaries (see Figure 5–21, page 178). As more blood flows through the lungs, more alveolar-capillary units become available for gas exchange. This provides a greater surface area through which oxygen can diffuse into the pulmonary capillary blood.

ALVEOLAR-ARTERIAL P_{O_2} DIFFERENCE

Normally, there is a mean alveolar-arterial oxygen tension difference $P_{(A-a)O_2}$ of about 10 mm Hg because of (1) mismatching of ventilation and perfusion, and (2) right-to-left pulmonary shunting of blood. In spite of increases in oxygen consumption ($\dot{V}_{O_2}$), alveolar ventilation, and cardiac output, the $P_{(A-a)O_2}$ remains essentially constant until 40 percent of the maximal $\dot{V}_{O_2}$ is reached. The $P_{(A-a)O_2}$ begins to increase when 40 percent of the maximal $\dot{V}_{O_2}$ is exceeded (Figure 14–6). An average $P_{(A-a)O_2}$ of 33 mm Hg has been reported for endurance runners who were exercising at their maximal $\dot{V}_{O_2}$.

Figure 14–6. *The alveolar-arterial oxygen tension difference $P_{(A-a)O_2}$ begins to increase when approximately 40 percent of the maximal $\dot{V}_{O_2}$ is exceeded.*

CIRCULATION

Heavy exercise is one of the most stressful conditions the circulatory system encounters. Blood flow to the working muscles may increase as much as 25-fold, and the total cardiac output may increase as much as 6-fold.

The ability of an individual to increase cardiac output to the muscles is the major factor that determines how long and to what intensity the exercise can be sustained. In fact, the speed of a marathon runner or swimmer is almost directly proportional to the athletes' ability to increase their cardiac output. Thus, the circulatory system is as important as the muscles themselves in setting the limits for exercise.

During exercise, three essential physiologic responses must occur in order for the circulatory system to supply the working muscles with an adequate amount of blood. These are: (1) sympathetic discharge, (2) increase in cardiac output, and (3) increase in arterial blood pressure.

SYMPATHETIC DISCHARGE

At the onset of exercise, the brain transmits signals to the vasomotor center in the medulla oblongata to trigger a sympathetic discharge. This sympathetic discharge has two circulatory effects: (1) the heart is stimulated to increase its rate and strength of contraction, and (2) the blood vessels of the peripheral vascular system constrict, except for the blood vessels of the working muscles, which strongly dilate in response to local vasodilators in the muscles themselves. The net result is an increased blood supply to the working muscles while the blood flow to nonworking muscles is reduced. It should be noted that vasoconstriction in the heart and brain does not occur during exercise, since both the heart and the brain are as important to exercise as the working muscles themselves.

INCREASED CARDIAC OUTPUT

The increased oxygen demands during exercise are met almost entirely by an increased cardiac output. Figure 14–7 shows that there is a linear relationship between the cardiac output and the intensity of exercise. The increased cardiac output during exercise results from (1) increased stroke volume, (2) increased heart rate, or (3) a combination of both.

Increased Stroke Volume

The increased stroke volume during exercise is primarily due to vasodilation in the working muscles. That is, the vasodilation in the working muscles increases the

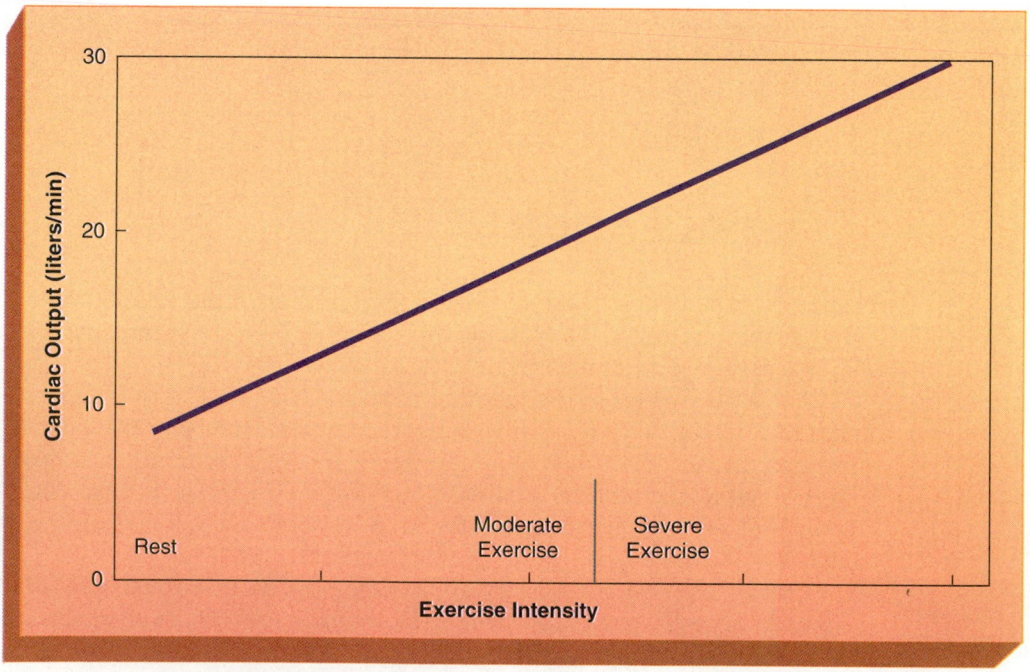

Figure 14–7. *There is a linear relationship between cardiac output and the intensity of exercise.*

venous return to the heart. The heart, in turn, pumps more oxygenated blood back to the working muscles. Thus, the degree of vasodilation in the working muscles directly influences the stroke volume and, therefore, the greater the vasodilation in the working muscles, the greater the stroke volume and cardiac output. Another factor that facilitates an increased venous return during exercise is the sympathetic discharge. This causes a constriction of all venous blood reservoirs and forces more blood out of the veins and toward the heart.

As discussed in Chapter 5, the ability of the heart to accommodate the increased venous return and, subsequently, increase the cardiac output is due to the Frank-Starling mechanism (see Figure 5–19, page 175). When more venous blood returns to the heart, the heart chambers increase in size to accommodate the increased volume. As the heart chambers increase in size, the force of the heart muscle contractions increase, which in turn increases the stroke volume.

In addition to the Frank-Starling mechanism, the heart is also strongly stimulated by the sympathetic discharge. Increased sympathetic stimulation causes (1) increased heart rate (as high as 200 beats per minute), and (2) increased strength of contraction. The combined effect of these two mechanisms greatly increases the heart's ability to pump blood beyond what could be accomplished by the Frank-Starling mechanism alone.

Increased Heart Rate

An individual's maximum heart rate is estimated by the following formula:

maximum heart rate = 220 − age

Thus, the maximum heart rate for a 45-year-old is about 175 (220 − 45 = 175).

Although the heart rate increases linearly with oxygen consumption, the magnitude of the change is influenced by the size of the stroke volume. That is, when the stroke volume decreases, the heart rate increases, and when the stroke volume increases, the heart rate decreases. The stroke volume, in turn, is influenced by (1) the individual's physical condition, (2) the specific muscles that are working, and (3) the distribution of blood flow. The body's ability to increase the heart rate and stroke volume during exercise progressively declines with age.

INCREASED ARTERIAL BLOOD PRESSURE

There is an increase in arterial blood pressure during exercise because of the (1) sympathetic discharge, (2) increased cardiac output, and (3) vasoconstriction of the blood vessels in the non-working muscle areas. Depending on the physical condition of the individual, as well as the intensity and duration of the exercise, the systolic arterial blood pressure may increase as little as 20 mm Hg or as much as 80 mm Hg.

PULMONARY VASCULAR PRESSURES

As oxygen consumption and cardiac output increase during exercise, the systolic, diastolic, and mean pulmonary arterial and wedge pressures also increase linearly (Figure 14–8, page 358). As discussed earlier, this mechanism enhances oxygen uptake by (1) distending the pulmonary capillaries, and (2) opening closed pulmonary capillaries.

Figure 14–8. *The systolic, diastolic, and mean pulmonary arterial and wedge pressures increase linearly as oxygen consumption and cardiac output increase.*

OPENING OF MUSCLE CAPILLARIES

At rest, approximately only 20 to 25 percent of the muscle capillaries are open. During heavy exercise, all these capillaries open up to facilitate the distribution of blood. This reduces the distance that oxygen and other nutrients must travel from the capillaries to the muscle fiber. At the same time, the blood vessels of the viscera and non-working muscles constrict.

The dilation of the blood vessels in the working muscles is caused primarily by local vasodilators acting directly on the arterioles. The most important local vasodilator effect is the reduction of oxygen in the working muscles. It is suggested that a diminished oxygen concentration in the muscles causes vasodilation because either (1) the vessels are unable to maintain contraction at low oxygen levels, or (2) low oxygen levels cause the release of vasodilator substances. The most likely vasodilator substance is *adenosine*. Other vasodilator substances include potassium ions, acetylcholine, adenosine triphosphate, lactic acids, and carbon dioxide. The precise role of each of these substances in increasing blood flow to working muscles is not known.

Finally, because the vasodilation of the major working muscle groups is greater than the vasoconstriction of the non-working muscle groups, the overall peripheral vascular resistance decreases. This is why highly trained athletes can increase their cardiac output substantially with only a slight increase in their mean systemic arterial blood pressure. Untrained individuals have a high peripheral vascular resistance and, therefore, high arterial blood pressure in response to modest increases in cardiac output during exercise.

INTERRELATIONSHIPS BETWEEN MUSCLE WORK, OXYGEN CONSUMPTION, AND CARDIAC OUTPUT

Figure 14–9 shows that muscle work, oxygen consumption, and cardiac output are all related to each other. Increased muscle work increases oxygen consumption and the increased oxygen consumption, in turn, dilates the intramuscular blood

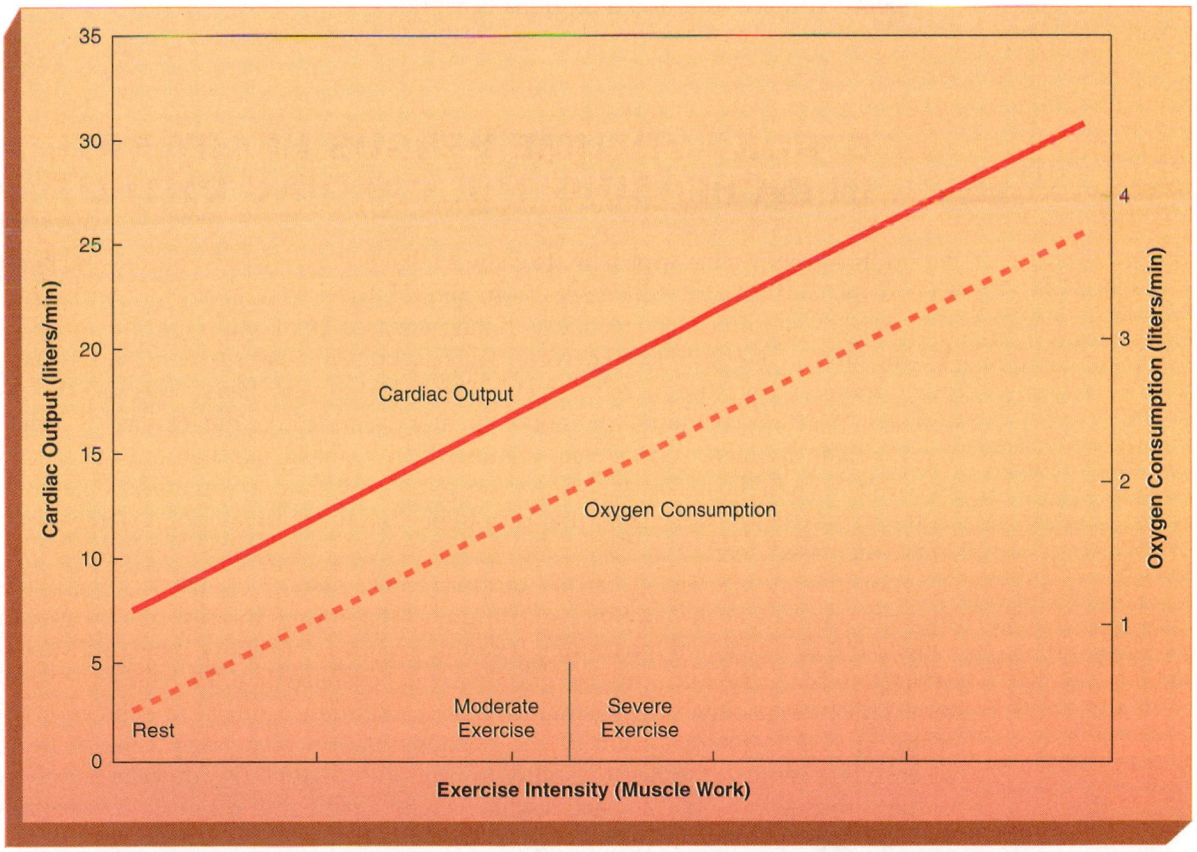

Figure 14–9. *Relationship between muscle work, oxygen consumption, and cardiac output.*

vessels. As the intramuscular blood vessels dilate, venous return increases, causing the cardiac output to rise. Marathon runners can have a cardiac output as great as 40 L per minute. The maximum cardiac output of a young, untrained individual is less than 25 L per minute.

THE INFLUENCE OF TRAINING ON THE HEART AND ON CARDIAC OUTPUT

The increased cardiac output seen in marathon runners results mainly from the fact that the heart chambers and heart mass increase as much as 40 percent. Cardiac enlargement and increased pumping ability occur only in the endurance type of athletic training and not in the sprint type of activity. The "athlete's heart" is an effective and physiologically sound heart. It should not be considered a pathologic heart. At rest, the cardiac output of the well-trained athletic is almost the same as that of the average untrained individual. The well-trained individual, however, has a greater stroke volume and a reduced heart rate.

STROKE VOLUME VERSUS HEART RATE IN INCREASING THE CARDIAC OUTPUT

Figure 14–10 shows the approximate changes that occur in stroke volume and heart rate as the cardiac output increases from about 5 L per minute to 30 L per minute in a marathon runner. The stroke volume increases from about 100 ml to about 150 ml, an increase of about 50 percent. The heart rate increases from 50 to 180 beats per minute, an increase of 260 percent. Thus, during very heavy exercise the increase in heart rate accounts for a much greater proportion of the increased cardiac output than the increase in stroke volume. In fact, the stroke volume reaches its maximum when the maximum cardiac output is only at approximately 50 percent. Thus, any further increase in cardiac output beyond the midway point is due solely to the increased heart rate.

At maximum exercise, cardiac output reaches about 90 percent of the maximum that can be achieved. Since maximum exercise taxes the respiratory system only about 65 percent of maximum, it can be seen that normally the cardiovascular system is a greater limiting factor on maximal exercise than the respiratory system. Thus, the maximum performance that a marathon runner can achieve is directly related to the condition of the cardiovascular system. Any type of heart disease that reduces the heart's ability to pump blood will also decrease an individual's muscle power. This partly explains why a patient in congestive heart failure may have difficulty in generating enough muscle power to climb out of bed, or to walk short distances.

Figure 14–10. *Approximate changes in stroke volume and heart rate that occur when the cardiac output increases from about 5 liters per minute to 30 liters per minute in a marathon runner.*

BODY TEMPERATURE/CUTANEOUS BLOOD FLOW RELATIONSHIP

During exercise, the body generates a tremendous amount of heat and heat production may increase as much as 20-fold. Although some of the heat is stored in the body during exercise, most of the heat is dissipated through the skin. This requires a substantial increase in blood flow to the body surface. Nevertheless, even during normal temperature and humidity conditions the body temperature may rise from its normal 98.6°F to 102° to 103°F (37°C to 40°C) during endurance athletics.

When exercise is performed during very hot and humid conditions, or without adequately ventilated clothing, heat loss may be impaired and an unusually large amount of blood may be distributed to the skin. During these conditions the body temperature can easily rise to 106° to 108°F. As much as 5 to 10 lb of body fluid can be lost in one hour. When this happens, a number of symptoms may appear, which collectively are referred to as **heat stroke**. These symptoms include:

- Profuse sweating, followed by no sweating
- Extreme weakness
- Muscle cramping

- Exhaustion
- Nausea
- Headache
- Dizziness
- Confusion
- Staggering gait
- Unconsciousness
- Circulatory collapse

Heat stroke can be lethal if not treated immediately. Even when the individual stops exercising, the temperature does not readily return to normal. This is because of (1) the temperature-regulating mechanism often fails at a very high temperature, and (2) the intracellular metabolism is much faster at higher temperatures, which in turn generates still more heat.

The primary treatment of heat stroke is to reduce the victim's body temperature as fast as possible. This is done by (1) spraying cool water on the victim's body, (2) continually sponging the victim with cool water, (3) blowing air over the body with a strong fan, or (4) a combination of all three.

CARDIOVASCULAR REHABILITATION

Cardiovascular rehabilitation is now a well accepted, multidisciplinary health care service. It provides cardiac patients with a process of developing and maintaining a desirable level of physical, social, and psychologic well-being. The prominent components of a cardiovascular rehabilitation program are patient education, counseling, nutritional guidance, and graded exercise training. The rehabilitative process for the cardiac patient is commonly divided into the following four phases:

PHASE I: ACUTE, IN-HOSPITAL

This phase consists of low-level exercise, patient and family education, group and individual counseling, and group discussion sessions.

PHASE II: OUTPATIENT, IMMEDIATELY AFTER HOSPITALIZATION

During this phase, the patient begins active range-of-motion exercises. Such exercises include work on the treadmill, air-dyne bike, arm ergometer, rowing machine, chest pulleys, and steps. The duration of phase II is between 2 and 4 months.

PHASE III: LONG-TERM OUTPATIENT

This phase includes the long-term aspects of cardiac rehabilitation. The primary objective during this phase is the conditioning of the cardiovascular system (aerobic) and skeletal muscles. Long-term graded exercises are emphasized, such as walking, walking/jogging, stationary bicycling, and/or swimming. The duration of phase III is between 6 and 24 months.

PHASE IV: MAINTENANCE

Phase IV of rehabilitation is the maintenance of the patient's physical condition. Components of phase IV include efforts to modify risk factors (e.g., control of blood lipids, cigarette smoking, hypertension, and obesity) and a routine program of physical activity. This phase should continue indefinitely. The patient commonly goes through a yearly evaluation, which includes graded exercise testing. Some patients may require more frequent evaluations.

The benefits from cardiac rehabilitation include improved exercise capacity and decreased angina pectoris, dyspnea, and fatigue. Patients involved in exercise training after myocardial infarction demonstrate a 20 to 25 percent reduction in mortality and major cardiac mishaps. Cardiac rehabilitation may improve oxygen transport, reduce the myocardial oxygen requirements during work, and reduce myocardial ischemia during physical activity. Finally, the efforts to modify risk factors during cardiac rehabilitation has clearly shown a reduction in the progression of coronary artery disease, morbidity, and mortality.

REVIEW QUESTIONS

1. During strenuous exercise, an adult's alveolar ventilation can increase as much as:
   a. 10-fold
   b. 20-fold
   c. 30-fold
   d. 40-fold
   e. 50-fold
2. The maximum alveolar ventilation generated during heavy exercise under normal conditions is about what percent of the maximum voluntary ventilation?
   a. 10–25%
   b. 20–35%
   c. 30–45%
   d. 40–55%
   e. 50–65%
3. During heavy exercise, the total cardiac output may increase as much as:
   a. 2-fold
   b. 4-fold
   c. 6-fold
   d. 8-fold
   e. 10-fold
4. At the onset of exercise, sympathetic discharge causes the:
   I. Heart rate to decrease

II. Peripheral vascular system to constrict

III. Heart to increase its strength of contraction

IV. Blood vessels of the working muscles to dilate

    a. I only

    b. III only

    c. II and IV only

    d. I and II only

    e. II, III, and IV only

5. During exercise, the stroke volume reaches its peak when the cardiac output is at about what percent of its maximum:

    a. 30%

    b. 40%

    c. 50%

    d. 60%

    e. 70%

6. During exercise, heat production may increase as much as:

    a. 10-fold

    b. 20-fold

    c. 30-fold

    d. 40-fold

    e. 50-fold

7. During exercise, the oxygen consumption ($\dot{V}_{O_2}$) of the skeletal muscles may account for more than:

    a. 55% of the total $\dot{V}_{O_2}$

    b. 65% of the total $\dot{V}_{O_2}$

    c. 75% of the total $\dot{V}_{O_2}$

    d. 85% of the total $\dot{V}_{O_2}$

    e. 95% of the total $\dot{V}_{O_2}$

8. During very heavy exercise, the:

    I. pH increases

    II. Pa_{CO_2} decreases

    III. Pa_{O_2} remains constant

    IV. pH decreases

    V. Pa_{CO_2} increases

      a. I and II only

      b. IV and V only

      c. II and IV only

      d. II, III, and IV only

      e. III, IV, and V only

9. During maximum exercise, the oxygen diffusion capacity may increase as much as:

    a. 3-fold

    b. 6-fold

    c. 9-fold

    d. 12-fold

    e. 15-fold

10. During exercise, the $P_{(A-a)O_2}$ begins to increase when the oxygen consumption reaches about what percent of its maximum?
    a. 10%
    b. 20%
    c. 30%
    d. 40%
    e. 50%

CHAPTER FIFTEEN

HIGH ALTITUDE AND ITS EFFECTS ON THE CARDIOPULMONARY SYSTEM

OBJECTIVES

By the end of this chapter, the student should be able to:

1. Describe the effects of high altitude on the following components of the cardiopulmonary system:
   —Ventilation
   —Red blood cell production
   —Acid-base status
   —Oxygen diffusion capacity
   —Alveolar-arterial oxygen tension difference
   —Ventilation-perfusion relationship
   —Cardiac output

   —Pulmonary vascular system
   —Myoglobin concentration
2. Describe other physiologic changes caused by high altitude, including:
   —Sleep
   —Acute mountain sickness
   —High-altitude pulmonary edema
   —High-altitude cerebral edema
   —Chronic mountain sickness
3. Complete the review questions at the end of this chapter.

HIGH ALTITUDE

The effects of high altitude on the cardiopulmonary system are of interest, since a better understanding of chronic oxygen deprivation can be applied to the treatment of chronic hypoxia caused by lung disease.

The barometric pressure progressively decreases with altitude (Figure 15–1). At an altitude of 18,000 to 19,000 ft, the barometric pressure is about half the sea level value of 760 mm Hg (380 mm Hg). The barometric pressure on the summit of Mount Everest (altitude: 29,028 ft) is about 250 mm Hg (the atmospheric P_{O_2}

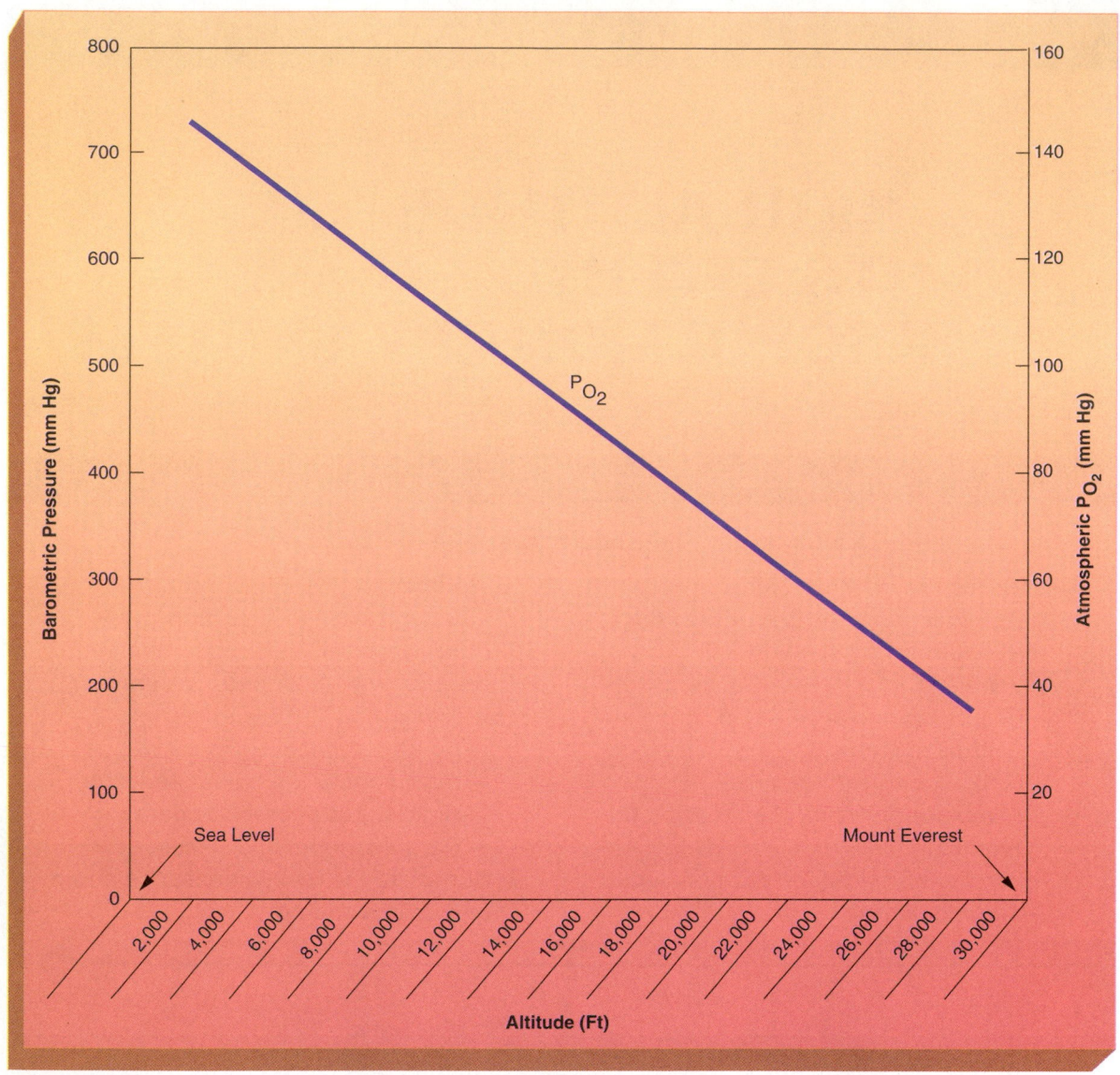

Figure 15–1. *The barometric pressure and the atmospheric P_{O_2} decrease linearly as altitude increases.*

is about 43 mm Hg). At an altitude of about 65,000 ft, the barometric pressure falls below the pressure of water vapor and tissue fluids begin to "boil" or "vaporize."

When an individual who normally lives near sea level spends a period of time at high altitudes, a number of compensatory responses develop—a process known as **acclimatization**. For example, it is an interesting fact that after a period of acclimatization, an individual may reach the summit of Mount Everest without supplementary oxygen. However, when an individual is suddenly exposed to the oxygen tension found at the summit of Mount Everest, a loss of consciousness occurs within minutes.

The following are some of the major cardiopulmonary changes seen after a period of acclimatization at high altitude.

VENTILATION

One of the most prominent features of acclimatization is increased alveolar ventilation. As already mentioned, when an individual ascends above the earth's surface, the barometric pressure progressively decreases and the atmospheric P_{O_2} declines. As the atmospheric P_{O_2} decreases, the individual's arterial oxygen pressure (Pa_{O_2}) also decreases. Eventually, the Pa_{O_2} will fall low enough (to about 60 mm Hg) to stimulate the carotid and aortic bodies, known collectively as the **peripheral chemoreceptors** (see Figure 10–3, page 284). When the peripheral chemoreceptors are stimulated, they transmit signals to the medulla to increase ventilation (see Figure 10–4). Because the peripheral chemoreceptors do not acclimate to a decreased oxygen concentration, increased alveolar ventilation will continue for the entire time the individual remains at the high altitude.

POLYCYTHEMIA

When an individual is subjected to a low concentration of oxygen for a prolonged period of time, the hormone *erythropoietin* from the kidneys stimulates the bone marrow to increase red blood cell (RBC) production. The increased hemoglobin available in polycythemia is an adaptive mechanism that increases the oxygen-carrying capacity of the blood. In fact, people who live at high altitudes often have a normal, or even above-normal, oxygen-carrying capacity, in spite of a chronically low Pa_{O_2} and oxygen saturation.

In lowlanders who ascend to high altitudes, the RBCs increase for about six weeks before the production rate levels off. As the level of RBCs increase the plasma volume decreases. Thus, there is no significant change in the total circulating blood volume. After six weeks, an average hemoglobin concentration of 20.5 g/dl has been observed in mountain climbers who were at altitudes greater than 18,000 ft.

ACID-BASE STATUS

Because of the increased ventilation generated by the peripheral chemoreceptors at high altitudes, the Pa_{CO_2} decreases, causing a secondary respiratory alkalosis. Over a 24- to 48-hour period, the renal system tries to offset the respiratory alkalosis by eliminating some of the excess bicarbonate. In spite of this mechanism, however, a mild respiratory alkalosis usually persists. In fact, even natives, who have been at high altitudes for generations, commonly have a mild respiratory alkalosis.

It is assumed that respiratory alkalosis may be advantageous for the transfer of oxygen across the alveolar-capillary membrane, since alkalosis increases the affinity of hemoglobin for oxygen. In other words, the alkalosis enhances the loading of oxygen to the hemoglobin as desaturated blood passes through the alveolar-capillary system (see Figure 7–9, page 218). It is also argued, however, that the increased affinity interferes with the unloading of oxygen at the cells (see Figure 7–10, page 219).

There is both experimental and theoretical evidence that the increased oxygen affinity at high altitude is beneficial. This is further supported by the fact that a mild respiratory alkalosis usually persists in mountain climbers, high-altitude natives, and even in animals who live in low-oxygen environments. The alkalosis persists even after the kidneys should have had more than enough time to fully eliminate the excess bicarbonate.

OXYGEN DIFFUSION CAPACITY

There is no significant change in the oxygen diffusion capacity of lowlanders who are acclimatized to high altitude. High-altitude natives, however, have been shown to have an oxygen diffusion capacity that is about 20 to 25 percent greater than predicted, both during rest and exercise. The increased oxygen diffusion may be explained by the larger lungs seen in the high-altitude natives. It is suggested that the larger lungs provide an increased alveolar surface area and a larger capillary blood volume.

This is further supported by studies that demonstrate that when animals are exposed to low-oxygen partial pressures during their active growth period, they develop larger lungs and greater diffusion capacity. On the other hand, animals exposed to a hyperoxic environment during their active growth period develop smaller lungs than expected.

ALVEOLAR-ARTERIAL P_{O_2} DIFFERENCE

At high altitude, oxygen diffusion across the alveolar-capillary membrane is limited and this results in an increased **alveolar-arterial oxygen tension difference** ($P_{(A-a)O_2}$). Figure 15–2 shows that under normal circumstances there is ample time for oxygen to equilibrate between the alveoli and the end-capillary blood. In contrast, Figure 15–3 (page 372) shows the estimated time necessary for oxygen to equilibrate for a climber at rest on the summit of Mount Everest. Note that the pulmonary blood enters the alveolar-capillary system with a P_{O_2} of about 21 mm Hg and slowly rises to about 28 mm Hg. As the blood leaves the alveolar-capillary system, there is thus a large $P_{(A-a)O_2}$ characteristic of oxygen diffusion-limitations. At high altitude, the $P_{(A-a)O_2}$ is further increased (1) during exercise—because of the increased cardiac output—and (2) in individuals with alveolar thickening caused by interstitial lung disease.

VENTILATION-PERFUSION RELATIONSHIP

At high altitude, the overall ventilation-perfusion ratio improves as a result of the more uniform distribution of blood flow that develops in response to the increased pulmonary arterial blood pressure. Under normal circumstances the better gas exchange that results from the improved ventilation-perfusion ratio is relatively insignificant.

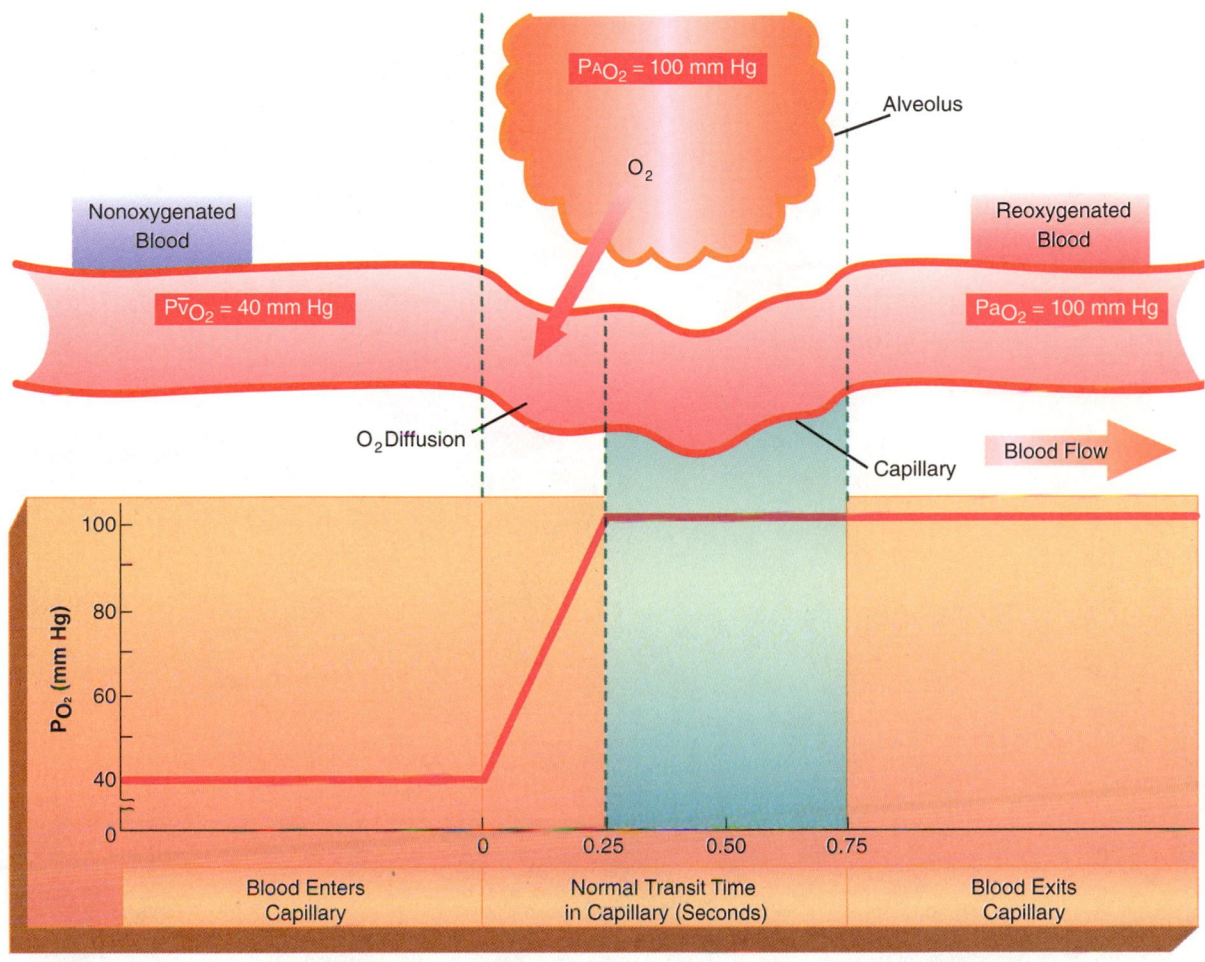

Figure 15–2. *Under normal resting conditions, blood moves through the alveolar-capillary membrane in about 0.75 second. The oxygen pressure (P$_{O_2}$) reaches equilibrium in about 0.25 second—one-third of the time available.*

CARDIAC OUTPUT

When an individual is acutely exposed to a hypoxic environment, the cardiac output during both rest and exercise increases, which increases the oxygen delivery to the peripheral cells. In individuals who have acclimatized to high altitude, however, and in high-altitude natives, increased cardiac output is not seen. Cardiac output and oxygen uptake are the same as at sea level. The precise reason for the return of the cardiac output and oxygen uptake to sea level values is unknown. It has been suggested that the polycythemia that develops in well-acclimatized subjects may play a role.

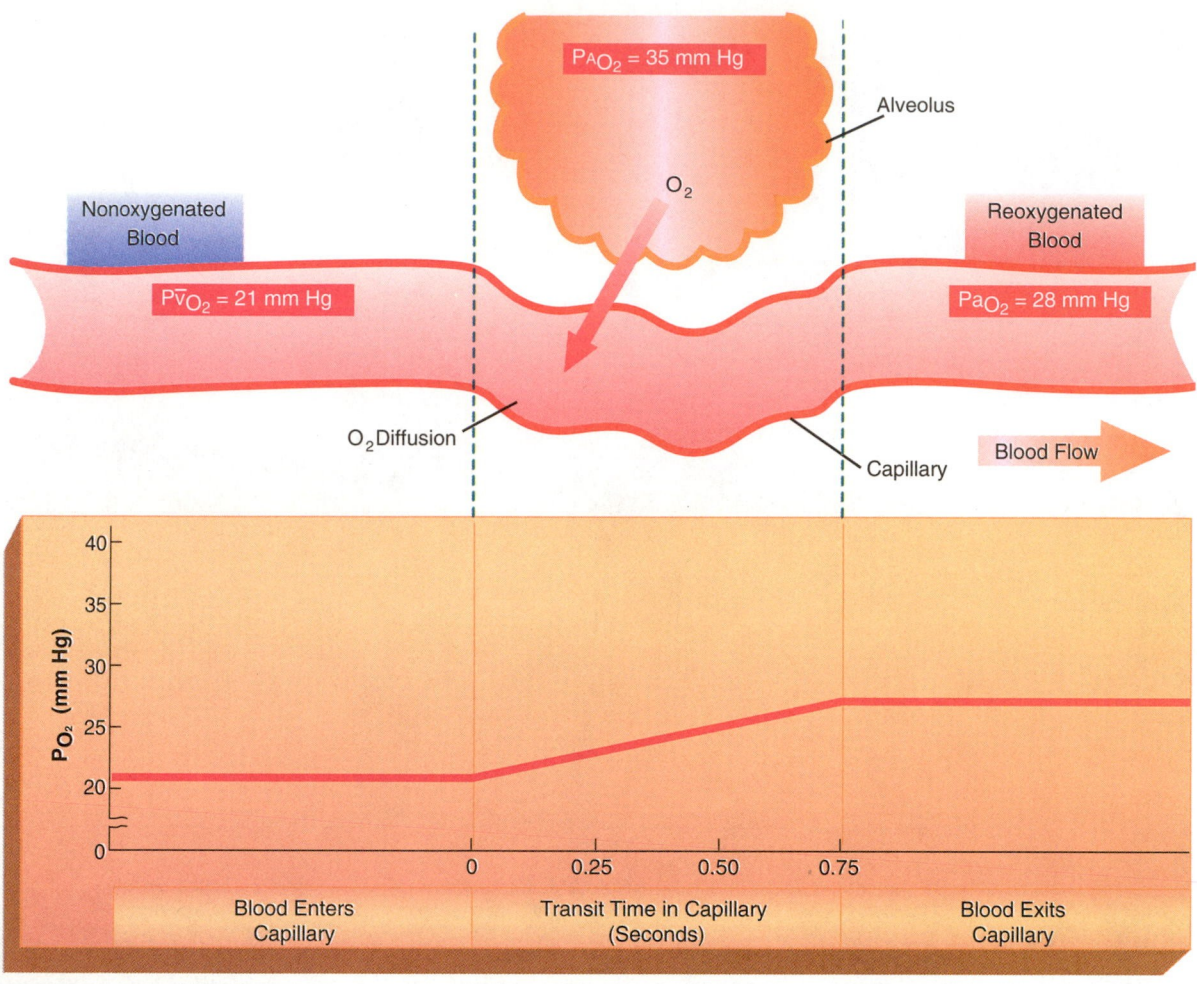

Figure 15–3. *Estimated time necessary for oxygen diffusion for a climber at rest on the summit of Mount Everest. As the blood leaves the alveolar-capillary system, there is a large alveolar-arterial oxygen tension difference $P_{(A-a)O_2}$.*

PULMONARY VASCULAR SYSTEM

As an individual ascends from the earth's surface, pulmonary hypertension progressively increases as a result of hypoxic pulmonary vasoconstriction. There is a linear relationship between the degree of ascent and the degree of pulmonary vasoconstriction and hypertension (Figure 15–4). The exact mechanism of this phenomenon is unclear. It is known, however, that it is the partial pressure of oxygen in the alveoli and not the partial pressure of arterial oxygen that chiefly controls this response.

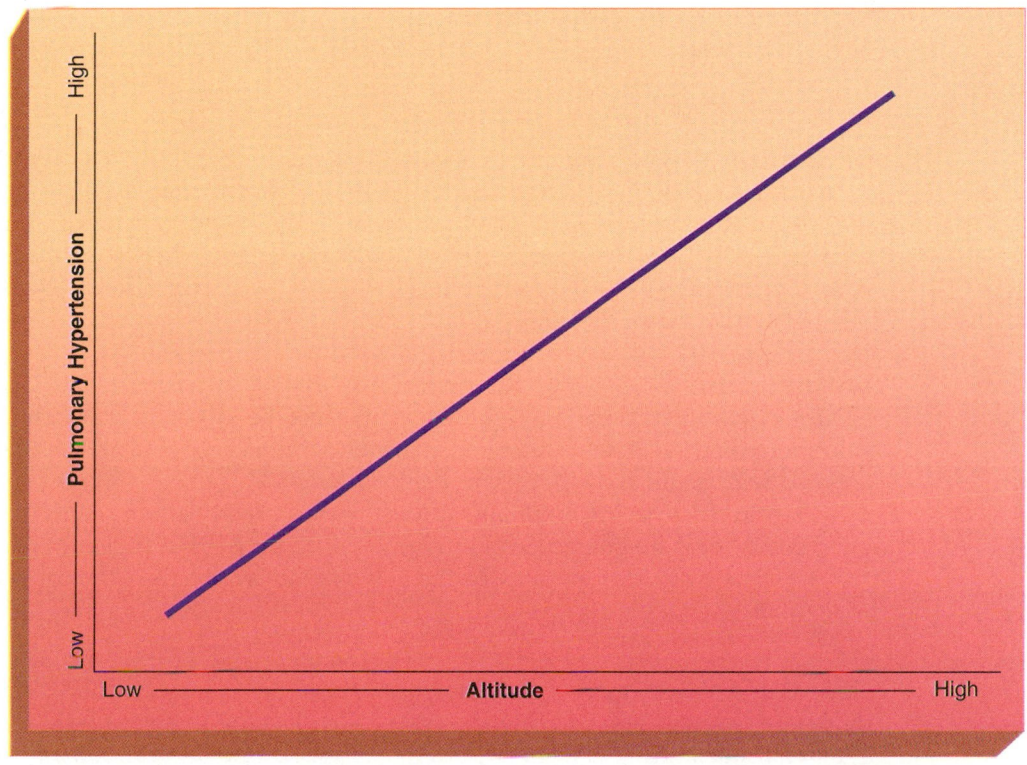

Figure 15–4. *Pulmonary hypertension increases linearly as altitude increases.*

 OTHER PHYSIOLOGIC CHANGES

SLEEP

During the first few days at high altitude, lowlanders frequently wake up during the night and complain that they do not feel refreshed when they awake in the morning. When sleeping, they commonly demonstrate breathing that waxes and wanes with apneic periods of 10 to 15 seconds duration (Cheyne-Stokes breathing). The arterial oxygen saturation (Sa_{O_2}) fluctuates accordingly.

MYOGLOBIN CONCENTRATION

The concentration of myoglobin in skeletal muscles is increased in high-altitude natives, and research in this group has shown a high concentration of myoglobin in the diaphragm, in the adductor muscles of the leg, in the pectoral muscles, and in the myocardium. Myoglobin enhances the transfer of oxygen between the capillary blood and peripheral cells, buffers regional P_{O_2} differences, and provides an oxygen storage compartment for short periods of very severe oxygen deprivation.

ACUTE MOUNTAIN SICKNESS

Newcomers to high altitude frequency experience what is known as acute mountain sickness. It is characterized by headache, fatigue, dizziness, palpitation, nausea, loss of appetite, and insomnia. Symptoms commonly do not occur until 6 to 12 hours after an individual ascends to a high altitude. The symptoms are generally most severe on the second or third day after ascent. Acclimatization is usually complete by the fourth or fifth day.

The precise cause of acute mountain sickness is not known. It is suggested that the primary cause is hypoxia, complicated by the hypocapnia and respiratory alkalosis associated with high altitude. It may also be linked to a fluid imbalance, since pulmonary edema, cerebral edema, and peripheral edema are commonly associated with acute and chronic mountain sickness.

Sensitivity to acute mountain sickness varies greatly among individuals. Being physical fit is no guarantee of immunity. Younger people appear to be more at risk. In some cases, descent may be the only way to reduce the symptoms.

HIGH-ALTITUDE PULMONARY EDEMA

High-altitude pulmonary edema is sometimes seen in individuals with acute mountain sickness. A typical scenario is as follows: A lowlander rapidly ascends to a high altitude and is very active during the trip, or upon arrival. Initially, the lowlander demonstrates shortness of breath, fatigue, and a dry cough. Physical signs include tachypnea, tachycardia, and crackles at the lung bases. Orthopnea (see page 98) is commonly present at this time. In severe cases, the lowlander may cough up large amounts of pink, frothy sputum. Death may occur.

The exact cause of high-altitude pulmonary edema is not fully understood. It may be associated with the pulmonary vasoconstriction that occurs in response to the alveolar hypoxia. It may also be associated with an increased permeability of the pulmonary capillaries. The best treatment of high-altitude pulmonary edema is rapid descent. Oxygen should be administered if available.

HIGH-ALTITUDE CEREBRAL EDEMA

High-altitude cerebral edema is a serious complication of acute mountain sickness. It is characterized by photophobia, ataxia, hallucinations, clouding of consciousness, coma, and, possibly, death. The precise cause of high-altitude cerebral edema is unclear. It is suggested that it may be linked to the increased cerebral vasodilation and blood flow that results from hypoxia. Oxygen should be administered if available.

CHRONIC MOUNTAIN SICKNESS

Chronic mountain sickness (also known as Monge's disease) is sometimes seen in long-term residents at high altitude. It is characterized by fatigue, reduced exercise tolerance, headache, dizziness, somnolence, loss of mental acuity, marked polycythemia, and severe hypoxemia. The severe oxygen desaturation and polycythemia causes a cyanotic appearance. Hematocrit of 83 percent and hemoglobin concentrations as high as 28 g/dl have been reported. As a result of the high hematocrit, the viscosity of the blood is significantly increased. Right ventricular hypertrophy is common.

REVIEW QUESTIONS

1. The barometric pressure is about half the sea level value of 760 mm Hg at an altitude of:
   a. 4,000–5,000 ft
   b. 9,000–10,000 ft
   c. 14,000–15,000 ft
   d. 18,000–19,000 ft
   e. 24,000–25,000 ft
2. The oxygen diffusion capacity of high-altitude natives is about
   a. 5–10% greater than predicted
   b. 10–15% greater than predicted
   c. 15–20% greater than predicted
   d. 20–25% greater than predicted
   e. 25–30% greater than predicted
3. Acute mountain sickness is characterized by:
   I. Insomnia
   II. Headache
   III. Dizziness
   IV. Palpitation
   V. Loss of appetite
      a. I and III only
      b. II and IV only
      c. III, IV, and V only
      d. II, III, and IV only
      e. I, II, III, IV, and V
4. The symptoms of acute mountain sickness are generally most severe on the:
   a. First or second day after ascent
   b. Second or third day after ascent
   c. Third or fourth day after ascent
   d. Fourth of fifth day after ascent
   e. Fifth or sixth day after ascent
5. When an individual is subjected to a high altitude for a prolonged period of time, which of the following is/are seen?
   I. An increased red blood cell production
   II. A decreased Pa_{CO_2}
   III. An increased $P_{(A-a)O_2}$
   IV. A decreased alveolar ventilation
      a. I and III only
      b. II and IV only

      c. III and IV only

      d. I, II, and III only

      e. I, III, and IV only

6. At high altitude, the overall ventilation-perfusion   True _____ False _____
ratio decreases.

7. In individuals who have acclimatized to a high   True _____ False _____
altitude, an increased cardiac output is seen.

8. There is a linear relationship between the degree   True _____ False _____
of ascent and the degree of pulmonary
vasoconstriction and hypertension.

9. Natives who have been at high altitudes for   True _____ False _____
generations commonly demonstrate a mild
respiratory alkalosis.

10. The concentration of myoglobin in skeletal   True _____ False _____
muscles is decreased in high-altitude natives.

CHAPTER SIXTEEN

HIGH-PRESSURE ENVIRONMENTS AND THEIR EFFECTS ON THE CARDIOPULMONARY SYSTEM

OBJECTIVES

By the end of this chapter, the student should be able to:

1. Describe how the following relate to the effects of high-pressure environments on the cardiopulmonary system:
   —Breath-hold diving
   —The CO_2–O_2 paradox
   —The dive response
   —Decompression sickness
   —Hyperbaric medicine
2. Complete the review questions at the end of this chapter.

High-pressure environments have a profound effect on the cardiopulmonary system. In general, high-pressure environments include recreational scuba diving, deep sea diving, and hyperbaric medicine. The effects of high-pressure environments on the cardiopulmonary system are typically studied in (1) actual dives in the sea, (2) hyperbaric chambers where the subject is exposed to mixtures of compressed gases (known as "simulated dry dives"), and (3) a water-filled hyperbaric chamber that can simulate any depth by adjusting the gas pressure above the water (known as "simulated wet dives").

DIVING

Because water is incompressible, the pressure increases linearly with depth. For every 33 feet (10 m) below the surface, the pressure increases 1.0 atmosphere (760 mm Hg). Thus, the total pressure at a depth of 33 feet is 2 atmospheres (1520 mm Hg)—1.0 atmosphere (1 atm) is due to the water column and 1.0 atmosphere pressure is due to the gaseous atmosphere above the water. At 66 feet (20 m) below the surface, the pressure is 3.0 atmospheres (2280 mm Hg) (Figure 16–1).

Figure 16–1. *Pressure increases linearly with depth. For every 33 feet (10 m) below sea level, the pressure increases 1.0 atmosphere.*

As an individual descends into water, the lung is compressed according to Boyle's law:

$$P_1 \times V_1 = P_2 \times V_2$$

where P_1 = the pressure prior to the dive, V_1 = the lung volume prior to the dive, P_2 = the pressure generated at a specific water depth, and V_2 = the lung volume at that water depth.

Thus, if an individual fully inhales to a total lung capacity of 6 liters at sea level, and dives to a depth of 33 feet, the lungs will be compressed to about 3 liters:

$$V_2 = \frac{P_1 \times V_1}{P_2}$$

$$= \frac{1 \times 6}{2}$$

$$= 3 \text{ liters}$$

At 66 feet, the lungs would be compressed to about 2 liters. At 99 feet, the lungs would be compressed to about 1.5 liters.

Boyle's law can also be used to calculate the pressure within a diver's lungs at a specific depth. For example, when the above diver descends from sea level to a depth of 33 feet (compressing the lung volume from 6 to 3 liters), the pressure within the diver's lungs will increase from 760 mm Hg to about 1520 mm Hg:

$$P_2 = \frac{P_1 \times V_1}{V_2}$$

$$= 760 \times 6\ 3$$

$$= 1520 \text{ mm Hg}$$

At 66 feet, the pressure within a diver's lungs will be about 2280 mm Hg. At 99 feet, the pressure will be about 3040 mm Hg.

BREATH-HOLD DIVING

Breath-hold diving is the simplest and most popular form of diving. The maximum time of a breath-hold dive is a function of (1) the diver's metabolic rate, and (2) the diver's ability to store and transport O_2 and CO_2. A delicate balance exists between the diver's O_2 and CO_2 levels during a breath-hold dive. For example, the P_{CO_2} must not rise too rapidly and reach the so-called respiratory drive "**breaking point**" (generally about 55 mm Hg) before the diver returns to the surface. On the other hand, the diver's P_{CO_2} must rise fast enough (relative to the decrease in O_2) to alert the diver of the need to return to the surface before loss of consciousness develops from hypoxia.

Voluntary hyperventilation can prolong the duration of a breath-hold dive. Hyperventilation reduces the diver's CO_2 stores and, therefore, increases the time before the CO_2 stores are replenished and the "breaking point" is reached. It should be noted, however, that hyperventilation prior to a breath-hold dive can be dangerous. The diver's oxygen stores may fall to a critically low level before the CO_2 "breaking point" is reached. Should this happen, the diver could lose consciousness before reaching the surface, and drown.

THE CO_2–O_2 PARADOX

When an individual breath-hold dives to a great depth, there is a so-called paradoxical reversal in the flow of CO_2 and O_2 between the alveoli and the pulmonary capillary blood. This **CO_2–O_2 paradox** is caused by the pressure changes that develop around the diver's body during the dive. The CO_2 paradox occurs as the diver descends, and the O_2 paradox occurs as the diver ascends.

The reason for the CO_2 paradox is as follows: As the diver descends, the lungs are compressed and the pressure in the lungs increases. In fact, the gas pressure in the lungs is about doubled when the diver reaches a depth of 33 feet (2 atm). Thus, assuming a normal $P_{A_{O_2}}$ of about 100 mm Hg and $P_{A_{CO_2}}$ of about 40 mm Hg, at a depth of 33 feet the $P_{A_{O_2}}$ will be about 200 mm Hg and the $P_{A_{CO_2}}$ will be about 80 mm Hg.

In view of these pressure increases, it can be seen that as a diver progressively descends, a CO_2 paradox will occur when the $P_{A_{CO_2}}$ becomes greater than the $P_{v_{CO_2}}$ of the pulmonary capillary blood (normally about 46 mm Hg). In other words, the CO_2 in the alveoli will move into the pulmonary capillary blood. As the diver returns to the surface, the alveolar air expands, causing the $P_{A_{CO_2}}$ to decrease. When this happens, the CO_2 from the pulmonary capillary blood will again move into the alveoli. It is suggested that this mechanism might work to relieve the respiratory CO_2 drive (breaking point) as the diver moves toward the surface.

The reason for the O_2 paradox is as follows: Like the $P_{A_{CO_2}}$, the $P_{A_{O_2}}$ increases as the diver descends, causing more O_2 to move from the alveoli into the pulmonary capillary blood. This mechanism provides more dissolved O_2 for tissue metabolism. However, this physiologic advantage is lost as the diver returns to the surface and the lungs expand and the $P_{A_{O_2}}$ decreases. If a good portion of the O_2 is taken up from the lungs during descent, the $P_{A_{O_2}}$ decline during ascent may be significant. In fact, the $P_{A_{O_2}}$ can fall below the $P_{v_{O_2}}$ of the pulmonary capillary blood. When this happens, the O_2 paradox occurs. That is, the O_2 in the pulmonary capillary blood moves into the alveoli. The fall in $P_{A_{O_2}}$ as a diver returns to the surface is also known as the **hypoxia of ascent**.

THE DIVE RESPONSE

The **dive response** consists of bradycardia, decreased cardiac output, and peripheral vasoconstriction elicited during a breath-hold dive. The dive response may partially explain the survival of numerous near-drowning cases in cold water after submersion lasting over 40 minutes. It is suggested that the peripheral vasoconstriction elicited during the dive response conserves oxygen for the heart and central nervous system by shunting blood away from less vital tissues.

DECOMPRESSION SICKNESS

During a deep dive, the dissolved gases in the diver's blood will also move into body tissues. The amount of dissolved gas that enters the tissues is a function of (1) the solubility of the gas in the tissues, (2) the partial pressure of the gas, and (3) the hydrostatic pressure in the tissue.

During ascent (decompression) the pressure around the diver's body falls. This reduces the hydrostatic pressure in the tissues and, therefore, the ability of the tissues to hold inert gases. When the decompression is performed at an appropriately slow rate, the gases leaving the tissues will be transported (in their dissolved state) by the venous blood to the lungs and exhaled. When the decompression is conducted too rapidly, the gases will be released from the tissue as bubbles. Depending on the size, number, and location of the bubbles, they can cause a number of signs and symptoms, collectively referred to as **decompression sickness**. Decompression sickness includes, but is not limited to, joint pains (the bends), chest pain and coughing (the chokes), paresthesia and paralysis (spinal cord involvement), circulatory failure, and, in severe cases, death.

 ## HYPERBARIC MEDICINE

The administration of oxygen at increased ambient pressures is now being used routinely to treat a variety of pathologic conditions. Clinically, this therapy is referred to as **hyperbaric medicine** and is accomplished by means of a compression chamber (also called a hyperbaric chamber). Most of the therapeutic benefits of hyperbaric oxygenation are associated with the increased oxygen delivery to the tissues.

As discussed in Chapter Seven, hemoglobin is about 97 percent saturated with oxygen at a normal arterial P_{O_2} of 80 to 100 mm Hg. Very little additional O_2 can combine with hemoglobin once this saturation level is reached. However, the quantity of dissolved O_2 will continue to rise linearly as the Pa_{O_2} increases. Approximately 0.3 ml of O_2 physically dissolves in each 100 ml of blood for every Pa_{O_2} increase of 100 mm Hg (Figure 16–2).

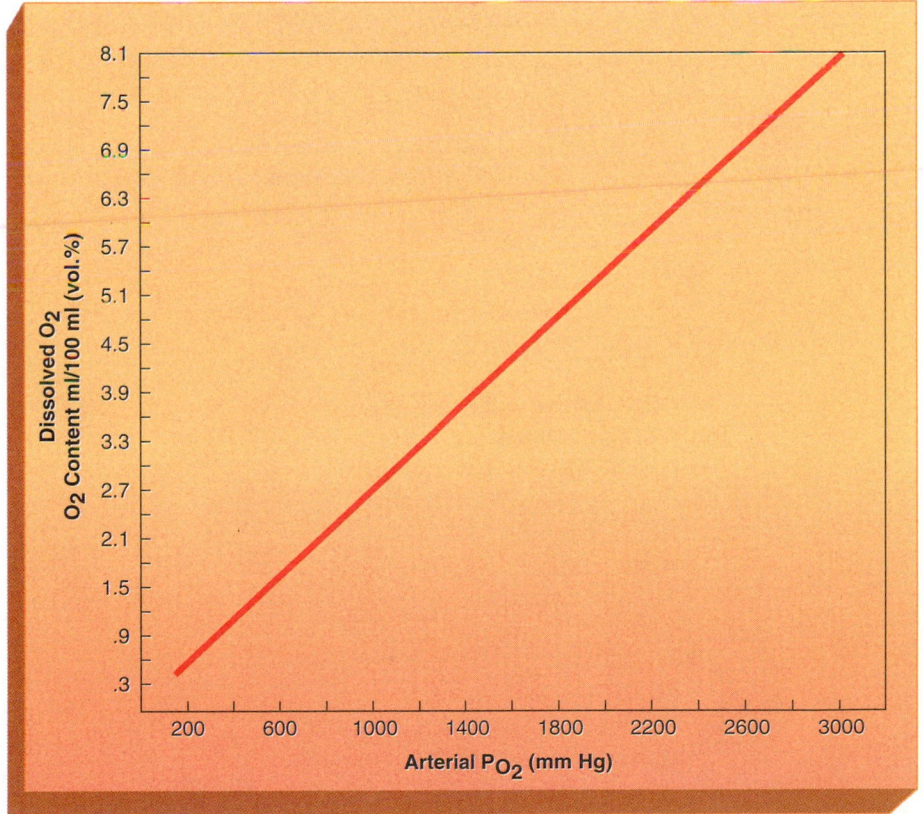

Figure 16–2. *The quantity of dissolved O_2 increases linearly as the Pa_{O_2} increases. About 0.3 ml of O_2 physically dissolves in each 100 ml of blood for every 100 mm Hg increase in Pa_{O_2}.*

INDICATIONS FOR HYPERBARIC OXYGENATION

As shown in Table 16–1, the administration of hyperbaric oxygen is now indicated for a number of clinical conditions. Hyperbaric oxygen has long been useful in the treatment of diseases such as decompression sickness and gas embolism. Regardless of the cause of the bubbles, hyperbaric oxygen is effective in reducing bubble size, accelerating bubble resolution, and maintaining tissue oxygenation.

Hyperbaric oxygen is used empirically to enhance wound healing in conditions associated with ischemic hypoxia. Clinically, such conditions include radiation necrosis of bone or soft tissue, diabetic microangiopathy, compromised skin grafts, crush wounds, acute traumatic ischemias, and thermal burns. It appears that hyperbaric oxygen not only increases tissue oxygenation in these conditions, but increases capillary density as well.

Clinical evidence supports the use of hyperbaric oxygen for the treatment of anaerobic infections, including clostridial myonecrosis (gas gangrene), a variety of necrotizing soft tissue infections, and chronic refractory osteomyelitis. Hyperbaric oxygen added to surgery and antibiotics in the treatment of clostridial myonecrosis increases tissue salvage and decreases mortality.

Hyperbaric oxygen is effective in the treatment of carbon monoxide poisoning. Carbon monoxide poisoning, which is commonly caused by defective indoor heaters, automobile exhaust systems, or smoke inhalation, is the leading cause of death by poisoning in the United States. The severity of intoxication is a function of both the level and duration of carbon monoxide exposure. The administration of

TABLE 16–1. Indications for Hyperbaric Oxygenation

GAS DISEASES
- Decompression Sickness
- Gas Embolism

VASCULAR INSUFFICIENCY STATES
- Radiation Necrosis of Bone or Soft Tissue
- Diabetic Microangiopathy
- Compromised Skin Grafts
- Crush Wounds
- Acute Traumatic Ischemias
- Thermal Burns

INFECTIONS
- Clostridial Myonecrosis
- Necrotizing Soft-tissue Infections
- Chronic Refractory Osteomyelitis

DEFECTS IN OXYGEN TRANSPORT
- Carbon Monoxide Poisoning

hyperbaric oxygen (1) increases the physically dissolved O_2 in the arterial blood, (2) increases the pressure gradient for driving oxygen into ischemic tissues, and (3) reduces the half-life of **carboxyhemoglobin** (CO_{Hb}). The CO_{Hb} half-life when a victim is breathing room air at 1 atmosphere is approximately 5 hours. That is, a CO_{Hb} of 20 percent will decrease to about 10 percent in 5 hours and 5 percent in another 5 hours. Breathing 100 percent oxygen at 1 atmosphere reduces the CO_{Hb} half-life to less than 1 hour.

REVIEW QUESTIONS

1. At what depth below the water surface does the pressure increase to 3.0 atmospheres?
   a. 13 feet
   b. 33 feet
   c. 66 feet
   d. 99 feet
   e. 132 feet

2. If an individual fully inhales to a total lung capacity of 5 liters at sea level (760 mm Hg), and dives to a depth of 66 feet, the lungs will be compressed to about:
   a. 0.5 liters
   b. 1.0 liters
   c. 1.5 liters
   d. 2.0 liters
   e. 2.5 liters

3. At sea level, a diver has:
   - Lung volume: 6 liters
   - Pressure within the lungs: 710 mm Hg

   If the above individual dives to a depth of 99 feet and compresses the lung volume to 2 liters, what will be the pressure within the diver's lungs?
   a. 960 mm Hg
   b. 1420 mm Hg
   c. 1765 mm Hg
   d. 2186 mm Hg
   e. 2615 mm Hg

4. The dive response consists of:
   I. Tachycardia
   II. Decreased cardiac output
   III. Bradycardia
   IV. Peripheral vasoconstriction
      a. I only
      b. II only
      c. III and IV only
      d. I and III only
      e. II, III, and IV only

5. The half-life of carboxyhemoglobin (CO_{Hb}) when a victim is breathing room air at 1 atmosphere is approximately:
   a. 1 hour
   b. 2 hours
   c. 3 hours
   d. 4 hours
   e. 5 hours

6. Hyperventilation prior to a breath-hold dive can be dangerous.   True _____ False _____

7. The fall in $P_{A_{O_2}}$ as a diver returns to the surface is known as the hypoxia of ascent.   True _____ False _____

8. Chest pain and coughing caused by decompression sickness is known as the bends.   True _____ False _____

9. The so-called P_{CO_2} respiratory drive "breaking point" during a dive is about 55 mm Hg.   True _____ False _____

10. Approximately 0.3 ml of O_2 is physically dissolved in each 100 ml of blood for every Pa_{O_2} increase of 100 mm Hg.   True _____ False _____

GLOSSARY

Abduct—to draw away from the median plane of the body or from one of its parts.

Acclimatization—physiological or psychological adjustment to a new environment.

Acetylcholine—a chemical found in most organs and tissues. Acetylcholine plays an important role in the transmission of parasympathetic nerve impulses at the synapses.

Acidemia—decreased pH and increased hydrogen ion concentration of the blood.

Acidosis—pathologic condition resulting from the accumulation of acid in, or loss of base from, the body.

Acinus (*pl.: acini*)—The smallest division of a gland; a group of secretory cells surrounding a cavity. The functional part of an organ. The respiratory acinus includes the respiratory bronchioles, alveolar ducts, alveoli, and all other structures within the acinus.

Acromion process—lateral portion of the spine of the scapula that forms the point of the shoulder. It articulates with the clavicle and gives attachment to the deltoid and trapezius muscles.

Acute—sharp, severe; of rapid onset and characterized by severe symptoms and a short course; not chronic.

Adrenergic—nerve fibers that, when stimulated, release epinephrine at their endings. Adrenergic fibers include nearly all sympathetic postganglionic fibers except those innervating sweat glands.

Afferent—carrying impulses toward a center.

Afferent nerves—nerves that carry impulses from the periphery to the central nervous system.

Affinity—attraction between two substances that, when united, form new substances (i.e., oxygen and hemoglobin form oxyhemoglobin).

Air trapping—the prevention of gas from leaving the alveoli during exhalation. This is usually caused by airway closure during exhalation.

Airway resistance—the pressure difference between the mouth and alveoli divided by flow rate.

Alkalemia—increased pH and decreased hydrogen ion concentration of the blood.

Allergen—any substance that causes an allergic reaction. It may or may not be a protein.

Allergy—acquired hypersensitivity to a substance (allergen) that normally does not cause a reaction.

Alpha receptor—site in the autonomic nerve pathways where excitatory responses occur when adrenergic agents such as norepinephrine and epinephrine are released.

Alveolus—a small, saclike structure. Often used interchangeably with acinus.

Amniotic fluid—liquid produced by the fetal membranes and the fetus; it surrounds the fetus throughout pregnancy, usually totaling about 1000 ml at term.

Analogous—similar in function but having a different origin or structure.

Anastomosis—joining of vessels, either naturally or surgically, to allow flow to other structures.

Anemia—disorder characterized by a decrease in hemoglobin in the blood to levels below the normal range.

Anoxia—deficiency of oxygen.

Anterior—indicating the front of a structure or body surface relative to other body parts.

Antibody—protein substance that develops in response to and interacts with an antigen. The antigen-antibody reaction forms the basis of immunity.

Antigen—substance that induces the formation of antibodies that interact specifically with it. The antigen-antibody reaction forms the basis for immunity.

Antitrypsin—inhibitor of trypsin; may be deficient in persons with emphysema.

Aperture—opening or orifice.

Apex—top end or tip of a structure.

Apnea—complete absence of spontaneous ventilation.

Arrhythmia—irregularity or loss of rhythm, especially of the heartbeat.

Arterial—pertaining to one artery or a network of arteries.

Arteriole—a very small artery, especially one that, at its distal end, leads into a capillary.

Arteriosclerosis—a common arterial disorder characterized by thickening, loss of elasticity, and calcification of arterial walls, resulting in a decreased blood supply.

Asphyxia—condition caused by an insufficient uptake of oxygen.

Aspiration—the act of inhaling. Pathologic aspiration of vomitus or other foreign substances into the respiratory tract.

Aspiration pneumonia—an inflammatory condition of the lungs and bronchi caused by the inhalation of foreign material or vomitus containing acid gastric contents.

Ataxia—an abnormal condition characterized by impaired ability to coordinate movement.

Atelectasis—collapse of the lung. May be caused by obstruction.

Atherosclerosis—a common arterial disorder characterized by yellowish plaques of cholesterol, lipids, and cellular debris in the medial layer of the walls of the large and medium-sized arteries.

Atmospheric pressure—pressure of the air on the earth at mean sea level; approximately 760 mm Hg (14.7 pounds per square inch).

Augment—to enlarge or increase in size, amount, or degree; make bigger.

Bacteriuria—the presence of bacteria in the urine.

Baroreceptor—a pressure sensor.

Basal—at the bottom; alkaline.

Basophil—a type of white blood cell that has a granular nucleus stained with basic dyes. These cells represent 1 percent or less of the total white blood cell count.

Beta receptor—site in autonomic nerve pathways where inhibitory responses occur when adrenergic agents, such as norepinephrine and epinephrine, are released.

Bicarbonate—the HCO_3^- anion or any salt containing the HCO_3^- anion.

Bifurcation—a separation into two branches; the point of forking.

Biot's breathing—short episodes of rapid, uniformly deep inspirations, followed by 10 to 30 seconds of apnea.

Blood–brain barrier—membrane between the circulating blood and the brain that prevents certain substances from reaching brain tissue and cerebrospinal fluid.

Bradykinin—a nonapeptide produced by activation of the kinin system in a variety of inflammatory conditions. It is an extremely potent vasodilator; it also increases vascular permeability, stimulates pain receptors, and causes contraction of a variety of extravascular smooth muscles.

Bronchoconstriction—narrowing of the pulmonary air passages.

Bronchodilation—widening of pulmonary air passages.

Bronchospasm—involuntary sudden movement or convulsive contraction of the muscular coats of the bronchus.

Calcification—process in which organic tissue becomes hardened by the deposition of lime salts in the tissue.

Calculus—a pathologic stone formed of mineral salts. Calculi are usually found within hollow organs or ducts.

Caliber—the inside diameter of a tube, commonly given in millimeters and fractions of an inch.

Canalicular—pertaining to a small channel or canal.

Capillary stasis—stagnation of normal flow of fluids or blood in capillaries.

Carbon dioxide (CO_2)—colorless, odorless, incombustible gas formed during respiration and combustion.

Cartilage—dense, firm, compact connective tissue capable of withstanding considerable pressure and tension. Located in the tracheobronchial tree, all true joints, the outer ear, and the movable sections of the ribs.

Catecholamines—biologically active amines that behave as epinephrine and norepinephrine.

Central venous pressure (CVP)—pressure within the superior vena cava, which reflects the pressure under which the blood is returned to the right atrium.

Cerebrospinal fluid (CSF)—fluid cushion that protects the brain and spinal cord from shock.

Chemoreceptor—sense organ or sensory nerve ending, located outside the central nervous system, which is stimulated by and reacts to chemical stimuli.

Cheyne-Stokes breathing—10 to 30 seconds of apnea, followed by a gradual increase in the volume and frequency of breathing, followed by a gradual decrease in the volume of breathing until another period of apnea occurs.

Chronic—denoting a process that shows little change and slow progression and is of long duration.

Cilia—small, hairlike projections on the surface of epithelial cells. In the bronchi they propel mucus and foreign particles in a whiplike movement toward the throat.

Clinical manifestations—symptoms or signs demonstrated by a patient.

Colloid—a state of matter composed of single large molecules or aggregations of smaller molecules of solids, liquids, or gases, in a continuous medium (dispersal medium), which also may be a solid, liquid, or gas.

Composition—makeup; what something is made of.

Compromise—a blending of the qualities of two different things; an unfavorable change.

Concave—a hollow surface, like the inside of a bowl.

Conception—the union of sperm and ovum.

Congenital—existing at and usually before birth; referring to conditions that are present at birth, regardless of their cause.

Congestion—excessive amount of blood or tissue fluid in an organ or tissue.

Congestive heart failure—myocardial insufficiency of the left ventricle that results in pulmonary congestion.

Consolidation—the process of becoming solid; a mass that has solidified.

Constrict—tighten or squeeze; making a part narrow.

Contiguous—being in actual contact; touching along a boundary or at a point.

Contusion—injury in which the skin is not broken; a bruise.

Convex—having a rounded, somewhat elevated surface, resembling a segment of the external surface of a sphere.

Cor pulmonale—failure of the right ventricle resulting from disorders of the lungs or pulmonary vessels.

Corpuscle—any small, rounded body; an encapsulated sensory nerve ending.

Cortex—the outer layer of an organ.

Crackles—abnormal, fine or medium crackling wet sounds typically heard during inspiration; also known as **rales**.

Creatinine—a substance formed from the metabolism of creatine, commonly found in blood, urine, and muscle tissue.

Deadspace ventilation—volume of gas that is ventilated, but not physiologically effective. There are three types of deadspace ventilation: *Anatomic dead space*—the volume of gas in the conducting airways: the nose, mouth, pharynx, larynx, and lower airways down to, but not including, the respiratory bronchioles. *Alveolar dead space*—alveoli that are ventilated, but not perfused with blood. *Physiologic dead space*—the sum of the anatomic dead space and alveolar dead space.

Density—mass of a substance per unit of volume (g/cm^3).

Deoxyribonucleic acid (DNA)—a nucleic acid containing deoxyribose as the sugar component and found principally in the nuclei of animal and vegetable cells, usually loosely bound to protein (hence termed dioxyribonucleoprotein). Considered to be the autoreproducing component of chromosomes and of many viruses, and the repository of hereditary characteristics.

Depolarize—to reduce to a nonpolarized condition; to reduce the amount of electrical charge between oppositely charged particles (*ions*).

Desquamation—the process in which the cornified layer of the epidermis is sloughed in fine scales.

Determinant—an element that identifies or determines the nature of something or that fixes or conditions an outcome.

Diabetes—a general term referring to a variety of disorders characterized by excessive urination (polyuria), as in diabetes mellitus and diabetes insipidus.

Diagnostic—pertaining to the use of scientific and skillful methods to establish the cause and nature of a sick person's disease.

Diastole—normal period in the heart cycle during which the muscle fibers lengthen, the heart dilates, and the chambers fill with blood.

Differentiate—to separate according to differences.

Diffusion—the movement of gas molecules from an area of relatively high concentration of gas to one of low concentration. Different gases each move according to their own individual partial pressure gradients. Diffusion continues until all the gases in the two areas are in equilibrium.

Digitation—a fingerlike projection.

Distal—away from or being the farthest from any point of reference.

Dorsal—pertaining to the back or to the posterior portion of a body.

Driving pressure—pressure difference between two areas in any vessel or airway.

Ductus arteriosus—vessel between the left pulmonary artery and the aorta that bypasses the lungs in the fetus.

Dyspnea—difficulty in breathing, of which the individual is aware.

Edema—a local or generalized condition in which the body tissues contain an excessive amount of extracellular fluid.

Efferent—carrying away from a central organ or section.

Efferent nerves—nerves that carry impulses from the brain or spinal cord to the periphery.

Elastance—the natural ability of matter to respond directly to force and to return to its original resting position or shape after the external force no longer exists. In pulmonary physiology, elastance is defined as the change in pressure per change in volume.

Electrocardiogram (ECG)—record of the electrical activity of the heart.

Electrolyte—an element or compound that, when melted or dissolved in water or other solvent, dissociates into ions and is able to conduct an electric current.

Elongation—the condition or process of being extended.

Embryonic—pertaining to the early stages (i.e., first three months) of fetal development.

End-expiration—the portion of a ventilatory cycle at which expiration stops (pre-inspiration).

End-inspiration—the portion of a ventilatory cycle at which inspiration stops (pre-expiration).

Endothelium—the layer of epithelial cells, originating from the mesoderm, that lines the cavities of the heart, the blood and lymph vessels, and the serous cavities of the body.

Endotracheal—within the trachea.

Eosinophil—a cell or cellular structure that stains readily with the acid stain eosin; specifically, a granular leukocyte.

Epinephrine—one of two active hormones (the other is norepinephrine) secreted by the adrenal medulla.

Epistaxis—bleeding from the nose, also called nosebleed.

Equilibrium—condition in which one or more forces are evenly balanced by opposite forces.

Erythrocyte—red blood cell (RBC).

Etiology—cause of disease.

Eupnea—normal, spontaneous breathing.

Excretion—elimination of waste products.

Excursion—the extent of movement from a central position or axis.

Expectoration—clearing the lungs by coughing up and spitting out matter.

Extra-alveolar—pertaining to the area outside of the alveoli.

Extracellular—outside a cell or in the cavities or spaces between cell layers or groups of cells.

Extravascular—outside a vessel.

Fascia—fibrous membrane that covers, supports, and separates muscles.

Fertilization—the union of sperm and ovum.

Fetus—the developing human *in utero* from the third month to birth.

Fibrin—whitish, filamentous protein formed by the action of thrombin on fibrinogen.

Fibroelastic—composed of fibrous and elastic tissue.

Fibrosis—formation of scar tissue.

Fissure—cleft or groove on the surface of an organ, often marking the division of the organ into parts, such as the lobes of the lung.

Fistula—abnormal passage or communication, usually between two internal organs or leading from an internal organ to the surface of the body.

Flail chest—a thorax in which multiple rib fractures cause instability in part of the chest wall and paradoxical breathing, with the lung underlying the injured areas contracting on inspiration and bulging on expiration.

Flex—to bend upon itself, as a muscle.

Foramen ovale—opening between the atria of the heart in the fetus. This opening normally closes shortly after birth.

Forced vital capacity—the maximum volume of gas that can be exhaled over a specific time period.

Functional residual capacity—the volume of air remaining in the lungs after a normal exhalation.

Functionally—according to its proper use or action; working as it should.

Gastrointestinal tract—the route taken by food from the stomach to the rectum.

Generation—the process of forming a new organism or part of an organism.

Gestation—the period of time from the fertilization of the ovum until birth.

Glomerulonephritis—inflammation of the glomerulus in the nephron of the kidney.

Glomerulus—a tuft or cluster; a structure composed of blood vessels or nerve fibers, such as a *renal glomerulus*.

Glossopharyngeal nerve—the 9th cranial nerve.

Glycoprotein—any of a class of conjugated proteins consisting of a compound of a protein with a carbohydrate group.

Goblet cell—a type of secretory cell found in the intestinal and respiratory tracts.

Gradient—a slope or grade; a difference in values between two points.

Hematocrit—volume of erythrocytes packed by centrifugation in a given volume of blood, is expressed as the percentage of total blood volume that consists of erythrocytes.

Hemoglobin—pigment of red blood cells containing iron.

Hemolysis—the breakdown of red blood cells and the release of hemoglobin.

Heparin—a polysaccharide produced by the mast cells of the liver and by basophil leukocytes that inhibits coagulation by preventing conversion of prothrombin to thrombin. It also inhibits coagulation by preventing liberation of thromboplastin from blood platelets.

Histamine—a substance that is normally present in the body and exerts a pharmacologic action when released from injured cells. It is produced from the amino acid *histidine*.

Hormone—a substance originating in an organ or gland that is conveyed through the body to another part of the body, which it stimulates by chemical action to increased functional activity and/or increased secretion.

Hydrostatic—pertaining to the pressure of liquids in equilibrium.

Hydrous—containing water, usually chemically combined.

Hypercapnia—greater than normal amount of carbon dioxide in the blood; also called *hypercarbia*.

Hyperchloremia—increased chloride level in the blood.

Hyperinflation—distension by air, gas, or liquid, as in the hyperinflation of the alveoli.

Hyperkalemia—increased amount of potassium in the blood.

Hyperpnea—increased depth (volume) of breathing, with or without an increased frequency.

Hypersecretion—substance or fluid produced by cells or glands in an excessive amount or more than normal.

Hypersensitivity—abnormal sensitivity to a stimulus of any kind.

Hypertension—higher than normal blood pressure.

Hyperthermia—higher than normal body temperature.

Hyperventilation—an increased alveolar ventilation.

Hypochloremia—a decreased amount of chloride in the blood.

Hypokalemia—a decreased amount of potassium in the blood.

Hypoperfusion—deficiency of blood coursing through the vessels of the circulatory system.

Hypothalamus—portion of the brain that controls certain metabolic activities.

Hypoventilation—a decreased alveolar ventilation.

Hypoxemia—below-normal oxygen content in blood.

Hypoxia—tissue oxygen deficiency.

Iliac crest—long curved upper margin of the hip bone.

Immaturity—the state of being not fully developed or ripened.

Immunoglobulin—one of a family of closely related but not identical proteins that are capable of acting as antibodies.

Immunologic mechanism—reaction of the body to substances that are foreign or are interpreted by the body as foreign.

Impede—to slow down; to stand in the way of; to fight against.

Inferior vena cava (IVC)—venous trunk for the lower extremities and the pelvic and abdominal viscera.

Inflammation—localized heat, redness, swelling, and pain as a result of irritation, injury, or infection.

Inguinal ligament—a fibrous band formed by the inferior border of the aponeurosis of the external oblique that extends from the anterior superior iliac spine to the pubic tubercle.

Inhibitory—repressive; tending to restrain a function.

Innervation—function of the nervous system that gives stimulation to a part of the body.

Inspiratory capacity—the volume of air that can be inhaled after a normal exhalation.

Interstitial—placed or lying between; pertaining to the interstices or spaces within an organ or tissue.

Intra-—prefix meaning within.

Intra-alveolar—within the alveoli.

Intrapleural—within the pleura.

Intrapulmonary—within the lungs.

Intrarenal—within the kidneys.

Intratubular—within a tube.

Intubation—passage of a tube into a body aperture; specifically, the insertion of a breathing tube through the mouth or nose or into the trachea.

Inverse—opposite in order, nature, or effect; being an inverse function.

Ion—atom, group of atoms, or molecule that has acquired a net electrical charge by gaining or losing electrons.

Ischemia—decreased blood supply to a body organ or part.

Isobar—a line on a map, chart, or nomogram connecting areas of equal pressure.

Kussmaul breathing—both an increased depth and rate of breathing.

Lactic acid—acid formed in muscles during activity by the breakdown of sugar without oxygen.

Ligamentum nuchae—upward continuation of the supraspinous ligament, extending from the 7th cervical vertebra to the occipital bone.

Linea alba—"white line" of connective tissue in the middle of the abdomen from sternum to pubis.

Linear response—a response or output that is directly proportional to the input.

Lipid—any of numerous fats generally insoluble in water that constitute one of the principal structural materials of cells.

Lobar—pertaining to a lobe, such as the lobes of the lung.

Lumen—inner open space of a tubular organ, such as a blood vessel or intestine.

Lung compliance—the change in lung volume per unit pressure change.

Magnitude—pertaining to size.

Malar—pertaining to the cheek or cheekbones.

Malformation—deformity; abnormal shape or structure, especially congenital.

Mastoid process—projection of the posterior portion of the temporal bone; gives attachment to the sternocleidomastoid, splenius capitis, and longissimus capitis muscles.

Mean—occupying a middle position; being near the average.

Mechanical—relating to physical properties.

Mechanoreceptor—receptor that receives mechanical stimuli such as pressure from sound or touch.

Medial—pertaining to the middle.

Mediated—between two parts or sides.

Medulla oblongata—vital part of the brain; contains the cardiac, vasomotor, and respiratory centers of the brain.

Mesoderm—the middle of the three cell layers of the developing embryo, which lies between the ectoderm and endoderm.

Metabolism—sum of all physical and chemical changes that take place within an organism; all energy and material transformations that occur within living cells.

Microvilli—minute cylindrical processes on the free surface of a cell (especially cells of the proximal convoluted renal tubule and those of the intestinal epithelium), which increase the surface area of the cell.

Molecular weight—weight of a molecule attained by adding the atomic weight of its constituent atoms.

Monocyte—a large, mononuclear leukocyte normally found in lymph nodes, spleen, bone marrow, and loose connective tissue.

Motor nerve—a nerve consisting of efferent fibers that conduct impulses from the brain or the spinal cord to one of the muscles or organs.

Mucous—pertaining to or resembling mucus; secreting mucus.

Mucus—the gel-like substance of the mucous membranes, composed of mucin (secreted by the mucus glands), along with various inorganic salts, desquamated cells, and leukocytes.

Myelin—the substance that constitutes the sheaths of various nerve fibers throughout the body. It is largely composed of fat, giving the fibers a white, creamy color.

Myoepithelial cells—spindle-shaped cells found around sweat, mammary and salivary glands. The myoepithelial cells are contractile and resemble smooth muscle cells.

Myoglobin—a ferrous globin complex consisting of one heme group and one globin polypeptide chain. It is responsible for the red pigment seen in skeletal muscle.

Necrosis—localized tissue death that occurs in groups of cells in response to disease or injury.

Neoplasms—a new and abnormal formation of tissue.

Neuropathy—any abnormal condition characterized by inflammation and degeneration of the peripheral nerves.

Nomogram—a graph consisting of several lines or curves (usually parallel) graduated for different variables in such a way that a straight line cutting the three lines gives the related values of the three variables.

Nonlinear—having or being a response or output that is not directly proportional to the input.

Norepinephrine—one of two active hormones (the other is epinephrine) secreted by the adrenal medulla. It is chiefly a vasoconstrictor and has little effect on cardiac output.

Occipital—referring to the back part or bone of the head.

Occlude—to close, obstruct, or join together.

Olfactory—pertaining to the sense of smell.

Oncotic pressure—osmotic pressure due to the presence of colloids in a solution.

Orthopnea—a condition in which an individual is able to breathe most comfortably only in the upright position.

Osmotic pressure—pressure that develops when two solutions with different concentrations of solutes are separated by a semipermeable membrane.

Oxygen content—total amount of oxygen in the blood.

Papillitis—an abnormal condition characterized by the inflammation of a papilla.

Paradoxical—occurring at variance with the normal rule.

Parasympathetic nervous system—a division of the autonomic nervous system that is mediated by the release of acetylcholine and primarily involves the protection, conservation, and restoration of body resources.

Parenchyma—essential parts of an organ that are concerned with its function.

Paroxysmal—concerning the sudden, periodic attack or recurrence of symptoms of a disease.

Parturition—the action or process of giving birth to offspring.

Pathogen—any agent causing disease, especially a microorganism.

Perfusion—passing of blood or fluid through a vascular bed.

Peribronchial—located around the bronchi.

Pericardium—a fibroserous sac that surrounds the heart and the roots of the great vessels.

Peripheral airways—small bronchioles on the outer sections of the lung.

Peristalsis—a progressive wave movement that occurs involuntarily in hollow tubes of the body, especially the intestines.

Perivascular—located around a vessel, especially a blood vessel.

Permeable—capable of allowing the passage of fluids or substances in solution.

pH—symbol for the logarithm of the reciprocal of the hydrogen ion concentration.

Phalanges—the bones of the fingers and toes.

Phosphate—a compound of phosphoric acid.

Photophobia—abnormal sensitivity to light, especially by the eyes.

Pituitary gland—a small, gray, rounded body attached to the base of the brain.

Pneumothorax—a collection of air or gas in the pleural space, causing the lung to collapse.

Posterior—back part of something; toward the back.

Prerenal—located in front of the kidneys.

Pressure—in physics, the quotient obtained by dividing a force by the area of the surface on which it acts.

Prognosis—prediction of outcome.

Proliferate—increasing or spreading at a rapid rate; the process or result of rapid reproduction.

Prostaglandins—a group of fatty acid derivatives present in many organs that affect the cardiovascular system and smooth muscle and stimulate the uterus to contract.

Prostate—a gland in males that surrounds the neck of the bladder and the urethra and elaborates a secretion that liquefies coagulated semen.

Prostatic hypertrophy—enlargement of the prostate gland.

Proximal—nearest the point of attachment, center of the body, or point of reference.

Pubic symphysis—junction of the pubic bones, composed of fibrocartilage.

Pulmonary—concerning or involving the lungs.

Pulmonary congestion—an abnormally large amount of fluid in the pulmonary system.

Pulmonary shunting—that portion of the cardiac output that enters the left side of the heart without exchanging gases with alveolar gases.

Pulmonary surfactant—a surfactant agent found in the lungs that functions to reduce the surface tension of the fluid on the surface of the cells of the lower respiratory system, enhancing the elasticity of the alveoli and bronchioles and thus the exchange of gases in the lungs.

Pulmonary vascular resistance (PVR)—pressure loss, per unit of blood flow, from pulmonary artery to the left ventricle.

Pyelonephritis—a diffuse pyogenic infection of the pelvis and parenchyma of the kidney.

Rales—abnormal dry or moist lung sounds, heard upon auscultation.

Reflex—an involuntary response to a stimulus.

Renal—pertaining to the kidneys.

Renal dysplasia—abnormal development of tissue in the kidneys.

Resonance—quality of the sound heard on percussion of a hollow structure such as the chest or abdomen.

Rhonchi—a dry, coarse rattling sound in the bronchial tubes, heard upon auscultation.

Semipermeable—permitting diffusion or flow of some liquids or solutes but preventing the transmission of others, usually in reference to a membrane.

Septic—pertaining to infection or contamination.

Septicemia—systemic infection in which pathogens and their toxins are present in the circulating blood stream, having spread from an infection in any part of the body.

Septum—wall dividing two cavities.

Serotonin—a potent vasoconstrictor that is present in platelets, gastrointestinal mucosa, mast cells, and carcinoid tumors.

Serum—clear watery fluid, especially that moistening surfaces of serous membranes or exuded inflammation of any of those membranes; the fluid portion of the blood obtained after removal of the fibrin clot and blood cells, sometimes used as a synonym for antiserum.

Shunt—to turn away from; to divert; an abnormal passage to divert flow from one route to another.

Sign—any objective evidence or manifestation of an illness or disordered function of the body.

Smooth muscle—muscle tissue that lacks cross-striations on its fibers, is involuntary in action, and is found principally in visceral organs.

Somatic nerve—nerve that innervates somatic structures, i.e., those constituting the body wall and extremities.

Somnolence—the condition of being sleepy or drowsy.

Spasm—involuntary sudden movement or convulsive muscular contraction.

Sputum—substance expelled by coughing or clearing the throat that may contain a variety of materials from the respiratory tract, including one or more of the following: cellular debris, mucus, blood, pus, caseous material, and microorganisms.

Stasis—stagnation of normal flow of fluids, as of the blood, urine, or intestinal mechanism.

Stroke volume—amount of blood ejected by the ventricle at each beat.

Subcutaneous—under the skin.

Sulfonamide—one of a large group of synthetic, bacteriostatic drugs that are effective in treating infections caused by many gram-negative and gram-positive microorganisms.

Superior vena cava—venous trunk draining blood from the head, neck, upper extremities, and chest.

Surfactant—a substance important in controlling the surface tension of the air–liquid emulsion in the lungs; an agent that lowers surface tension.

Sympathetic nervous system—a division of the autonomic nervous system that accelerates the heart rate, constricts blood vessels, and raises blood pressure.

Sympathomimetic—producing effects resembling those resulting from stimulation of the sympathetic nervous system.

Symptom—any perceptible change in the body or its functions that indicates disease or the type or phases of disease. Symptoms may be classified as objective, subjective, cardinal, and sometimes constitutional.

Systemic—pertaining to the whole body rather than to one of its parts.

Systemic reaction—whole body response to a stimulus.

Systole—that part of the heart cycle in which the heart is in contraction.

Systolic pressure—maximum blood pressure; occurs during contraction of the ventricle.

Tachycardia—an abnormal circulatory condition in which the myocardium contracts regularly but at a rate of greater than 100 beats per minute.

Tachypnea—a rapid rate of breathing.

Thoracolumbar—relating to the thoracic and lumbar portions of the vertebral column.

Tidal volume—the volume of air that normally moves into and out of the lungs in one quiet breath.

Tone—that state of a body or any of its organs or parts in which the functions are healthy and normal.

Total lung capacity—the maximum amount of air that the lung can accommodate.

Transairway pressure—the barometric pressure difference between the mouth pressure and the alveolar pressure.

Transient—passing especially quickly into and out of existence; passing through or by a place with only a brief stay.

Transpulmonary pressure—the difference between the alveolar pressure and the pleural pressure.

Transthoracic pressure—the difference between the alveolar pressure and the body surface pressure.

Trimester—one of the three periods of approximately three months into which pregnancy is divided.

Unilateral renal agenesis—failure of development of one of the kidneys.

Vagus—the 10th cranial nerve. It is a mixed nerve, having motor and sensory functions and a wider distribution than any of the other cranial nerves.

Vascular—relating to or containing blood vessels.

Vasoconstriction—decrease in the caliber of blood vessels.

Vasodilation—widening of blood vessels, especially the small arteries and arterioles.

Venous—pertaining to a vein or veins.

Venous return—the amount of blood returning to the atria of the heart.

Ventilation—the mechanical movement of air into and out of the lungs in a cyclic fashion. It is the mechanism by which oxygen is carried from the atmosphere to the alveoli and by which carbon dioxide is carried from the lungs to the atmosphere.

Ventral—pertaining to the anterior portion or front of the body.

Ventricle—either of two lower chambers of the heart.

Viscosity—stickiness or gumminess; internal friction resistance offered by a fluid to change of form or relative position of its particles due to attraction of molecules to each other.

Viscous—sticky; gummy; gelatinous.

Viscus—any organ enclosed within a cavity, such as the thorax or abdomen.

Vital capacity—the maximum volume of air that can be exhaled after a maximal inspiration.

Volume percent (Vol%)—the number of milliliters (ml) of a substance contained in 100 ml of another substance.

SYMBOLS AND ABBREVIATIONS

The symbols and abbreviations listed below are commonly used in respiratory physiology.

Primary Symbols

GAS SYMBOLS		BLOOD SYMBOLS	
P	Pressure	Q	Blood volume
V	Gas volume	$\dot{Q}$	Blood flow
$\dot{V}$	Gas volume per unit of time, or flow	C	Content in blood
F	Fractional concentration of gas	S	Saturation

Secondary Symbols

GAS SYMBOLS		BLOOD SYMBOLS	
I	Inspired	a	Arterial
E	Expired	c	Capillary
A	Alveolar	v	Venous
T	Tidal	$\bar{v}$	Mixed venous
D	Deadspace		

Abbreviations

LUNG VOLUME

VC	Vital capacity
IC	Inspiratory capacity

LUNG VOLUME (cont'd.)

IRV	Inspiratory reserve volume
ERV	Expiratory reserve volume
FRC	Functional residual capacity
RV	Residual volume
TLC	Total lung capacity
RV/TLC(%)	Residual volume to total lung capacity ratio, expressed as a percentage
V_T	Tidal volume
V_A	Alveolar ventilation
V_D	Deadspace ventilation
V_L	Actual lung volume

SPIROMETRY

FVC	Forced vital capacity with maximally forced expiratory effort
FEV_T	Forced expiratory volume timed
$FEF_{200-1200}$	Average rate of airflow between 200–1200 ml of the FVC
$FEF_{25\%-75\%}$	Forced expiratory flow during the middle half of the FVC (formerly called the maximal midexpiratory flow or MMF)
PEFR	Maximum flow rate that can be achieved
$\dot{V}_{max\ x}$	Forced expiratory flow related to the actual volume of the lungs as denoted by subscript x, which refers to the amount of lung volume remaining when measurement is made
MVV	Maximal voluntary ventilation as the volume of air expired in a specified interval

MECHANICS

C_L	Lung compliance; volume change per unit of pressure change
R_{aw}	Airway resistance; pressure per unit of flow

DIFFUSION

DL_{CO}	Diffusing capacity of carbon monoxide

BLOOD GASES

PA_{O_2}	Alveolar oxygen tension
P_{CO_2}	Pulmonary capillary oxygen tension
Pa_{O_2}	Arterial oxygen tension
$P\bar{v}_{O_2}$	Mixed venous oxygen tension
PA_{CO_2}	Alveolar carbon dioxide tension
Pc_{CO_2}	Pulmonary capillary carbon dioxide tension
Pa_{CO_2}	Arterial carbon dioxide tension
Sa_{O_2}	Arterial oxygen saturation

(*continues*)

BLOOD GASES (cont'd)

$S\bar{v}_{O_2}$	Mixed venous oxygen saturation
pH	Negative logarithm of the H+ concentration used as a positive number
HCO_3^-	Plasma bicarbonate concentration
mEq/L	The number of grams of solute dissolved in a normal solution
Ca_{O_2}	Oxygen content of arterial blood
Cc_{O_2}	Oxygen content of capillary blood
$C\bar{v}_{O_2}$	Oxygen content of mixed venous blood
$\dot{V}/\dot{Q}$	Ventilation-perfusion ratio
$\dot{Q}s/\dot{Q}_T$	Shunt
$\dot{Q}_T$	Total cardiac output

OXYGEN TRANSPORT STUDIES

$C(a - \bar{v})_{O_2}$	Arterial-venous oxygen content difference
$\dot{V}_{O_2}$	Oxygen consumption (oxygen uptake)
O_2ER	Oxygen extraction ratio
D_{O_2}	Total oxygen delivery

Hemodynamic Measurement Abbreviations

DIRECT MEASUREMENTS

CVP	Central venous pressure
RAP	Right atrial pressure
$\overline{PA}$	Mean pulmonary artery pressure
PCWP	Pulmonary capillary wedge pressure
PAW	Pulmonary artery wedge
PAO	Pulmonary artery occlusion
CO	Cardiac output

INDIRECT MEASUREMENTS

SV	Stroke volume
SVI	Stroke volume index
CI	Cardiac index
RVSWI	Right ventricular stroke work index
LVSWI	Left ventricular stroke work index
PVR	Pulmonary vascular resistance
SVR	Systemic vascular resistance

Metric Measurement Abbreviations

VOLUME MEASUREMENTS

L	Liter
dl	deciliter (1×10^{-1})
ml	milliliter (1×10^{-3})
μl	microliter (1×10^{-6})
nl	nanoliter (1×10^{-9})

LINEAR MEASUREMENTS

m	meter
cm	centimeter ($m \times 10^{-2}$)
mm	millimeter ($m \times 10^{-3}$)
μ or μm	micrometer ($m \times 10^{-6}$)

WEIGHT MEASUREMENTS

g	gram
mg	milligram ($g \times 10^{-3}$)
μg	microgram ($g \times 10^{-6}$)
ng	nanogram ($g \times 10^{-9}$)

UNITS OF MEASUREMENT

Metric Weight

GRAMS	CENTIGRAMS	MILLIGRAMS	MICROGRAMS	NANOGRAMS
1	100	1000	1,000,000	1,000,000,000
.01	1	10	10,000	10,000,000
.001	.1	1	1000	1,000,000
.000001	.0001	.001	1	1000
.000000001	.0000001	.000001	.001	1

Metric Liquid

LITER	CENTILITER	MILLILITER	MICROLITER	NANOLITER
1	100	1000	1,000,000	1,000,000,000
.01	1	10	10,000	10,000,000
.001	.1	1	1000	1,000,000
.000001	.0001	.001	1	1000
.000000001	.0000001	.000001	.001	1

Metric Length

METER	CENTIMETER	MILLIMETER	MICROMETER	NANOMETER
1	100	1000	1,000,000	1,000,000,000
.01	1	10	10,000	10,000,000
.001	.1	1	1000	1,000,000
.000001	.0001	.001	1	1000
.000000001	.0000001	.000001	.001	1

Weight Conversions (Metric and Avoirdupois)

GRAMS	KILOGRAMS	OUNCES	POUNDS
1	.001	.0353	.0022
1000	1	35.3	2.2
28.35	.02835	1	$\frac{1}{16}$
454.5	.4545	16	1

Weight Conversions (Metric and Apothecary)

GRAMS	MILLIGRAMS	GRAINS	DRAMS	OUNCES	POUNDS
1	1000	15.4	.2577	.0322	.00268
.001	1	.0154	.00026	.0000322	.00000268
.0648	64.8	1	$\frac{1}{60}$	$\frac{1}{480}$	$\frac{1}{5760}$
3.888	3888	60	1	$\frac{1}{8}$	$\frac{1}{96}$
31.1	31104	480	8	1	$\frac{1}{12}$
373.25	373248	5760	96	12	1

Approximate Household Measurement Equivalents (Volume)

1 tsp = 5 ml
1 tbsp = 3 tsp = 15 ml
1 fl oz = 2 tbsp = 6 tsp = 30 ml
1 cup = 8 fl oz = 240 ml
1 pt = 2 cups = 16 fl oz = 480 ml
1 qt = 2 pt = 4 cups = 32 fl oz = 960 ml
1 gal = 4 qt = 8 pt = 16 cups = 128 fl oz = 3840 ml

Weight

METRIC	APPROXIMATE APOTHECARY EQUIVALENTS
Grams	**Grains**
.0002	$\frac{1}{300}$
.0003	$\frac{1}{200}$
.0004	$\frac{1}{150}$
.0005	$\frac{1}{120}$
.0006	$\frac{1}{100}$
.001	$\frac{1}{60}$
.002	$\frac{1}{30}$
.005	$\frac{1}{12}$
.010	$\frac{1}{6}$
.015	$\frac{1}{4}$
.025	$\frac{3}{8}$
.030	$\frac{1}{2}$
.050	$\frac{3}{4}$
.060	1
.100	1½
.120	2
.200	3
.300	5
.500	7½
.600	10
1	15
2	30
4	60

Liquid Measure

METRIC	APPROXIMATE APOTHECARY EQUIVALENTS
Milliliters	
1,000	1 quart
750	1½ pints
500	1 pint
250	8 fluid ounces

(continues)

Liquid Measure (cont'd)	
METRIC	**APPROXIMATE APOTHECARY EQUIVALENTS**
Milliliters	
200	7 fluid ounces
100	3½ fluid ounces
50	1¾ fluid ounces
30	1 fluid ounce
15	4 fluid drams
10	2½ fluid drams
8	2 fluid drams
5	1¼ fluid drams
4	1 fluid dram
3	45 minims
2	30 minims
1	15 minims
0.75	12 minims
0.6	10 minims
0.5	8 minims
0.3	5 minims
0.25	4 minims
0.2	3 minims
0.1	1½ minims
0.06	1 minim
0.05	¾ minim
0.03	½ minim

Volume Conversions (Metric and Apothecary)

MILLILITERS	MINIMS	FLUID DRAMS	FLUID OUNCES	PINTS
1	16.2	.27	.0333	.0021
.0616	1	$\frac{1}{60}$	$\frac{1}{480}$	$\frac{1}{7680}$
3.697	60	1	$\frac{1}{8}$	$\frac{1}{128}$
29.58	480	8	1	$\frac{1}{16}$
473.2	7680	128	16	1

LITERS	GALLONS	QUARTS	FLUID OUNCES	PINTS
1	.2642	1.057	33.824	2.114
3.785	1	4	128	8
.946	$\frac{1}{4}$	1	32	2
.473	$\frac{1}{8}$	$\frac{1}{2}$	16	1
.0296	$\frac{1}{128}$	$\frac{1}{32}$	1	$\frac{1}{16}$

Length Conversions (Metric and English System)

UNIT	MILLIMETERS	CENTIMETERS	INCHES	FEET	YARDS	METERS
1 Å =	$\frac{1}{10,000,000}$	$\frac{1}{100,000,000}$	$\frac{1}{254,000,000}$	$\frac{1}{3,050,000,000}$	$\frac{1}{9,140,000,000}$	$\frac{1}{10,000,000,000}$
1 nm =	$\frac{1}{1,000,000}$	$\frac{1}{10,000,000}$	$\frac{1}{25,400,000}$	$\frac{1}{305,000,000}$	$\frac{1}{914,000,000}$	$\frac{1}{1,000,000,000}$
1 μ =	$\frac{1}{1,000}$	$\frac{1}{10,000}$	$\frac{1}{25,400}$	$\frac{1}{305,000}$	$\frac{1}{914,000}$	$\frac{1}{1,000,000}$
1 mm =	1.0	0.1	0.03937	0.00328	0.0011	0.001
1 cm =	10.0	1.0	0.3937	0.03281	0.0109	0.01
1 in =	25.4	2.54	1.0	0.0833	0.0278	0.0254
1 ft =	304.8	30.48	12.0	1.0	0.333	0.3048
1 yd =	914.40	91.44	36.0	3.0	1.0	0.9144
1 m =	1000.0	100.0	39.37	3.2808	1.0936	1.0

POISEUILLE'S LAW

POISEUILLE'S LAW FOR FLOW REARRANGED TO A SIMPLE PROPORTIONALITY

$$\dot{V} \simeq \Delta Pr^4, \text{ or rewritten as } \frac{\dot{V}}{r^4} \simeq \Delta P.$$

When ΔP remains constant, then

$$\frac{\dot{V}_1}{r_1^{\ 4}} \simeq \frac{\dot{V}_2}{r_2^{\ 4}}$$

Example 1. If the radius (r_1) is decreased to one-half its previous radius $(r_2 = \frac{1}{2} r_1)$, then

$$\frac{\dot{V}_1}{r_1^{\ 4}} \simeq \frac{\dot{V}_2}{(\frac{1}{2}r_1)^4}$$

$$\frac{\dot{V}_1}{r_1^{\ 4}} \simeq \frac{\dot{V}_2}{(\frac{1}{16}r_1)^4}$$

$$(r_1^{\ 4})\frac{\dot{V}_1}{r_1^{\ 4}} \simeq (r_1^{\ 4})\frac{\dot{V}_2}{(\frac{1}{16})r_1^{\ 4}}$$

$$\dot{V}_1 \simeq \frac{\dot{V}_2}{\frac{1}{16}}$$

$$(\tfrac{1}{16})\dot{V}_1 \simeq (\tfrac{1}{16})\frac{\dot{V}_2}{\frac{1}{16}}$$

$$(\tfrac{1}{16})\dot{V}_1 \simeq \dot{V}_2$$

then gas flow $(\dot{V}_1)$ is reduced to $\frac{1}{16}$ its original flow rate $[\dot{V}_2 \simeq (\frac{1}{16})\dot{V}_1]$.

Example 2. If the radius (r_1) is decreased by 16% ($r_2 = r_1 - 0.16\,r_1 = 0.84r_1$), then

$$\frac{\dot{V}_1}{r_1{}^4} \simeq \frac{\dot{V}_2}{r_2{}^4}$$

$$\frac{\dot{V}_1}{r_1{}^4} \simeq \frac{\dot{V}_2}{(0.84r_1)^4}$$

$$\dot{V}_2 \simeq \frac{(.084r_1)^4\,\dot{V}_1}{r_1{}^4}$$

$$\dot{V}_2 \simeq \frac{0.4979\,\cancel{r_1{}^4}\,\dot{V}_1}{\cancel{r_1{}^4}}$$

$$\dot{V}_2 \simeq \tfrac{1}{2}\,\dot{V}_1$$

then the flow rate ($\dot{V}_1$) would decrease to one-half the original flow rate ($\dot{V}_2 \simeq \tfrac{1}{2}\dot{V}_1$).

(Courtesy of Des Jardins, *Clinical Manifestations of Respiratory Disease*, 2nd ed. © 1990 by Mosby Year Book Medical Publishers, Inc., Chicago.)

POISEUILLE'S LAW FOR PRESSURE REARRANGED TO A SIMPLE PROPORTIONALITY

$$P \simeq \frac{\dot{V}}{r^4}\text{, or rewritten as } P \cdot r^4 \simeq \dot{V}$$

when $\dot{V}$ remains constant, then

$$P_1 \cdot r_1{}^4 \simeq P_2 \cdot r_2{}^4$$

Example 1. If the radius (r_1) is reduced to one-half its original radius [$r_2 = (\tfrac{1}{2})\,r_1$], then

$$P_1 \cdot r_1{}^4 \simeq P_2 \cdot r_2{}^4$$

$$P_1 \cdot r_1{}^4 \simeq P_2[(\tfrac{1}{2})r_1]^4$$

$$P_1 \cdot r_1{}^4 \simeq P_2 \cdot (\tfrac{1}{16})r_1{}^4$$

$$\frac{P_1 \cdot \cancel{r_1{}^4}}{\cancel{r_1{}^4}} \simeq \frac{P_2 \cdot (\tfrac{1}{16})\cancel{r_1{}^4}}{\cancel{r_1{}^4}}$$

$$P_1 \simeq P_2 \cdot (\tfrac{1}{16})$$

$$16\,P_1 \simeq \cancel{16} \cdot P_2 \cdot \cancel{(\tfrac{1}{16})}$$

$$16\,P_1 \simeq P_2$$

then the pressure (P_1) will increase to 16 times its original level ($P_2 \simeq 16 \cdot P_1$).

Example 2. If the radius (r_1) is decreased by 16% ($r_2 = r_1 - .16\,r_1 = 0.84 r_1$), then

$$P_1 \cdot r_1^{\,4} \simeq P_2 \cdot r_2^{\,4}$$

$$P_1 \cdot r_1^{\,4} \simeq P_2 (0.4979) r_1^{\,4}$$

$$\frac{P_1 r_1^{\,4}}{(0.4979 r_1)^4} = P_2$$

$$2\,P_1 = P_2$$

then the pressure (P_1) would increase to twice its original pressure ($P_2 \simeq 2 \cdot P_1$).

(Courtesy of Des Jardins, *Clinical Manifestations of Respiratory Disease*, 2nd ed. © 1990 by Mosby Year Book Medical Publishers, Inc., Chicago)

DUBOIS BODY SURFACE CHART

Directions

To find body surface of a patient, locate the height in inches (or centimeters) on Scale I and the weight in pounds (or kilograms) on Scale II and place a straight edge (ruler) between these two points which will intersect Scale III at the patient's surface area.

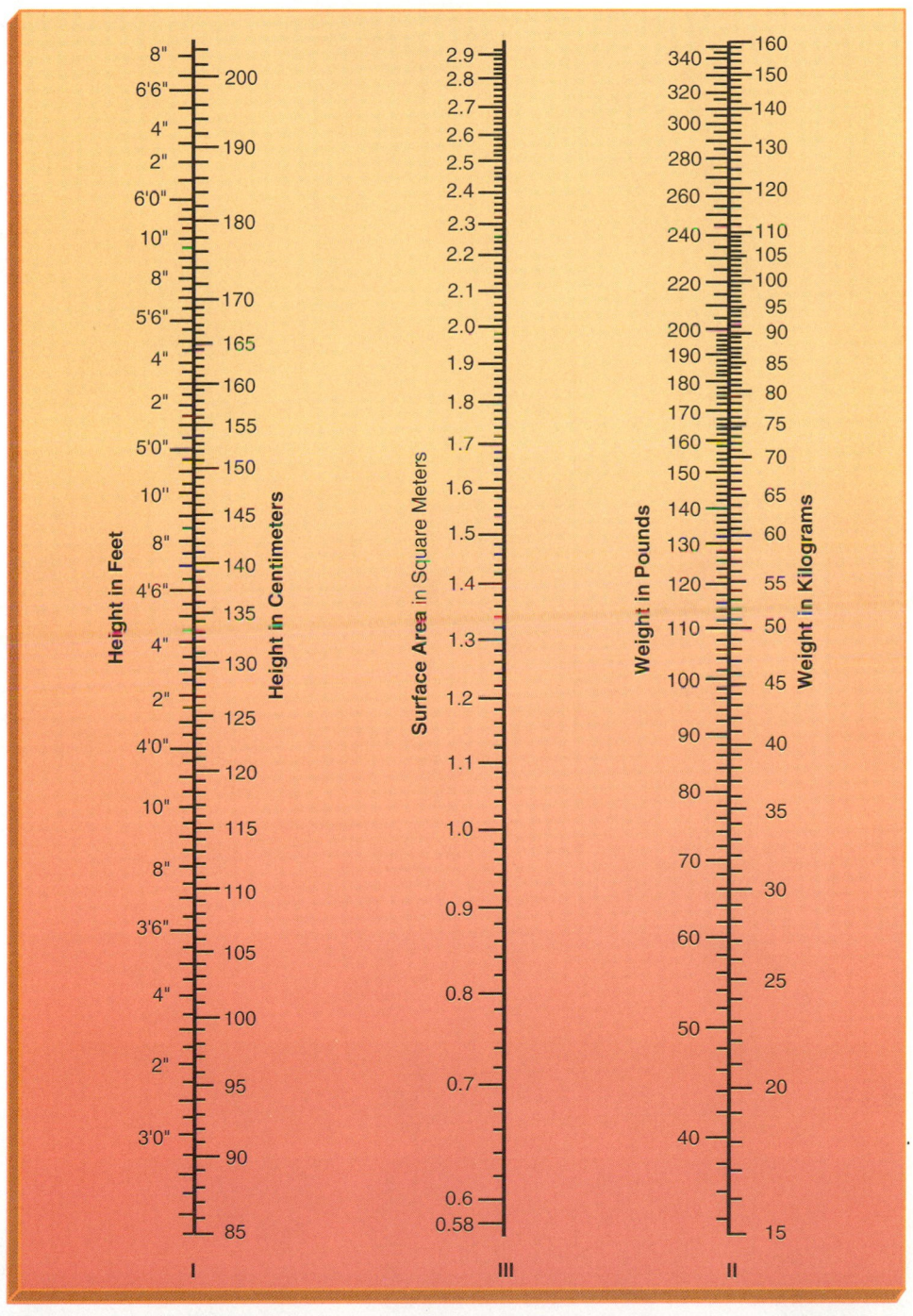

Adapted from DuBois, Eugene F.: *Basal Metabolism in Health and Disease.* Philadelphia: Lea and Febiger, 1924.

CARDIOPULMONARY PROFILE

A representative example of a cardiopulmonary profile sheet used to monitor the critically ill patient. See Chapters 5, 6, and 7 for explanations of the various components presented in this sample cardiopulmonary profile. Areas shaded in pink represent normal ranges.

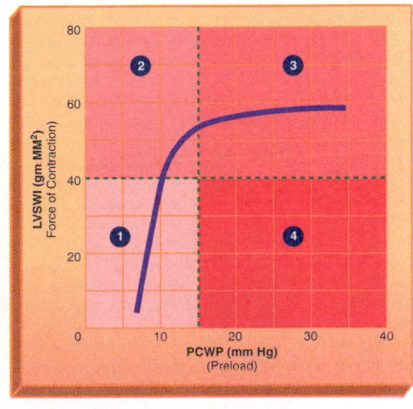

Quadrant 1: Hypovolemia
Quadrant 2: Optimal Function
Quadrant 3: Hypervolemia
Quadrant 4: Cardiac Failure

Temperature: _____

Heart Rate: _____

Cardiac Output: _____

Medications: _____

_____

Blood Gas Values

pH _____

Pa_{CO_2} _____

HCO_3^- _____

Pa_{O_2} _____ $P\bar{v}_{O_2}$ _____

Sa_{O_2} _____ % $S\bar{v}_{O_2}$ _____ %

FI_{O_2} _____   Hb _____

Mode(s) of Ventilatory

Support: _____
_____
_____
_____
_____
_____

Shaded areas
represent
normal
ranges.

Patient's Name _____

Date _____

Time _____

P$_{CO_2}$/HCO$_3^-$/pH NOMOGRAM

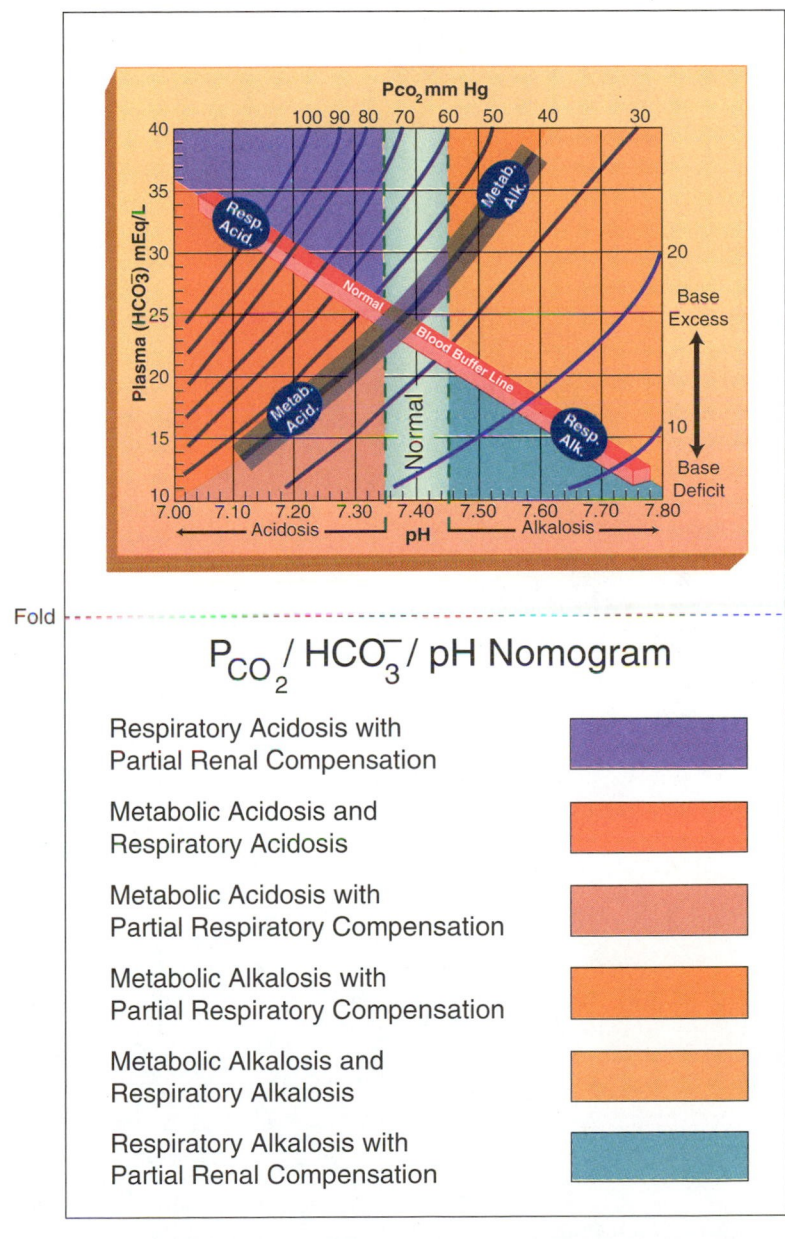

P$_{CO_2}$ / HCO$_3^-$ / pH Nomogram

Respiratory Acidosis with Partial Renal Compensation	
Metabolic Acidosis and Respiratory Acidosis	
Metabolic Acidosis with Partial Respiratory Compensation	
Metabolic Alkalosis with Partial Respiratory Compensation	
Metabolic Alkalosis and Respiratory Alkalosis	
Respiratory Alkalosis with Partial Renal Compensation	

Copy the above P$_{CO_2}$ / HCO$_3^-$/ pH Nomogram and have it laminated for use as a handy, pocket-size reference tool.

See Chapter 8 on how to use the P$_{CO_2}$ / HCO$_3^-$/ pH Nomogram in the clinical setting.

BIBLIOGRAPHY

GENERAL ANATOMY AND PHYSIOLOGY

Anthony, C.P., and Thibodeau, G.A. *Anthony's Textbook of Anatomy and Physiology.* 15th ed. St. Louis: C.V. Mosby Co., 1996.

Clemente, C.D. *Anatomy: A Regional Atlas of the Human Body.* 3rd ed. Philadelphia. Wilkins/Wilcox, 1987.

Crouch, J.E. *Functional Human Anatomy.* 4th ed. Philadelphia: Lea and Febiger, 1985.

Gray, H. *Anatomy of the Human Body.* 38th ed. Philadelphia: Lea and Febiger, 1995.

Hole, J.W. *Essentials of Human Anatomy and Physiology.* 4th ed. Dubuque, Iowa: Wm. C. Brown Co., 1992.

Maried, E.N. *Human Anatomy and Physiology.* 3rd ed. Redwood City, Calif.: Benjamin/Cummings, 1995.

McMinn, R.M.H., and Hutchings, R.T. *Color Atlas of Human Anatomy.* 3rd ed. Chicago: Mosby-Year Book Medical Publishers, 1993.

McMinn, R.M.H.; Gaddum-Rosse, Penelope Gadum; Hutchings, R.T.; and Logan, B.M. *McMinn's Functional and Clinical Anatomy.* St. Louis, Mosby-Year Book, 1995.

Snell, R.S. *Clinical Anatomy for Medical Students.* 5th ed. Boston: Little, Brown and Co., 1995.

Thibodeau, G.A., and Patton, K. *Anatomy and Physiology,* 2nd ed. St. Louis: 1992, Mosby-Year Book., 1992.

Thibodeau, G.A. *Structure and Function of the Body,* 9th ed. St. Louis: Mosby-Year Book, 1992.

Tortora, G.J., and Anagnostakos, N.P. *Principles of Anatomy and Physiology.* 7th ed. New York: Harper Collins, 1995.

VanDeGraaff, K.M. *Human Anatomy.* 4th ed. Dubuque, Iowa: Wm. C. Brown Co., 1995.

Vander, A.J.; Sherman, J.H.; and Luciano, D.S. *Human Physiology: The Mechanisms of Body Function.* 5th ed. New York: McGraw-Hill Book Co., 1990.

Woodburne, R.T. *Essentials of Human Anatomy.* 9th ed. Oxford, England: Oxford University Press, 1994.

CARDIOPULMONARY ANATOMY AND PHYSIOLOGY

Braun, H.A.; Cheney, F.W., Jr.; and Loehnen, C.P. *Introduction to Respiratory Physiology.* 2nd ed. Boston: Little, Brown and Co., 1980.

Campbell, E.J.M.; Agostoni, E.; and Newsom-Davis, J.N. *The Respiratory Muscles: Mechanics and Neural Control.* Philadelphia: W.B. Saunders Co., 1970.

Cherniack, R.M., and Cherniack, L.C. *Respiration in Health and Disease.* 3rd ed. Philadelphia: W.B. Saunders Co., 1983.

Comroe, J.H. *Physiology of Respiration.* 2nd ed. Chicago: Mosby-Year Book Medical Publishers, 1974.

Daily, E.K., and Schroeder, J.S. *Techniques in Bedside Hemodynamic Monitoring.* 5th ed. St. Louis: C.V. Mosby Co., 1994.

Davenport, H.W. *ABC of Acid-Base Chemistry.* 7th ed. Chicago: University of Chicago Press, 1978.

Fraser, R.G., and Pare, J.A.P. *Organ Physiology: Structure and Function of the Lung.* 2nd ed. Philadelphia: W.B. Saunders Co., 1977.

Green, J.F. *Fundamental Cardiovascular and Pulmonary Physiology.* 2nd ed. Philadelphia: Lea and Febiger, 1987.

Huber, Gary L. *Arterial Blood Gas and Acid-Base Physiology.* A Scope Current Concepts Publication. Kalamazoo: Upjohn Company, 1978.

Jacques, J.A. *Respiratory Physiology.* New York: McGraw-Hill Book Co., 1979.

Jones, N.L. *Blood Gases and Acid-Base Physiology.* 2nd ed. New York: Thieme-Stratton, 1987.

Leff, A.R., and Schumacker, P.T. *Respiratory Physiology: Basics and Applications.* Philadelphia: W.B. Saunders, 1993.

Levitzky, M.G. *Pulmonary Physiology.* 4th ed. New York: McGraw-Hill Book Co., 1995.

Matthews, L.R. *Cardiopulmonary Anatomy and Physiology.* Philadelphia: Lippincott, 1996.

Mines, A.H. *Respiratory Physiology.* 3th ed. New York: Lippincott-Raven Press, 1993.

Murray, J.F. *The Normal Lung,* 2nd ed. Philadelphia: W.B. Saunders Co., 1986.

Netter, F.H. *The CIBA Collection of Medical Illustrations.* Vol. 7, *Respiratory System*, pp. 3–43. Summit, N.J.: CIBA Pharmaceutical Products, 1979.

Oblouk Darovic, G: *Hemodynamic Monitoring: Invasive and Noninvasive Clinical Application*, 2nd ed., Philadelphia: W.B. Saunders, 1995.

Rosendorff, C. *Clinical Cardiovascular and Pulmonary Physiology.* New York: Raven Press, 1983.

Schweiss, J.F. *Continuous Measurement of Blood Oxygen Saturation in the High Risk Patient.* Vol. 1. San Diego: Beach International, 1983.

Shapiro, B.A.; Harrison, R.A.; Roy, C.D.; and Rozanna, T. *Clinical Application of Blood Gases.* 5th ed. Chicago: Year Book Medical Publishers, 1993.

Slonim, N.B., and Hamilton, L.H. *Respiratory Physiology.* 5th ed. St. Louis: C.V. Mosby Co., 1987.

West, J.B. *Respiratory Physiology, The Essentials.* 4th ed. Baltimore: Williams and Wilkins Co., 1990.

West, J.B. "State of the Art: Ventilation-Perfusion Relationships." *Am. Rev. Respir. Dis.* 116(1977):919–943.

SUPPLEMENTARY ANATOMY AND PHYSIOLOGY OF THE CARDIOVASCULAR SYSTEM

Berne, R.M., and Levy, M.N. *Cardiovascular Physiology.* 6th ed. St. Louis: C.V. Mosby Co., 1992.

Braunwald, E. "Regulation of the Circulation." *N. Engl. J. Med.* 290(1974):1124, 1420.

Conover, M.H., and Zalis, E.G. *Understanding Electrocardiography: Physiological and Interpretive Concept.* 7th ed. St. Louis: C.V. Mosby Co., 1995.

Honig, C.R. *Modern Cardiovascular Physiology.* 2nd ed. Boston: Little, Brown and Co., 1988.

Hurst, J.W., and Logue, R.B., eds. *The Heart.* 7th ed. New York: McGraw-Hill Book Co., 1987.

Mohrman, D.E., and Heller, L.J. *Cardiovascular Physiology.* 3rd ed. New York: McGraw-Hill Book Co., 1991.

Netter, F.H. *The CIBA Collection of Medical Illustrations.* Vol. 5, *The Heart.* Summit, N.J.: CIBA Pharmaceutical Products, 1969.

Smith, J.J., and Kampine, J.P. *Circulatory Physiology: The Essentials.* 3rd ed. Baltimore: Williams and Wilkins, 1990.

RENAL SYSTEM

Coltman, K. "Urinary Tract Infections: New Thoughts on an Old Subject." *Practitioner* 223(1979):351.

Grob, P.R. "Urinary Tract Infections in General Practice." *Practitioner* 221, no. 8(1978):237–244.

Kunin, C. *Detection, Prevention and Management of Urinary Tract Infections.* 4th ed., pp. 41, 99, 157. Philadelphia: Lea and Febiger, 1987.

Leaf, A., and Cotran, R. *Renal Pathophysiology,* 3rd ed., pp. 167, 204. New York: Oxford University Press, 1985.

Marsh, D.J. *Renal Physiology.* New York: Raven Press, 1983.

Porth, C. *Pathophysiology—Concepts of Altered Health States.* 4th ed. Philadelphia: J.B. Lippincott, 1994.

Rose, B.D. *Clinical Physiology of Acid-Base and Electrolyte Disorders.* 3rd ed. New York: McGraw-Hill Book Co., 1989.

Sullivan, L.P., and Grantham, J.J. *Physiology of the Kidney.* 2nd ed. Philadelphia: Lea and Febiger, 1982.

Turek, M. "Urinary Tract Infections." *Hosp. Pract.* 15, no. 1(1980): 49–58.

Valtin, H. *Renal Function.* 3rd ed. Boston: Little, Brown and Co., 1994.

Vander, A.J. *Renal Physiology.* 5th ed. New York: McGraw-Hill Book Co., 1994.

Zeluff, G.W.; Eknoyan, G.; and Jackson, D. "Pericarditis in Renal Failure." *Heart and Lung* 8, no. 6(1979): 1139.

AGING AND THE CARDIOPULMONARY SYSTEM

Cassel, C.K., and Walsh, J.R. *Geriatric Medicine.* New York: Springer-Verlag, 1996.

Ebersole, P., and Hess, P. *Toward Healthy Aging.* 4th ed. St. Louis: C.V. Mosby Co., 1994.

Fitzgerald, P.L. "Exercise for the Elderly." *Medical Clinics of North America* 69, no. 1(1985): 189–196.

Gioiella, E.C., and Bevil, C.W. *Nursing Care of the Aging Client—Promoting Healthy Adaptation*. Norwalk, Conn.: Appleton-Century-Crofts, 1985.

Holm, K., and Kirchoff, K.T. "Perspective on Exercise and Aging." *Heart and Lung* no. 5(1984): 13, 519–524.

McBee, S. "Here Come the Baby-Boomers." *U.S. News and World Report*. (Nov. 5, 1984), 68–73.

Newton, K.D. *Making the Mid-Years the Prime of Life*. Chicago: Budlong Press Co., 1978.

Powell, S. "Measuring Impact of the 'Baby Bust' on U.S. Future." *U.S. News and World Report* (Dec. 16, 1985), 66–67.

Riffer, J. "Elderly 21 Percent of Population by 2040." *Hospital* (March 1, 1985), 41–44.

Shepherd, R.J. *Physical Activity and Aging*. 2nd ed. Gaithersburg, M.D.: Aspen, 1987.

Sivy, M. "The Middle-Aged Shape of Things to Come." *Money*, (Nov. 1985), 66- 72.

Stengel, R. "Snapshot of a Changing America—The U.S. Population is Growing Older and Thinking Smaller." *Time*, (Sept. 2, 1985), 16–18.

CARDIOPULMONARY ANATOMY AND PHYSIOLOGY OF THE FETUS AND THE NEWBORN

Aloan, C.A. *Respiratory Care of the Newborn—A Clinical Manual*. 2nd ed. Philadelphia: J.B. Lippincott Co., 1994.

Avery, M.E.; Wang, N.; and Taeusch, H.W. "The Lung of the Newborn Infant." *Scientific American* 228(April 1973):74–85.

Barnhart, S.L., and Czervinske, M.P. *Perinatal and Pediatric Respiratory Care*. Philadelphia: W.B. Saunders Co., 1995

Bodegard, G. "Control of Respiration in Newborn Babies." IV, *Acta Paediatr. Scand.* 65(1976):257.

Charnock, E.L., and Doershuk, C.F. "Development Aspects of the Human Lung." *Pediatr. Clin. North Am.* 20(1973):275.

Crelin, E.S. "Development of the Lower Respiratory System." *Clin. Symp.* 27, no. 4(1975):3.

James, L.S., and Adamsons, K., Jr. "Respiratory Physiology of the Fetus and Newborn Infant." *N. Engl. J. Med.* 271(1964):1352–1409.

Klaus, M.H., and Fanaroff, A.A. *Care of the High-risk Neonate*. 4th ed. Philadelphia: W.B. Saunders Co., 1993.

Koff, P.B.; Eitzman, D.; and Neu, J. *Neonatal and Pediatric Respiratory Care*. 2nd ed. St. Louis, Mosby-Year Book, 1993.

Korones, S.B. *High-Risk Newborn Infants*. 4th ed. St. Louis: C.V. Mosby Co., 1986.

Lubchenco, L.O. *The High Risk Infant*. Philadelphia: W.B. Saunders Co., 1976.

Strang, L.B. "The Lungs at Birth." *Arch. Dis. Child.* 40(1965):575.

Walsh, S.Z.; Meyer, W.W.; and Lind, J. *The Human Fetal and Neonatal Circulation*. Springfield, Ill.: Charles C. Thomas, 1974.

Wells, L.J., and Boyden, E.A. "The Development of the Bronchopulmonary Segments in Human Embryos of Horizons XVII to XIX." *Am. J. Anat.* 95(1954): 163.

EXERCISE AND ITS EFFECTS ON THE CARDIOPULMONARY SYSTEM

Appenzeller, O., and Atkinson, R., eds. *Health Aspects of Endurance Training*. New York: S. Karger, 1978.

Apple, D.F., Jr., and Cantwell, J.D. *Medicine for Sport*. Chicago: Year Book Medical Publishers, 1980.

Bevegard, G.B.S., and Shepherd, J.T. "Regulation of the Circulation during Exercise in Man." *Physiol. Rev.*, 47(1967):178.

Clarke, D.H. *Exercise Physiology*. Englewood Cliffs, N.J.: Prentice-Hall, 1975.

Fox, E.L. *Sports Physiology*. 3rd ed. Philadelphia: W.B. Saunders. 1992.

Rasch, P.J., and Burke, R.K. *Kinesiology and Applied Anatomy: The Science of Human Movement*. 7th ed. Philadelphia: Lea & Febiger, 1989.

Strauss, R.H., ed. *Sports and Medicine and Physiology*. 2nd ed. Philadelphia: W.B. Saunders, 1991.

Wyndham, C.H. "The Physiology of Exercise under Heat Stress." *Annu. Rev. Physiol.*, 35(1973):193.

HIGH ALTITUDE AND ITS EFFECTS ON THE CARDIOPULMONARY SYSTEM

Cassin, S.R.; Gilbert, D; Bunnell, C.F.; and Johnson, E.M. "Capillary Development during Exposure to Chronic Hypoxia." *Am. J. Physiol.* 220(1971):448–451.

DeGraff, A.C.; Grover, R.F.; Johnson, R.L.; Hammond, J.W.; and Miller, J.M. "Diffusing Capacity of the Lung in Caucasians Native to 3100 m." *J. Appl. Physiol.* 29(1970):71–76.

Frisancho, A.R. "Functional Adaptation to High Altitude Hypoxia." *Science* 187 (1975): 313.

Groves, B.M.; Reeves, J.T.; Sutton, J.R.; Wagner, P.D.; Cymerman, A.; Malconian, M.K.; Rock, P.B.; Young, P.M.; and Houston, C.S. "Operation Everest II: Elevated High-altitude Pulmonary Resistance Unresponsive to Oxygen." *J. Appl. Physiol.* 63(1987):521–530.

Guleria, J.S.; Pande, J.N.; Sethi, P.K.; and Roy, S.B. "Pulmonary Diffusing Capacity at High Altitude." *J. Appl. Physiol.* 31(1971):536–543.

Kreuzer, F.; Van Lookeren; and Champagne, P. "Resting Pulmonary Diffusing Capacity for CO and O_2 at High Altitude." *J. Appl. Physiol.* 20(1965):519–524.

Lahiri, S. "Physiological Responses and Adaptations to High Altitude." *Int. Rev. Physiol.* 15(1977):217.

Oelz, O.; Howald, H.; diPrampero, P.E.; Hoppeler, H.; Claassen, A.H.; Jenni, R.; Biihlmann, A.; Ferretti, G.; Bruckner, J.C.; Veicsteinas, A.; Gussoni, M.; and Certetelli, P. "Physiological Profile of World-class High-altitude Climbers." *J. Appl. Physiol.* 60(1986):1734–1742.

Reite, M.; Jackson, D.; Cahoon, R.L.; and Weil, J.V. "Sleep Physiology at High Altitude." *Electroencephalogr. Clin. Neurophysiol.* 38(1975):463–471.

Reynafarje, B. "Myoglobin Content and Enzymatic Activity of Muscle and Altitude Adaptation." *J. Appl. Physiol.* 17(1962):301–305.

Schoene, R.B.; Lahiri, S.; Hackett, P.H.; Peters, R.M., Jr.; Milledge, J.S.; Pizzo, C.J.; Sarnquist, F.H.; Boyer, S.J.; Graber, D.J.; Maret, K.H.; and West, J.B. "Relationship of Hypoxic Ventilatory Response to Exercise Performance on Mount Everest." *J. Appl. Physiol.: Respir. Environ. Exercise Physiol.* 56(1984):1478–1483.

Singh, I.; Khanna, P.K.; Srivastava, M.C.; Lai, M.; Roy, S.B.; and Subramanyam, C.S.V. "Acute Mountain Sickness." *N. Engl. J. Med.* 280(1969):175–184.

Vogel, J.A., and Harris, C.W. "Cardiopulmonary Responses of Resting Man during Early Exposure to High Altitude." *J. Appl. Physiol.* 22(1967):1124–1128.

Vogel, J.A.; Hartley, L.H.; and Cruz, J.C. "Cardiac Output during Exercise in Altitude Natives at Sea Level and High Altitude." *J. Appl. Physiol.* 36(1974): 173–176.

Wagner, P.D.; Saltzman, H.A.; and West, J.B. "Measurement of Continuous Distributions of Ventilation-Perfusion Ratios: Theory." *J. Appl. Physiol.* 36(1974): 588–599.

Ward, M.P.; Milledge, J.S.; and West, J.B. *High Altitude Medicine and Physiology*, 2nd ed. London: Chapman & Hall Medical, 1989.

Weil, J.V.; Kryger, M.H.; and Scoggin, C.H. "Sleep and Breathing at High Altitude. In: *Sleep Apnea Syndromes*, edited by C. Guilleminault and W. Dement, New York: Alan R. Liss. 1978. pp. 119–136.

West, J.B.; Peters, R.M., Jr.; Aksnes, G.; Maret, K.H.; Milledge, J.S.; and Schoene, R.B. "Nocturnal Periodic Breathing at Altitudes of 6300 meters and 8050 meters." *.J Appl. Physiol.* 61(1986):280–287.

West, J.B. "Climbing Mt. Everest without Supplementary Oxygen: An Analysis of Maximal Exercise during Extreme Hypoxia." *Respir. Physiol.* 52(1983):265–279.

West, J.B. "Diffusing Capacity of the Lung for Carbon Monoxide at High Altitude." *J. Appl. Physiol.* 17(1962):421–426.

West, J.B.; Boyer, S.J.; Graber, D.J.; Hackett, P.H.; Maret, K.H.; Milledge, J.S.; Peters, R.M., Jr.; Pizzo, C.J.; Samaja, M.; Sarnquist, F.H.; Schoene, R.B.; and Winslow, R.M. "Maximal Exercise at Extreme Altitudes on Mount Everest." *J. Appl. Physiol.: Respir. Environ. Exercise Physiol.* 55(1983):688–698.

West, J.B.; Lahiri, S.; Maret, K.H.; Peters, R.M., Jr.; andPizzo, C.J. "Barometric Pressures at Extreme Altitudes on Mt. Everest: Physiological Significance." *J. Appl. Physiol.: Respir. Environ. Exercise Physiol.* 54(1983):1188–1194.

Winslow, R.M., and Monge, C.C. *Hypoxia, Polycythemia, and Chronic Mountain Sickness*. Washington, D.C.: Johns Hopkins University Press, 1987; pp. 184–196.

HIGH PRESSURE ENVIRONMENTS AND THEIR EFFECT ON THE CARDIOPULMONARY SYSTEM

Bakker, D.J. "Clostridial Myonecrosis." In: *Problem Wounds: The Role of Oxygen*, edited by J.C. Davis and T.K. Hunt, pp. 153–172.. New York: Elsevier, 1988.

Craig, A.B., Jr. "Depth Limits of Breath-hold Diving (An Example of Fennology)." *Respir. Physiol.* 5(1968):14–22.

Davis, J.C.; Dunn, J.M.; and Heimbach, R.D. "Hyperbaric Medicine: Patient Selection, Treatment Procedures, and Side-Effects." In: *Problem Wounds: The Role of Oxygen*, edited by J.C. Davis and T.K. Hunt, pp. 225–235. New York; Elsevier, 1988.

Davis, J.C. and Hunt, T.K., eds. *Problem Wounds. The Role of Oxygen*. New York: Elsevier, 1988.

Gamarra, J.A. *Decompression Sickness*. Hagerstown, Md.: Harper & Row, 1974.

Hempelman, H.V., and Lockwood, A.P.M. *The Physiology of Diving in Man and Other Animals*. London: Edward Arnold, 1978.

Lundgren, C.E.G., and Farhi, L.E. "Pulmonary Circulation in Diving and Hyperbaric Environment." In: *Pulmonary Vascular Physiology and Pathophysiology, Lung Biology in Health and Disease,* edited by E.K. Weir and J.T. Reeves, pp. 199–240. New York: Marcel Dekker, 1989.

Mader, J.T., ed. *Hyperbaric Oxygen Therapy Committee Report*. Bethesda, Md.: Undersea and Hyperbaric Medical Society, 1989.

Marx, R.E., and Johnson, R.P. "Problem Wounds in Oral and Maxillofacial Surgery: The Role of Hyperbaric Oxygen." In: *Problem Wounds. The Role of Oxygen,* edited by J.C. Davis and T.K. Hunt, pp. 65–123. New York: Elsevier, 1988.

Nemiroff, M.J.; Saltz, G.R.; and Weg, J.G. "Survival after Cold-water Near-drowning: The Protective Effect of the Diving Reflex." *Am. Rev. Respir. Dis.* 115(1977): 145.

Olszowka, A.J., and Rahn, H. "Breath Hold Diving." In: *Hypoxia and Cold,* edited by J.R. Sutton, C.S. Houston, and G. Coates, pp. 417–428. New York: Praeger, 1987.

Schaefer, K.E.; Allison, R.D.; Dougherty, J.H., Jr.; Carey, C.R.; Walker, R.; Yost, F.; and Parker, D. "Pulmonary and Circulatory Adjustments Determining the Limits of Depths in Breathhold Diving." *Science* 162(1968):1020–1023.

Shilling, C.W., and Beckett, M.W. (eds.). *Underwater Physiology IV*. Bethesda, Md.: Federation of American Societies for Experimental Biology, 1978.

Thom, S.R. "Hyperbaric Oxygen Therapy." *J. Intensive Care Med.* 4(1989):58–74.

Undersea and Hyperbaric Medical Society. "The Physiological Basis of Decompression." In: *Proceedings of 38th Undersea and Hyperbaric Medical Society Workshop,* edited by R.D. Vann, p. 437. Bethesda, Md.: Undersea and Hyperbaric Medical Society, 1989.

———. "Physiological and Human Engineering Aspects of Underwater Breathing Apparatus." In: *Proceedings of 38th Undersea and Hyperbaric Medical Society Workshop,* edited by C. Lundgren and D. Warkander, p. 270. Bethesda, Md.: Undersea and Hyperbaric Medical Society, 1989.

CARDIOVASCULAR REHABILITATION

American Association of Cardiovascular and Pulmonary Rehabilitation. "Scientific Evidence of the Value of Cardiac Rehabilitation Services with Emphasis on Patients following Myocardial Infarction. Section I. Exercise Conditioning Component (position paper). *J. Cardiopulm. Rehabil.* 10(1990):79–87.

Burgess, A.W.; Lerner, D.J.; D'Agostino, R.B.; Vokonas, P.S.; Hartman, C.R.; and Gaccione, P. "A Randomized Control Trial of Cardiac Rehabilitation." *Soc. Sci. Med.* 24(1987):359–370.

DeBusk, R.F.; Haskell, W.L.; Miller, N.H.; Berra, K.; Taylor, C.B.; Berger, W.E., III; and Lew, H. "Medically Directed At Home Rehabilitation soon after Clinically Uncomplicated Acute Myocardial Infarction: A New Model for Patient Care." *Am. J. Cardiol.* 55(1985):251–257.

Ehsani, A.A.; Martin, W.H., III; Health, G.W.; and Coyle, E.F. "Cardiac Effects of Prolonged and Intense Exercise Training in Patients with Coronary Artery Disease. *Am. J. Cardiol.* 50(1982):246–254.

Froelicher, V.; Jensen, D.; Genter, F.; Sullivan, M.; McKirnan, M.D.; Witztum, K.; Scharf, J.; Strong, M.L.; and Ashburn, W. "A Randomized Trial of Exercise Training in Patients with Coronary Heart Disease. *JAMA* 252(1984) :1291–1297.

Health and Public Policy Committee, American College of Physicians. "Cardiac Rehabilitation Services" (position paper). *Ann. Intern. Med.* 109(1988):671–673.

O'Connor, G.T.; Buring, J.E.; Yusuf, S.; Goldhaber, S.Z.; Olmstead, E.M.; Paffenbarger, R.S., Jr.; and Hennekens, C.H. "An Overview of Randomized Trials of Rehabilitation with Exercise after Myocardial Infarction." *Circulation* 80(1989): 234–244.

Paffenbarger, R.S., Jr., and Hyde, R.T. "Exercise in the Prevention of Coronary Heart Disease." *Prev. Med.* 13(1984):3–22.

"Rehabilitation: Status, 1990." *May. Clin. Proc.* 65(1990):731–755.

Squires, R.W.; Gau, G.T.; and Orszulak, T.A. "Cardiac Rehabilitation: Benefits of a Structured, Brief Inpatient Program after Coronary Bypass Surgery (abstract)." *Med. Sci. Sports Exerc.* 19 (Suppl)(1987): S20.

Squires, R.W., and Lavie, C.J. "New Trends in Cardiac Rehabilitation Exercise." *Cardio.* 5(July 1988):85–87; 91–92; 112.

Sullivan, M.J.; Higginbotham, M.B.; and Cobb, F.R. "Exercise Training in Patients with Severe Left Ventricular Dysfunction: Hemodynamic and Metabolic Effects. *Circulation* 78(1988):506–515.

Thompson, P.D. "The Benefits and Risks of Exercise Training in Patients with Chronic Coronary Artery Disease." *JAMA* 259(1988):1537–1540.

Williams. R.S. "Exercise Training of Patients with Ventricular Dysfunction and Heart Failure. *Cardiovasc. Clin.* 15 (no. 2)(1985): 219–231.

SUPPLEMENTARY RESPIRATORY CARE

Burton, G.G.; Hodgkin, J.E.K; and Ward, J.J. *Respiratory Care: A Guide to Clinical Practice.* 4th ed. Philadelphia: J.B. Lippincott Co., 1997.

Rau, J.L. *Respiratory Care Pharmacology.* 4th ed. Chicago: Mosby-Year Book Medical Publishers, 1993.

Ruppel, G. *Manual of Pulmonary Function.* 6th ed. Mosby-Year Book, Inc., 1994.

Shapiro, B.A.; Kacmark, R.M.; Cane, R.D.; and Hauptman, D. *Clinical Application of Respiratory Care.* 4th ed. Chicago: Mosby-Year Book, Inc., 1991.

INDEX